THE BEST SKIN OF YOUR LIFE STARTS HERE

BUSTING BEAUTY MYTHS SO YOU KNOW WHAT TO USE AND WHY

PAULA BEGOUN
BRYAN BARRON
DESIREE STORDAHL

Editors: John Hopper and Elaine Trumpey
Research Editor: Nathan Rivas
Research Assistants: Mercedes Santaella-Lam and Vanessa Lucas
Art Direction, Cover Design and Typography: Erin Bloom and Andrew Eder
Layout: Anita L. Elder
Project Manager: Karen Link
Printing: RR Donnelley

Copyright © 2015, Paula's Choice, LLC
Publisher: Beginning Press
Seattle, WA

1st Edition Printing: November, 2015

ISBN: 978-1-877988-40-0

This book is distributed to the United States book trade by:
Publishers Group West
1700 Fourth Street
Berkeley, California 94710

And to the Canadian book trade by:
Raincoast Books Dist. Ltd.
2440 Viking Way
Richmond, British Columbia, V6V1N2 CANADA

And in Australia and New Zealand by:
Peribo Pty Limited
58 Beaumont Road
Mount Kuring-Gai NSW 2080 AUSTRALIA

Authors' Disclaimer

The intent of this book is to present the authors' ideas and perceptions about the marketing, selling, and use of cosmetics, as well as to present consumer information and advice regarding the purchase of makeup and skin-care products. The information and recommendations presented in this book strictly reflect the authors' opinions, perceptions, and knowledge about the subject and products mentioned.

It is everyone's unalienable right to judge products and information such as this by their own criteria and to disagree with the authors. More importantly, because everyone's skin can and probably will, react to an external stimulus at some time, any product can cause a negative reaction on skin at one time or another. If you develop skin sensitivity to a cosmetic, stop using it immediately and consult your physician.

If you need medical advice about your skin, you should consult a dermatologist or physician. The authors are not medical doctors, nor are they professional healthcare providers and do not provide medical advice or medical diagnosis. This book does not offer medical advice, or attempt to diagnose or treat any skin problem, disease, or skin condition or any other health or medical problem or condition. If you have a medical condition or problem with your skin, please make an appointment to see a dermatologist or physician in your area.

Do not use or rely on the statements in this book for medical advice or to treat any medical condition or as an alternative to medical advice from your doctor or other professional healthcare provider. Consult a doctor or other professional healthcare provider with any questions about any medical matter and seek immediate medical attention if you believe you or others may be suffering from any medical condition.

Any information provided by the authors is, at best, of a general nature and cannot substitute for the advice of a medical professional (for instance, a qualified doctor/physician, dermatologist, nurse, or pharmacist). All products mentioned should be used as directed on the product container or on the website from where such products were purchased. Discontinue using any product that causes irritation (e.g., redness, itching, burning, scaling, soreness, or other symptoms).

DO NOT DELAY SEEKING MEDICAL ADVICE, DISREGARD MEDICAL ADVICE, OR DISCONTINUE MEDICAL TREATMENT BECAUSE OF INFORMATION OR STATEMENTS PROVIDED IN THIS BOOK.

TABLE OF CONTENTS

PREFACE

The One Constant Is Change

One of the most incredible aspects of the cosmetics industry, especially surrounding skincare products, is how rapidly the technology and our understanding of the physiology and biology of skin has changed and evolved. Over the past 30 years, we have been amazed by how the research and serious investigations into how skin functions have shed new light on the best possible ways to take care of skin. We have watched with awe and respect as new ingredients, new combinations of ingredients, and the promising hopes of new scientific discoveries have transformed what cosmetics products can do.

In our constant quest to seek out new data and studies on skin and skincare, we use those findings to update our Expert Advice articles and Cosmetic Ingredient Dictionary. We want to emphasize our steadfast use of research-based information because we know how easy it is to be lured in by a new miracle product or by an ingredient that the cosmetics industry serves up as the next best thing. Unfortunately, succumbing to such seductions can be detrimental for your skin. We've seen fad ingredients come and go, some that linger longer than others and some that just won't go away despite their negative effects on skin.

Cutting through the hype and finding out exactly what the growing scientific and professional communities and substantiated studies have to say about skin and skincare can play a major role in getting you the best skin of your life. We have been providing that information for 30 years and are devoted to continuing to do so. After you've read this book, you can continue to stay up-to-date on the latest research and what does (and doesn't) work for skin by visiting us at BeautyMythBusters.com. We are committed to helping you have the best skin of your life *now*, in the *future*, and *every step* along the way!

CHAPTER 1

The Best Skin of Your Life Starts Here and Now...

A MESSAGE FROM US

The title of this book and the name of this chapter make bold statements, yet we make them with the utmost confidence. That's because the information you'll find on every page is based on what current research shows can help you solve your skin concerns using a step-by-step cohesive skincare system you can understand and put into action. By doing this we know you can have and maintain the beautiful skin you've always wanted! All the details, recommendations, and encouragement we present throughout this book are what you need to get yourself on the fast track to finding the best products and best answers for your skin.

ABOUT PAULA

As one of the authors of this book, I'm the one with the dubious distinction of being in the world of cosmetics and writing books about beauty the longest. If you're not familiar with my work, I've been studying, reviewing, and researching scientific and medical journals about skincare for over 35 years. I have a background in science from my university studies, and I was a lifestyle reporter in Seattle for four years. Starting in 1985—and now with this book—I've written 21 books on beauty, skincare, makeup, and hair care (the first entitled *Blue Eyeshadow Should Be Illegal*), most of them more than 500 pages and some more than 1,000 pages, with millions of copies sold around the world.

By the way, of those 21 books, I've written eight with my co-author Bryan Barron, and two with my other co-author Desiree Stordahl. Together we have also written endless articles on skin and skincare.

I am also founder of Paula's Choice Skincare, which I launched in 1995, a collection of products I formulated with options for practically every skin type and skin concern. Of course, I love my products. But, because there are many great products from other lines and because my mission has always been to help you get the best skin of your life, my goal is for you to understand how to take the best care of you skin, what you should and shouldn't do AND to find the products that are ideal for your skin type and your skin concerns.

To that end, since creating Paula's Choice Skincare, my team and I have formulated over 100 skincare products, and we're still doing so today. My teams have grown to include some of the best talent in the industry, which means we leave no stone unturned to get you the most current information and research about skincare available. We are exclusively interested in facts and truth about skin. We will never waste your time on fabrication or guile.

PAULA'S JOURNEY: THE WAY-BACK-WHEN MACHINE!

I've had a love-hate relationship with the cosmetics industry from the very beginning. It started with an intense curiosity and passion for skincare, make-up, and hair care when I was very young. My passion wasn't because I was fixated on buying cosmetics for a lark; rather, it was about trying to take care of my problem skin that progressively got worse and worse no matter what I used or what expert I consulted. It was emotional torture for me as a teenager. To this day, it is still painful for me to recount the stress and embarrassment of dealing with the unsightly skin problems I suffered through as a youth.

At the age of 11, I started suffering from acne and super-oily skin along with debilitating eczema over 60% of my body (in school I had to wear gloves to hold a pencil because my hands were so raw and sore from my incessant scratching of the eczema-caused itching). All I wanted at the time were effective products that would do as they claimed. This didn't seem like too much to ask, right? Given how many times I was told month after month, year after year, how different products would end my struggle, surely something would work. However, over the next several years, no matter where I turned, whether to cosmetics counters, drugstores, spas, or even doctors' offices, almost every product I tried led to disappointment. Despite the promises and claims, my skin rarely showed any signs of improvement, and it gradually just got worse! I felt helpless! I was in a frustrating cycle of trying to find products that worked—but every time it led to disappointment, and continued suffering. Yet, like most women, that didn't stop me from trying again and again.

Finally, in early adulthood, I came to the realization that most skincare claims were either seriously misleading, just plain wrong, or, at best, delusional. I was determined and resolute to find out the truth about skin and skincare—it became a compulsion, eventually leading me to take my first steps into a career in the world of cosmetics. It was by no means a straight path, and I had no idea that it would lead me to where I am today; I only knew I was on a mission, and I have never wavered from that mission throughout all the years I've been doing this.

From my first book to thousands of media interviews and appearances, to presentations to women's groups around the world, and to the products I've formulated, I have been, and continue to be, determined to change the face of beauty for myself, for the people I know, and for people everywhere. I didn't want anyone to go through what I went through ever again. In looking over my evolving career, I believe I've accomplished much of what I set out to do. But I'm not quitting! There's still a lot of work and research yet to be done.

PAULA'S LIFE-CHANGING MOMENT!

I started my cosmetics career back in 1977. During my early years working as a makeup artist as well as selling skincare and makeup products, I didn't know many of the technical details of why so many skincare and makeup products failed abysmally to live up to their claims; I just knew they didn't work as advertised. More often than not, the claims made for the products and what they were supposed to do rarely matched their performance, or even came close, but at the time I had no way to confirm my suspicions; there was no Internet as we know it today and no one had personal computers.

It was about that time one of the most historic advancements in the world of cosmetics was taking place. In 1977, the U.S. Food and Drug Administration (FDA) finalized the Fair Packaging and Labeling Act, a piece of cosmetic regulation that was about to change the face of beauty forever, and my future as well. What took place—after many years of legal wrangling and deliberation—was the mandatory requirement for all cosmetics to include a complete list of ingredients printed on the product's packaging and presented in descending order of content. The ingredients first on the list were there in the largest amounts and the ingredients at the end were present in the tiniest amounts.

It's difficult to imagine now how significant and radical an event that was. The United States passed this regulation in 1977; the next country to mandate cosmetic ingredient labeling (Australia) didn't enact it until 1995! Other countries didn't follow suit until 2000 through 2009.

Needless to say, I was very pleased to finally know what was in a cosmetic, but, at the same time, it was a disappointment because so many of the ingredient names were indecipherable (and they still are to this day). Here was this amazing information on the label, but I had no idea what I was reading and, on top of that, there were (and are) thousands of different ingredients that a cosmetics chemist can use to make a product. It made my head spin, but it also spurred the beginning of my quest to learn what it all meant and to then spread the word—that is where my books and, eventually, Paula's Choice would play a critical role.

With a background in science from my university days and access to scientific journals (all in hard copy in libraries, as there was no Google back then), my search began. I immersed myself in biology and physiology books and the scientific and medical journals on skin (something I still do with my team today, albeit with much easier access).

JUST KNOWING INGREDIENTS ISN'T ENOUGH

As fascinating as it was to finally know what products actually contain, whether those ingredients were actually effective or beneficial (or how problematic they were), it wasn't enough. In other words, although I now knew the function of an ingredient in a formula, fundamental and complicated questions remained. I still needed to know which ingredients, in what amounts, and in what types of products they would work best for which skin type and which skin concerns, from acne to wrinkles, dry skin, rosacea, oily skin, combination skin, sun damage, loss of firmness, blackheads, and on and on. Moreover, what should be done if someone had multiple problems, like oily skin and wrinkles with occasional breakouts, or dry skin with rosacea and sun damage? Many people, including me, deal with frustrating combinations like this, and it can be incredibly confusing to know how to treat seemingly contradictory skin concerns.

It was overwhelming, just imagining the vast amount of scientific and medical literature I would have to tackle to accomplish what I'd set out to do. There were myriad questions that needed answers.

The most basic question of all, however, was what kinds of products, among other elements of a skincare routine, could be combined into a cohesive routine that takes into account everything someone needs—and that excludes what is absolutely not needed—to have beautiful, healthy skin?

An even more complex problem is that most ingredients have nuances that affect their degree of benefit (or their potential for damage) to skin. For example, not all ingredients can be stable in the same formula, but those same ingredients can sometimes be combined with the right formulary considerations. There's also the issue of how much of any specific ingredient is needed to get the best results.

When it comes to plant extracts, it gets even more complicated because different parts of a plant can have different attributes. Take green tea for example, which would be listed on a product as *Camellia sinensis*. Research is clear that green tea is a good skincare ingredient, but which part of the plant is the best? Do you want the leaves, flower, roots, or stem of the plant? Eventually, I was to learn that this nuance applied to most ingredients.

I went back to the library, spending endless days searching for answers to these questions. Over a period of five years, I assembled enough data and details to realize what formulations would be best for skin, for different skin types, different skin concerns, and perhaps most importantly, which ones would present a serious risk of irritation to skin.

All this culminated in my first book, *Blue Eyeshadow Should Be Illegal,* which was published in 1985. Two years later I appeared on *The Oprah Winfrey Show* for the first time and would go on to make 14 more appearances on her show during the years it aired.

ANCIENT WISDOM WAS NOT VERY WISE

...At least not when it came to skincare! With each book I wrote, I thought I had really, this time, finally said it all, and that now people would find their way, as I had, to having the best skin possible and I would never have to write another book. Obviously, that wasn't the case, as I went on to write many more books and articles. I would have loved it if my first book could have covered everything, but as countless new studies were conducted and scientific discoveries were published, knowledge about skincare progressed and changed, and so did our conclusions and recommendations about what would (and wouldn't) work for skin.

As the research evolved, so did our work, as we needed to incorporate what the most current research demonstrated to be true for skin. Each new book reflected the recent significant and meaningful information so you would stay informed and be able to take the best care of your skin. And, as with every book before it, beautiful skin is what this book (and Paula's Choice Skincare) is all about!

Many people ask us: Why does skincare have to be so complicated? Believe us, we wish it weren't, but it is, although some people understandably still doubt us. Women sometimes tell us, "Well, my grandmother just used bar soap and she looked great!" We have no doubt grandma was a beautiful woman, but we would no sooner expect you to use a typewriter rather than your laptop computer—or a hard-wired landline rather than a smart phone—just because that worked well for your grandmother. Like laptops and smart phones, advances in skincare reflect the same concept in terms of the innovative and cutting-edge technology used to develop today's best products.

Taking care of your skin can seem as complicated as rocket science, but as multifaceted and complex as skincare is, we can bring it down to earth for you so you can make the best decisions for your skin.

With all due respect to previous generations and ancient cultures, the often-disastrous skincare routines and products used throughout history were not necessarily beautiful, and they certainly were not solutions. Don't cheat your skin by accepting myths about skincare. Even as little as 20 years ago, there was little to no information about sun protection, antioxidants, increasing collagen production, preventing environmental damage, and so on.

It's also important to remember that there are no miraculous ingredients when it comes to skincare. This is one of the more difficult facts to get across in this book, and you may find it hard to accept because cosmetics companies endlessly parade new ingredients with elaborate and enticing fabricated stories about their amazing effects on skin. It is not easy to ignore that barrage of inducements. Please try to resist being seduced by yet another rare plant extract, exotic plant oil, or some scientifically manufactured ingredient because, without exception, this belief will be a disaster for your skin. It's not that new ingredients are not interesting and potentially beneficial for skin, but skin is too complicated for any single ingredient to be enough. If anything, just the opposite is true: Skin needs a vast array of substances to be healthy, to heal, to stay young looking, to feel smoother, and to look flawless.

THE GENESIS OF PAULA'S CHOICE

Paula's Choice Skincare was launched in 1995 and I am very proud of the products we've created. That was almost ten years to the day from when my first book was published. What a remarkable journey it has been and continues to be!

Creating my own line of skincare products was controversial given that I had been such a strong and vocal critic of the cosmetics industry. Wasn't I sleeping with the enemy and going over to the dark side? How could I ever be impartial again? Anyone who is familiar with my work over the years knows that I haven't compromised my principles or integrity for one moment—you will find just the opposite is true. The more my team and I learned by formulating products and working with brilliant cosmetics chemists, the more in-depth knowledge we gained about skincare and skincare products. All this reinforced my drive to not just create great products but also to put forth reliable, research-supported information.

My reason for starting Paula's Choice Skincare was in large part due to pressure from my friends, family, and readers of my books. They kept asking me to make my own products that didn't have all the "buts" and warnings of the other products I reviewed. They would say, "You always write 'this product is good...—but it's too expensive for what you get, —but it has too much fragrance, —but it's in unstable packaging, —but there are better products out there." They'd practically yell at me, exclaiming: "Just make your own products so we know what to use, because otherwise it's overwhelming and there's no way to know what's best!" I understood precisely what they were talking about.

There was also another reason I considered starting Paula's Choice Skincare, though I'm a bit reluctant to admit it. The plain truth is I also started my own line of products because I didn't want to write any more books. Each new book was bigger and bigger, requiring hours of exhaustive research and energy. It seemed relatively easier to put my energy, time, and what I knew about skincare into my own products—no more books.

So, in 1993, after all the cajoling and encouragement from people in my life and after overcoming self-doubt, it dawned on me that "Yes, I could indeed make state-of-the-art products that left out all the 'buts' and that were loaded with ingredients research showed were beneficial for skin." The idea for Paula's Choice Skincare was born; the first products began arriving nearly two years later!

Obviously, as you now know, my enthusiasm for writing books didn't go away! I couldn't give up what I had been doing for the previous ten years of my life. Skincare information is not only my mission and heritage; it is also my legacy.

I also want to set the record straight for those who think I hate the cosmetics industry and/or I like only my own products; nothing could be further from the truth. I am and have always been in constant awe of what well-formulated beauty products can do, no matter who they're from. However, what I do hate are the ludicrous claims, misinformation, and poorly-formulated products that can hurt or mislead consumers into taking poor care of their skin and wasting their money. And, while I definitely love my own products as you will see throughout this book, I definitely do not ignore alternative options.

IT TAKES A VILLAGE...

In the beginning, I used to handle all of the writing and research myself, but fortunately, my co-authors Bryan and Desiree joined me, along with formula experts, researchers, and others to help publish our books and articles and maintain our website PaulasChoice.com, which is one of the best and most frequently updated sources for complete skincare information in the world.

Together, this amazing team accomplishes time after time what most would say is the impossible. As a result, each subsequent edition of our books has achieved a higher level of excellence in providing you with an unparalleled, easy-to-understand resource about skincare and makeup. Without question, this book would not be possible without the hard work and dedication of the entire Paula's Choice Research Team. Each one of us has taken the information, research, and philosophy to new heights of dedication and responsibility.

Together, we search out and analyze endless studies on skincare and ingredients, pore over fashion magazines, and spend hours upon hours researching what works and what doesn't, and in finding ways to help as many people as possible navigate the often-confusing world of skincare and makeup.

I always say it takes a village of enthusiastic and educated people to do the work we do at Paula's Choice—to write books like this one, and to ensure the quality of the products we create for Paula's Choice Skincare. Through it all, my team and I remain steadfast in our mission to provide current and insightful information about skincare and makeup.

SHARING OUR PURSUIT FOR TRUTH

I have always worked hard in trying to find the best way to help people see the difference between fact and fiction when it comes to taking care of their skin. In the beginning, I feared I was being too critical. Indeed, I was often told I just had a vendetta against the cosmetics industry, and would I please just stop being so critical.

Nowadays, if you Google my name you will see that very few people are neutral about my work—they either hate it or love it. You'll read statements claiming that I'm not a dermatologist, I'm not a scientist, I'm biased, I'm critical of other products just to push my own, I'm not really objective ... and on and on. You'll also see lots of positive comments, such as praise for my 35 years of work, which speaks for itself, the fact that I've changed my views in response to new research findings, that I've helped their skin in ways they never thought possible, and that my team and I provide one-of-a-kind information you can't find anywhere else in the world.

People also wonder about other companies; that is, if what we say here at Paula's Choice Skincare is true, then why don't the other companies know the same things? Why don't they follow suit? The answer is: We don't know. The research and studies my team and I cite throughout all our books and articles are accessible to everyone. There are no secrets in the world of skincare because all the validated published research, scientific journals, and medical textbooks are only a click away on your computer, and even on mobile devices these days—though sometimes fees are involved and the studies can be difficult to decipher. The point is that the research and its results are not secrets, and there are no patented secrets either as the legality of a patent worldwide means that every minute detail of the ingredient and the formula must be disclosed and available to the public.

Regardless of whether or not you agree with everything this book has to say, you will at least have someone else's voice whispering in your ear, saying, "Here is the research showing why doing this is best for your skin" or "Given the physiology of skin, this is why a product can't work or can work as claimed." We believe this is a far better way to make decisions about how to take care of your skin than relying on a never-ending litany of misleading claims and flawed information that prevail throughout much of the cosmetics industry.

SKIN FRUSTRATIONS ARE UNIVERSAL

Paula's Choice Skincare products are sold in over 50 countries around the world. This has given me the opportunity to give hundreds of media interviews and to hold speaking engagements in places such as Jakarta, Indonesia; Seoul, South Korea; Stockholm, Sweden; Mexico City, Mexico; Singapore; Sydney and Melbourne, Australia; Kuala Lumpur, Malaysia; Amsterdam, The Netherlands; Moscow, Russia; Taipei, Taiwan; Toronto, Edmonton, and Vancouver, Canada; and, of course, almost every major city in the United States.

What I've learned is that the business of beauty is universally crazy. There's no place in the world where people aren't frustrated about how to take the best care of their skin. No matter where I've been in the world, people are equally concerned about looking younger and having picture-perfect skin. As a result, I am asked the same questions wherever I go and I rarely have to change my responses!

People want to know why a product they bought didn't work. Why didn't their deep wrinkles go away? Why didn't their red marks from acne fade? Why wasn't their skin lifted? Why didn't their skin discolorations change? Why are they still breaking out or just starting to break out? Why do they still have dry, flaky skin after buying so many products promising to make things better? Why is their skin so red and irritated? What is the best anti-aging ingredient? Do I know about a recently launched product with a supposed miracle ingredient and does it work? What about ingredients from Morocco, the Amazon, India, China, or some other far-flung place?

During my presentations, I've come to expect a look of understanding gradually wash over the audience member's faces as they begin to grasp how myths have taken over the facts about what is best for skin.

What people everywhere want is to take the best care of their skin, look younger and have an even skin tone, with no breakouts, smaller pores, and on and on. In each country I visit, without fail, beauty ideals revolve entirely around youth and flawless skin, and how to get there. That last point—how to get there—is inevitably accompanied by shared confusion, worldwide. My team and I want to clear up that confusion for you here and now! We don't want you to take our word for it. We want you to know all the facts.

WANTING BEAUTIFUL SKIN

We understand the distress that skin problems can cause. Many of us feel a blow to our self-esteem when our skin doesn't look and feel beautiful. At any age, that can be crushing. On top of that, what makes this utterly maddening, for us and for you, is that solutions can seem impossible to find. That's not because solutions don't exist, but rather because too often the truth or reality is mired in misleading information, myths, false pretext, and poor product formulations.

You're often told that all-natural is the way to go, or that there is a new miracle ingredient that is best for your skin, or that this one product is the answer, or that whatever product the celebrity you admire is using is what you should be using, and on and on. The industry uses all of these methods to assure you that you will be doing the best thing for your skin, and that you won't be hurting your skin … and then the next promises and miracle products or plant extracts start gaining attention in traditional and social media … and the cycle continues.

We understand why all that marketing makes it tempting and how easy it is to be seduced by it. All of us here at Paula's Choice Skincare have gone through this ourselves. That's why we are so dedicated to researching and discovering what really works and what doesn't work for skin based on scientific studies and medical textbooks, not on fabrications or made-up claims. This is how all of us here at Paula's Choice Skincare have resolved our skin problems, and how we've helped millions of people around the world address their problems. For that, we are not only proud, but also privileged to have lived our dream and to continue to do so every day.

We can assure you with complete certainty that the results for all of us have been nothing short of astounding—and we know you can experience the same real results without all the puffery or pretense! We know those are bold statements, but hang in there with us—you'll find it well worth your while.

WE WORRY ABOUT YOU

Why are we worried? Because we know how much of the information you've read or heard about skincare is more often than not incomplete, one-sided, just plain wrong, or what amounts to nothing more than fear-mongering. That makes us worry about how you will decide what to use and what not to use on your skin. You can't get the best skin of your life based on myths and fabrications. It's absolutely frustrating to us to see consumers stuck in the middle, being pushed and pulled by such disparate, maddening information and hoping the next product they buy, or facial they get, or medical procedure they have will finally be the answer. It's a vicious merry-go-round that isn't all that merry and is hard to get off.

Much of the information out there is unreliable and spurious, and not only won't help you take the best care of your skin, but can also make matters worse and consistently waste your money, two things we can't abide.

We could wax poetic about the past and present senseless, impractical myths and bad skincare advice that has and still does run rampant in every corner of the cosmetics industry. Everything we reveal in this book will help you find your way through and come out of the maze of confusion. You will be empowered to start doing what is best for your skin! This book factually demonstrates exactly how you can do that, whether you use Paula's Choice Skincare products or someone else's. If we've succeeded, perhaps you'll even have a little fun along the way! But first, a bit more background....

AGE, SKIN COLOR, AND RACE ARE NOT SKIN TYPES!

There are several aspects to understanding your skin type, but first you must understand that your age, skin color, and race are not as important as other factors. I know that may be hard to believe, especially considering how often you've read statements to the contrary, but it's 100% true. It isn't that older skin isn't different from younger skin or that darker skin color isn't different from lighter skin color, it's just that when it comes to how you take care of your skin and what you should and shouldn't do, these factors—age of your skin and color of your skin—don't matter.

What does matter are the skin concerns you're dealing with and your skin type. You can be 60 and have oily skin with breakouts and sun damage, but understand that someone can have the exact same issues at age 30.

The types of ingredients and products that treat dry skin, oily skin, rosacea, wrinkles, acne, blackheads, skin discolorations, uneven skin tone, red marks from breakouts, sensitive skin, sun damage (everyone has sun damage), eczema, combination skin, and on and on are essentially the SAME (with only minor exceptions) for everyone.

Think about it like your diet. What's healthy or unhealthy to eat is generally the same for everyone. Adding more green, leafy vegetables and fruit to your diet is healthy, regardless of your age or race. Likewise, chocolate cake and hydrogenated fats can't be considered health foods for anyone, regardless of their age or race.

Research has clearly established the types of skincare formulas that can work wonders and likewise those that are badly formulated and can make matters worse. This is true no matter who you are, how old you are, what race you are, or where you live. We discuss skin type further in Chapter 3, *Skin Type vs. Skin Concern*.

SETTING REALISTIC EXPECTATIONS AND GOALS

This section of our book may not be easy for some of you because we're about to discuss the limitations of skincare. People do want to believe in miracle products and in miracle ingredients that will replace the need for cosmetic surgery or cosmetic corrective procedures. We wish we could tell you otherwise, but such products just don't exist. It's not that there aren't brilliantly formulated, remarkable products to consider—it's just that they all have limitations (and that includes my products).

It's our devout promise that we will never mislead you or exaggerate the truth. Unfortunately—and we know from our own experience—it's far easier to believe in the exaggerations and the hype hoping, just hoping, that there is some truth in it. So, while the information we present in this section may be somewhat disappointing for you, it is vitally important for you to stop the endless search for and temptation to buy yet another product claiming miraculous results.

It's important to realize that skincare products have limitations, despite the claims made in the advertisements you've seen, articles you've read, or what you've been told by salespeople, dermatologists, aestheticians, or your friends. Skincare products cannot replace what cosmetic corrective procedures or face-lifts can do. They can make a phenomenal difference, especially when you consistently use great products and keep your skin protected from the sun (daylight) 365 days a year, but they cannot give you the kind of results you keep pinning your hopes on.

Skincare products can't stop time and they can't dramatically turn the clock back. You aren't going to lift a sagging neck, jaw line, or under-eye area with skincare products. You also aren't going to erase deep wrinkles or the effects of advanced sun damage. Again, skincare can provide impressive improvements, but it's always within the parameters of physiological reality. Understanding the limitations and knowing what's possible (and not possible) will not only save you from one disappointment after another, but also keep you from wasting a lot of money along the way. We discuss this in greater detail and provide key information about cosmetic corrective and surgical procedures in Chapter 13, *Botox, Fillers, Lasers, and Surgery.*

You've probably heard the saying that if you repeat a lie often enough it becomes accepted as fact. Well, the beauty industry is no exception. Throughout this book you will learn only the facts about what research says is best for your skin, in ways that will surprise you and often give you dramatic results (almost overnight), especially once you stop using products that are useless (or actually bad) for your skin.

SURPRISES AWAIT...

We present a lot of information in this book, but the following list gives you an overview of some of the more salient, universal points we want you to keep in mind as you peruse these pages. In *The Best Skin of Your Life Starts Here*, you'll find discussions and explanations of the following facts:

» Why you should avoid jar packaging
» Why many natural ingredients are bad for skin (really, really bad)
» Why spending more money on skincare isn't necessarily better
» How irritating ingredients damage skin
» Why your skin doesn't always let you know when it's being irritated or damaged
» Why and how some anti-acne products can actually cause more breakouts
» Why some eye creams are a problem for the eye area
» How fragrance (whether natural or synthetic) damages skin
» Why some "essential" oils are unessential and, in fact, seriously problematic for skin
» Why antiwrinkle creams can't work like Botox, dermal fillers, lasers, or light treatments
» Why sunscreen is the most important part of a daily skincare routine
» Why terms like "hypoallergenic," "non-comedogenic," "patented ingredients," "dermatologist-approved," and "cosmeceutical" are meaningless, and, in fact, are seen on some of the worst products you'll ever use

» Why there are no miracle skincare ingredients (just lots of great ones)
» Why your skin doesn't "adapt to" the skincare products you are using
» How you might be causing a skin type or concern you don't want
» Which cosmetic ingredients you must avoid and what to use instead (and not based on the typical synthetic-versus-natural argument)
» Why the best approach to makeup is to learn techniques that really make sense and really work, not just buying more products
» And much, much more

WHAT ARE THE BEST INGREDIENTS?

My team and I are continually asked which ingredients in skincare products are the best. If there's a new ingredient being touted, we're asked if it's now "the answer" to their specific skincare woes, especially when it comes to wrinkles.

Aside from the fact that there are literally thousands of different ingredients that can be included in a skincare product, there's no all-inclusive way to sum up which are the best. Actually, to even suggest there's any one ingredient that will solve your skincare woes is just plain silly. Everyone is looking for a magic bullet from that one does-it-all product, but such a product just doesn't exist in the world of skincare.

We wish skincare were as easy as finding the consummate skincare ingredient that can do it all, but it's not … not even close. Skin, the largest organ of the body, has a vast range of substances and is the site of multiple hormonal and molecular interactions that keep it young, radiant, smooth, healthy, breakout-free, and even-toned. As you might suspect, countless things can go wrong when these systems become damaged or start slowing down.

When skin's natural restoring system of antioxidants and skin-repairing ingredients are abundant and working correctly, your skin has a far better chance of healing and staying younger, longer. But when sun damage, age, hormonal changes, environmental damage, and other factors cause those substances to break down and those systems to slow down or change, you must provide your skin with what it needs to repair itself and prevent further problems. That repair can never be solved with any one ingredient or any one product.

Just like your body requires you to eat a complex assortment of beneficial foods to keep you healthy, your skin requires a similarly complex array of ingredients. In addition, different skin types require different products to meet different needs, such as oily, dry, or combination skin, skin that is affected by rosacea, sun damage, brown spots, red marks, acne, wrinkles, and so on. One ingredient may help some of these concerns, but certainly not all of them.

The good news is that there are hundreds of great good-for-your-skin ingredients. On the other hand, there also are dozens of ingredients (both synthetic and natural) that are a serious problem for skin. Whenever you read that some vitamin, plant oil or plant extract is the "best" ingredient for skin, ignore it. Think about it like this, green tea may be healthy for you to drink, but if you drink only green tea you soon will become unhealthy and even risk your life. Think of your skin the same way; it needs a range of substances naturally found in skin to keep "feeding it" day in and day out to be as healthy as possible. Unfortunately, that makes skincare complicated, but we have information and answers for you to help simplify it to the extent possible.

WHAT ABOUT NATURAL INGREDIENTS?

Natural or naturally derived and organic ingredients are a polarizing topic. Some people enjoy the idea of using only skincare products that contain natural or organic ingredients, but there's no benefit to using natural ingredients if those ingredients are going to damage your skin. (Natural does not always mean better—after all, cyanide, lead and snake venom are all perfectly natural substances!) The question we always ask when evaluating any ingredient is: what potential benefit does it have for skin versus its potential to do harm? If it has the potential to irritate or damage skin, how strong is that potential, and is there an alternative ingredient that provides the same benefit without such concerns?

You will be shocked to learn how many natural ingredients can be a problem for skin, and actually damage it. Not all natural skincare ingredients are beneficial. Many companies touting their natural ingredients are not telling the truth when they suggest that synthetic ingredients are inherently bad for skin because, in fact, many are actually brilliant for skin.

In short, there are good and bad natural or naturally-derived ingredients and good and bad synthetic ingredients. That's why we continually pore through the research literature, to help you find the products that contain more of what's proven to help skin and avoid those loaded with irritating, harmful ingredients or over-glorified ingredients that can't perform as you've been told.

To make it easier for you to understand what you'll see on ingredient lists, we include in this book a portion of our Cosmetic Ingredient Dictionary, which you'll find in Chapter 16. It highlights some of the more typical (and controversial) ingredients you'll find in skincare products. This resource explains what an ingredient is and does based on published research, not on hype or fanciful storytelling.

DON'T TRY THIS ON YOURSELF

We're often asked why someone shouldn't just try a product to see if they like it or just rely on someone else's experience with a product to determine if it would work for their needs. We can't think of a bigger mistake for your skin than to rely solely on personal assessment, whether yours or someone else's, to determine the benefit and/or quality of a product. Even here at Paula's Choice Skincare we don't personally test all our own formulas to determine efficacy. It's not that you shouldn't use a product you like, but you should make your selection only from the best-formulated products, those that are right for your skin type and that have the best ingredients research has shown to provide incredible results. How a product feels on your skin alone doesn't give you the vital information you need about the quality of any formula.

So, what's wrong with applying a product to see if it works? Just because you apply a skincare product, even for a relatively long period, doesn't mean that you'll be able to tell if it's helping or hurting your skin. This is true for many reasons.

First, there is an incredible risk to skin from using (or even "just trying") a badly-formulated product. Just because someone likes a product they personally tested doesn't mean it's a good product, for them or for you. They may like the feel or the look of the product, but that doesn't tell you anything about whether or not it is beneficial for skin or harmful for skin.

When it comes to skincare, and even to one's diet, people often "like" what isn't good for them in the short term and, even more important, over the long term. As for skincare, it is difficult, if not impossible, to tell whether a product is good or bad just from applying it. The product may be packaged in a jar, which weakens the beneficial ingredients; it may contain problematic ingredients and so cause damage when used over the long term; it may contain nothing useful at all for repairing more advanced skin concerns; or it may be a daytime moisturizer that doesn't contain sunscreen.

Think about it this way: Just because someone swears by smoking for keeping their weight down doesn't make smoking good for you. It's important to realize that many skincare products have positive or negative results that can be ongoing and/or that can take years to manifest. The benefit of a healthy diet doesn't always show up immediately and the same is true for a terrible diet; it can be years before you see the resulting damage. This also holds true for badly-formulated skincare products: The harm would be ongoing and you wouldn't know because the damage is taking place in the lower layers of skin, beyond what you can see. It can also take years before you see the damage on the surface of skin. I don't want any of us to wait years only to find out that what we were using on our skin all along was detrimental.

It also isn't necessary to test drive a product to know its strengths or weaknesses because the research on most ingredients has already been carried out so the information is readily available, just as it is for food or medicine. You don't need to eat processed foods to know how unhealthy they are for you or smoke cigarettes to find out years later that was a bad choice. A vast amount of research has already been done to determine what those results will be, and the same is true for skincare ingredients.

How skincare ingredients are combined and how they work in products is well known from research in the cosmetic, medical, and biological sciences. There's also extensive, documented medical and scientific research about how different ingredients affect skin. Our information about ingredients is based on that research, which is why our recommendations can really help you find products that work for your skin type, your skin concerns and that you will enjoy using—because they really work! Now that's a concept all of us can agree on, right?

CAN YOU READ AN INGREDIENT LABEL?

I wish I could teach everyone how to read an ingredient label because therein lies the basic, but fundamental, information for determining the effectiveness and functionality of almost any skincare product (makeup is an entirely different matter, which we get to in Chapter 15). The ingredient list is the key to understanding whether or not a product's claims make any sense and whether it's problematic or beneficial for your skin. But, deciphering the ingredient list is not easy, especially if you don't have a background in cosmetic science or cosmetic formulation.

The first and foremost complicating factor is the sheer number of ingredients available that can be included in a formulation. There are literally thousands of ingredients and thousands upon thousands of potential mixtures of those ingredients. The current International Nomenclature of Cosmetic Ingredients (INCI) comprises four huge printed volumes and an online subscription costs thousands of dollars.

Even more confounding are the chemical names of the ingredients, at times far too technical to understand. How can the average consumer ever hope to comprehend what polymethylsilsesquioxane, palmitoyl hexapeptide-12, or cetyl ricinoleate are, let alone understand what they do? Even plant extracts have names that are unpronounceable, such as *Gaultheria procumbens* or *Simmondsia chinensis.* Vitamin C is one of the many great ingredients for skin, but even that has over a dozen different forms with overly-technical names on an ingredient label, and each one has its own benefit and usefulness in a formulation.

In addition to the difficulty of untangling an ingredient label and all the claims espousing an ingredient's or product's benefits, there are also all the horror stories about some ingredients you encounter on the Internet and from other sources. Almost without exception, the fear-mongering you've read about such ingredients as parabens, silicones, mineral oil, sulfates, and so on is just plain wrong. Sometimes the statements made about these types of ingredients (and many others) are taken out of context from research, leading to irrelevant and silly conclusions, or the statements are made up out of thin air, derived or extrapolated from unrelated sources, and/or have no scientific basis.

Any ingredient can be made to sound scary by manipulating the facts. For example, water's chemical name is *Dihydrogen monoxide,* which has been confused repeatedly with the dangerous carbon monoxide because the two have similar-sounding names—not to mention that as innocuous as water seems, drinking too much water within a short period of time can cause serious health problems.

To highlight how this fear-mongering works, we'll use mineral oil as an example. There are those who want to scare you into believing that mineral oil is bad for you, but research reveals just the opposite. Not only is mineral oil natural (it begins as petroleum from the earth), but also the research makes it crystal clear that it's one of the gentlest and safest cosmetic ingredients out there, especially for wound healing and dry skin. In some ways, it's safer than water!

Other examples of ingredients that have been subject to fear-mongering include silicones, which are a brilliant group of ingredients that have been used in hospital burn units around the world for decades; sulfates, which are not problematic and do not cause cancer; and parabens, which are some of the safest, most non-irritating preservatives ever used in cosmetics.

The authentic scientific and balanced information is out there, but it's been a lifelong pursuit for us to filter through the research, not something a consumer can easily pick up or find the time to figure out; even many people within the cosmetics industry have difficulty in this area, and so fall prey to misleading or completely false information. Now it's time for us to give you the facts about skincare and about how to take the best care of your skin.

CHAPTER 2

Skincare Facts Everyone Needs to Know

WHY YOU MIGHT NOT HAVE YOUR BEST SKIN YET

There are many reasons you may not have the skin you want: sun damage, genetics, skin disorders, aging, hormone loss, health issues, pollution, skincare products that contain irritating ingredients, and on and on. To one degree or another, all of these factors are responsible for free-radical damage, a complex and continual process of molecular deterioration that occurs both inside and outside the body, often accompanied and/or caused by inflammation.

In addition to the free-radical damage and inflammation occurring internally in your body causing aging and disease, the same sort of progressive deterioration is occurring on and within your skin. Over time, this ongoing process creates and re-creates inflammation, which slowly decreases skin's ability to keep itself young, healthy, even-toned, firm, and breakout-free. Inflammation can also trigger excess oil production and keep skin from looking smooth. No matter how you look at it, inflammation is just bad news!

Although all the factors mentioned above play havoc with your body and skin due to the inflammation they trigger, what you put on your skin can have the same effect, and often plays a significant role in what is going wrong. Skincare products can cause irritation, which in turn produces inflammation, resulting in problems—problems that you'll try to fix with skincare products and cosmetic corrective procedures. [1]

Understanding what your skin needs for your skin type and skin concerns is vital, but it's equally important to know what your skin *doesn't* need. That's critical because the very skincare products you are using may, in fact, be exacerbating the problems you're trying to fix.

Given our cumulative years of looking at skincare formulations, it still shocks us that many of the products people buy to treat a specific skin condition actually make it worse. For example, products you've purchased claiming to control oily skin often contain ingredients that make the skin even more oily. Products claiming to be oil-free often contain ingredients that nonetheless make the skin feel greasy. Products claiming they won't cause breakouts may contain pore-clogging, emollient ingredients that don't sound like they would be a problem because we don't recognize the names on the ingredient label. Countless skincare products contain irritating ingredients that further damage your skin with each use. Those are the sorts of things we address in this chapter.

IRRITATION IS YOUR SKIN'S WORST ENEMY

We cannot stress this enough: Irritation and inflammation are bad for skin—really, really bad! Daily assaults from unprotected sun exposure, splashing the face with hot water, and applying skincare products that contain irritating ingredients have a harsh and inflammatory effect. These types of attacks reduce the skin's ability to heal, break down the skin's chief support substances (collagen and elastin), weaken skin's outer protective layer, and can cause many other complications. [2,3]

For those with oily skin, it's especially important to know that irritation triggers the nerve endings in the pore that, in turn, trigger the production of androgens, hormones that increase oil production and make pores bigger! [3,4] That is not good for any skin type!

It turns out that much of what we know about skin aging, wrinkles, brown spots, skin healing, and acne has evolved from our increased understanding of skin's inflammatory reaction to sun exposure (UV radiation), pollution, cigarette smoke, and even irritation from skincare products. These all trigger an inflammatory process that leads to cumulative damage within skin, resulting in the deterioration of collagen and elastin, depletion of disease-fighting cells, and out-of-control free-radical damage. [5,6,7]

SKIN'S SILENT KILLER

It would probably be easier for those who smoke cigarettes to stop smoking if the damage it was causing on the inside showed itself instantly on the outside. Regrettably, that isn't the case; as we now know, it can take years for the damage to show up. Interestingly, the same can be said for skin damage.

People often assume their skincare products aren't hurting their skin because they don't feel or see any negative reactions. BUT, although we may not see or feel anything, the damage is taking place beneath the surface of the skin, from things we apply to it or do to it; eventually (perhaps years from now), it will show up on the surface, and it won't be pretty. [2]

You can get a clearer idea of how this hidden, underlying damage from irritating skincare routines or from specific products takes place by imagining what happens to the skin in reaction to unprotected sun exposure. The sun is a major cause of free-radical damage and inflammation. These effects cause brown spots, wrinkling, skin cancer, and other degenerative issues. Yet, other than the (hopefully) rare occasion when you get sunburned, you don't feel or even see the damage done to your skin from the sun, until—you guessed it— years later. Even more shocking is that the most damaging rays of the sun can penetrate windows—now that really is a silent killer! [8,9]

FRAGRANCE: SMELLS LIKE TROUBLE FOR YOUR SKIN

We are all attracted to a pleasing fragrance. In fact, the first thing most people do when considering just about any skincare product is smell it. As nice as it is to have a product with a wonderful aroma, it just doesn't make sense for good skincare. Whether the fragrance in the product is from a plant or a synthetic source, with very few exceptions what pleases your nose is a problem for your skin.

The way most fragrance ingredients impart scent is through a volatile re-action, which on your skin causes irritation and at least some inflammation. Research has established that fragrant ingredients in skincare products are among the most common cause of sensitizing and allergic reactions.

That means that daily use of products that contain a high amount of fra-grance, whether the fragrant ingredients are synthetic or natural, will lead to chronic irritation that can damage healthy collagen production, lead to or worsen dryness, and impair your skin's ability to heal. Fragrance-free is the best way to go for all skin types. [5,6,10,11,12]

Unfortunately, your nose cannot determine from the smell of a product whether or not it contains irritating fragrant ingredients. Many beneficial skincare ingredients (antioxidants, for example) have a natural fragrance, and some even smell great! However, distinguishing between the potent antioxi-dants that actually reduce inflammation and the ingredients that are added to make you "shop with your nose" and that can cause irritation, isn't easy.

Like anything in skincare, the basic information is on the ingredient label, but because those ingredients read like a college chemistry course, they are a challenge to decipher, especially if fragrant plant oils are listed only by their Latin names in place of the more obvious "fragrance."

EVERYONE HAS SENSITIVE SKIN

Most of us, to one degree or another, have sensitive skin; that is, our skin reacts negatively to the environment and can react negatively to what we put on it. Regardless of your skin type or concerns, irritation inflames the skin, and that's always damaging, regardless of what the source of the irritation happens to be and whether or not you see a reaction on the surface. [2,5,7] Lots of things irritate our skin; some we can avoid and some we can't, but we can mitigate much of it by using great skincare products and being smart about avoiding sun damage.

No matter how you think your skin reacts to different aspects of the environment and to the products you use, we are all sensitive to irritation and inflammation, and the resulting damage.

As mentioned above, whether you know it or not, you have sensitive skin. If you are going to take the best possible care of your skin, it's essential you take the same precautions that someone with more obviously sensitive skin takes: Regardless of your skin type, treat your skin as gently as you possibly can. Whether you think of your facial skin as normal, oily, dry, or acne-prone, you still need to be gentle and avoid things that cause irritation as much as possible. Doing so is a key step to getting and keeping the skin you want!

YOU HAVE TO BE GENTLE

Everyone's skin will react negatively to irritating skincare ingredients. So, for the overall health of your skin (and because irritation is so terrible for skin), anything you can do to treat yours gently is a very good thing. We mention this many times throughout this book, not to be repetitive, but so it really sinks in—being gentle is truly that important!

Always keep in mind that treating skin gently and using well-formulated, non-irritating skincare products encourages normal collagen production, helps maintain a smooth and radiant surface, helps the skin better protect itself from environmental damage, prevents or reduces excess oil production, and makes enlarged pores smaller. The chapters that follow explain exactly how that works for each skin type and skin concern. In the meantime, we guarantee you will see potentially dramatic improvements to your skin simply by avoiding irritating products and learning to be gentle.

RULES FOR SKINCARE SUCCESS

One of the most important ways to achieve the best skin of your life is to follow the fundamental rules of great skincare.

Be consistent. For best results, a great skincare routine should be carried out regularly. Some products you'll use once or twice daily, others every other day, or once a week, but consistency is the key. It's also important to use products in the right order. For example, sunscreen should be the last skincare product you apply before makeup so as not to dilute it with other skincare products; we explain this more in Chapter 6, *Sun Damage and Sunscreen Questions Answered.*

Don't expect instant results. Although there are products that can have dramatic, overnight results, they are the exception; it takes time for most products to really make a difference. Even more important, continued use is necessary to maintain the results. For example, products for skin discolorations take at least three to six weeks to begin showing results assuming, of course, that the product is well-formulated and that you're using a sunscreen every day. Because sunscreen protects skin every day and prevents damage, you won't see a dramatic difference in skin discolorations if you don't apply it daily. Many skincare products are about long-terms benefits and preventing what would happen if you didn't use the products.

Your skin must be "fed" daily. As you age, and mostly because of sun damage, your skin can't naturally replenish the substances it needs to be healthy. Great skincare products give those substances back to skin, but they get used up quickly and must be replenished on a constant, daily basis. Don't cheat your skin by not giving it the ingredients it needs to maintain a beautiful, healthy appearance, now and years from now.

Skin doesn't repair itself only at night. We hear this repeatedly—"that skin repairs itself only at night"—we discuss it here because it is sheer nonsense! All of our skincare woes are happening all day long, whether from the environment, sunlight, aging, health, or endlessly fluctuating hormones. Skin needs help, day and night, to repair and soothe this damage for it to be healthy and to prevent more damage from taking place. Your skin needs brilliantly formulated products day and night, with the only difference being that for daytime one of those products must be a well-formulated sunscreen with SPF 30 or higher.

One product can't do it all. All skin types (especially if you have multiple concerns) require a variety of products to give you the best skin of your life. Aside from the basics (such as a cleanser, toner, exfoliant, sunscreen, and moisturizer), if you have breakouts, rosacea, very dry skin, extremely sun-damaged skin, combination skin, skin discolorations, or other concerns, you will need to address those with treatment products designed for that specific problem.

Don't skip using a leave-on exfoliant. We explain this more in Chapter 4, *Which Skincare Products You Need and Which Ones to Avoid*, but the gist of it is that the benefit to your skin can be astounding. A leave-on exfoliant is one of the few products that can produce dramatic results overnight, and every night of your life, for that matter. Helping skin shed the excess buildup of accumulated skin cells, caused mostly from sun damage or having oily/combination or breakout-prone skin, can make all the difference in the world. It isn't a cure; think of it as maintenance that you perform consistently to take excellent care of your skin.

Do consider a retinol product. There are so many reasons to apply a well-formulated retinol product it's hard to know where to begin. We discuss how retinol relates to specific skin types and concerns in subsequent chapters, but for now, just know that this cell-communicating ingredient helps all skin types generate healthy cells, unclog pores, smooth skin, and reduce wrinkles and breakouts. If there were a single, "miracle" ingredient in skincare, this would be at or near the top of the list. Just to be clear, retinol is not the only ingredient skin needs, but it is one of those ingredients with special properties that work for everyone, and the results can be fairly immediate.

Pay attention when your skin changes. There are all sorts of things that can cause your skin to change seemingly overnight. Many women know what can happen to their skin when they get their period. For others they experience skin changes during perimenopause or menopause. For both genders, seasonal weather shifts, traveling to a different climate, and extreme stress can all change what is happening to your skin. Given that your skin is changing, you may need to adapt your skincare routine accordingly. For example, even though you may never have had a breakout growing up or experienced oily skin, random hormonal changes between the ages of 30 and 60 can change all that and you'll need to consider different skincare products—even if your skin is also showing signs of aging.

Everyone needs the same basic ingredients to obtain healthy, younger, smoother, and breakout-free skin. We can't stress this enough. As we explain in Chapter 3, *Skin Type vs. Skin Concern*, all skin types—and we mean ALL skin types—need the same vitally important skincare ingredients, which include antioxidants, skin-repairing ingredients (sometimes called barrier-repair ingredients or skin-identical ingredients), and cell-communicating ingredients. Each of these is mandatory, and we mean imperative, if you are to obtain the best skin of your life, and that goes for everyone on the face of the earth.

Knowing how to balance the needs of your skin type with the needs of your skin concerns is how you create the best skincare routine possible. Identifying skin type is the first part of putting together a great skincare routine because your skin type determines the kinds of product textures you should be using for your core skincare routine. Cleanser, toner, exfoliant, moisturizer, and sunscreen are the core skincare products everyone needs with the basic ingredients we mentioned above, but depending on your skin type they will have different textures (which we explain in the next rule).

Once you understand that aspect of skincare, the next step is to determine what skin concerns you have, which can be one or a combination of problems such as skin discolorations, breakouts, wrinkles, uneven skin tone, very dry skin, very oily skin, acne, blackheads, sun damage, and so on. These concerns will determine what additional treatment products you may need. Balancing the core products you need for your skin type with the treatment products you need for your skin concerns are the pieces of the puzzle whose answers will enable you to create the best skincare routine for you.

Product texture is everything. Now that you know everyone needs the same fundamental, crucial ingredients for their skin (antioxidants, skin-repairing ingredients, and cell-communicating ingredients) the next step is to understand how skin type determines the texture of the products you need to deliver those ingredients to your skin.

In short, as mentioned above, the texture of a product is determined by your skin type. That means if you have normal to dry skin, you should generally be using lotion- to cream-textured products. If you have very dry skin, you should be using very emollient, richly textured products. If you have normal to oily/combination skin, you should be using only gels, liquids, lightweight serums, or thin-textured lotions. If you have very oily skin all over, liquids and gels will probably feel the best. The same vital ingredients should be present, but the products should have different textures based on skin type.

Treatment products that address your skin concerns should have lighter-weight textures because they are inserted into your core skincare routine.

Layering products can make all the difference. It is possible to maintain and achieve great skin with a relatively simple skincare routine, but that's true only if you have few or no skincare problems or concerns. If you are not one of those lucky few, than layering skincare products can make all the difference in the world. We describe layering more in Chapter 3, but for now just be aware that specialty treatment products for advanced sun damage, oily areas, rosacea, extremely dry skin, breakout-prone skin, blackheads, and many other problems will require a more advanced skincare routine.

Diet plays a role. It's hard to have the best skin of your life without paying attention to your diet. Ample research shows how an unhealthy diet loaded with sugars, processed foods, saturated animal fats, and too much alcohol are all pro-aging for your body and for your skin. A poor diet can even make acne-prone skin worse, because so many foods that aren't good for us cause inflammation. When it comes to skin aging, the damage may not show up when you're young, but the calamity for skin is certain if you keep eating an unhealthy diet—in the long run your skin will pay for it. On the other hand, a diet rich in antioxidants, omega-3 and omega-6 fatty acids, whole grains, and many other healthy food groups, can be anti-aging and anti-acne. Without question your skin, heart, and your entire body will thank you for it.

Sunscreen. By the end of this book you will surely be tired of hearing this, but nothing is as vital as sun protection. Despite the abundant research showing how damaging unprotected sun exposure is and how tanning causes irreparable harm to skin, less than 20% of the population wears sunscreen on a regular basis (which just causes our jaws to hit the floor). That's why we keep repeating this: Sunscreen is a cornerstone of getting the best skin of your life now and forever!

CHAPTER 3

Skin Type vs. Skin Concern

One of the more confusing aspects of developing an effective skincare routine is finding products that work for your skin type and that also address your skin concerns. It's important to understand exactly what you should be using for each (skin type and skin concern) and why. Here's how it works.

Skin type is the primary feel of your skin: how dry, oily, combination (meaning oily in some areas dry in others), or normal it is (normal meaning neither oily nor combination nor dry, just normal). Some people would add sensitive skin as a skin type, but because the research shows that skin is reactive to the environment and to everything we apply to it, whether we feel it or not, everyone truly has sensitive skin and must treat it as such.

Once you've determined what your skin type is and you know whether it's normal, dry, oily, or combination, you can then determine what type of products you will need for your core skincare routine. You must look for products that are identified as being appropriate for your skin type. Products for the core routine include cleansers, toners, exfoliants, moisturizers, and sunscreens. These products, with textures appropriate for your skin type, will meet the basic needs of your skin every day of your life. Creamy, rich-textured products will be best for dry skin, lotions for normal skin, and gels and watery serums or liquids for oily/combination skin.

Next, identify your skin concerns so you can add the appropriate treatment products to address those needs. The most typical skin concerns are wrinkles, loss of firmness, brown spots, red spots, sun damage, advanced sun damage, blackheads, acne, occasional breakouts, rough skin, patches of flaky skin, redness, rosacea, keratosis pilaris, and sebaceous hyperplasia.

Because you will use your treatment products in conjunction with your core skincare routine, the textures of the treatment products should generally be lighter weight so as to not feel heavy on skin. They can be absorbent serums, liquids, light lotions, or fluids.

Once you've determined your skin type along with your skin concerns, you can begin assessing what types of products and formulas you can combine to get the best results.

Not every skin concern will need a separate treatment product because many treatment products can address more than one concern, and sometimes your core skincare routine is just right to achieve unbelievable results. But, the more concerns you have or the more stubborn they are, it can take multiple products to get your skin concerns under control. This is especially true if you're dealing with multiple concerns, such as breakouts, wrinkles, advanced sun damage, and skin discolorations.

To sum up: If you have oily/combination skin, you should be using products with a liquid, gel, lightweight serum or thin, matte-finish lotion texture. If you have dry skin, you should be using rich emollient creams and lotions. If you have normal skin, the product textures you should be looking for are soft-feeling lightweight lotions.

Keeping these factors in mind, use them as your guideline to assemble a skincare routine that addresses your skin's everyday needs. Your skin type is the basis for a routine that should include a cleanser, toner, AHA (alpha hydroxy acid) or BHA (beta hydroxy acid) exfoliant, daytime moisturizer with sunscreen, and a moisturizer without sunscreen for use at night.

Now that you have your basic routine, it's time to identify your skin concerns and determine what additional targeted treatment products, if any, are necessary. For example, in some cases, a concern (such as clogged pores) might be handled beautifully by one of the products in your basic skincare routine, such as a BHA exfoliant. However, if you also have brown spots, you'll want to add a skin-lightening treatment to your regular routine to address the discolorations in a more targeted manner than merely using an AHA or BHA exfoliant.

WHAT EVERY SKIN TYPE NEEDS

We touched on this topic in Chapter 2, *Skincare Facts Everyone Needs to Know*, but now we'll expand a bit on the critical types of ingredients that all skin types need. These substances occur naturally in skin, but due to sun damage, age, skin disorders such as acne or rosacea, and other issues, they gradually become depleted and eventually skin stops producing them. Providing these integral substances to your skin daily can make all the difference in the long-term health and appearance of your skin. Of course, to keep these vital ingredients protected sunscreen is equally important, just in a different way. (We talk at length about the need for sunscreen in Chapter 6, *Sun Damage and Sunscreen Questions Answered*.)

Antioxidants are a group of natural and synthetic ingredients that reduce free-radical damage and environmental damage. Why is this important? Antioxidants can prevent some of the degenerative effects in skin caused by sun exposure, and can reduce inflammation within skin. [13,14] Inflammation is deadly for skin because it causes the destruction of collagen and elastin, prevents the skin from healing, and thins the layers of skin. [5,6,15] Anything you can do to reduce inflammation is incredibly beneficial, and antioxidants are definitely one group of ingredients that are fundamental for doing that.

The best moisturizers (lotions for normal skin, creams for dry skin, and gels and liquids for oily/combination skin) are formulated with a potent blend of antioxidants that help your skin reduce inflammation and act younger. It's also critical for these antioxidants to be housed in packaging that will ensure they remain effective, which means they should not be packaged in a jar or in clear packaging because antioxidants break down in the presence of light and air. [5,6,15]

Skin-identical and skin-repairing ingredients are substances between skin cells that keep those cells connected (think of mortar between bricks) to help maintain skin's barrier. A healthy, intact barrier allows skin to look smooth, soft, and radiant. It also allows skin to repair itself, which is critical for healing breakouts and red marks and preventing environmental damage. There are many skin-identical ingredients, including such well-known substances as hyaluronic acid, sodium hyaluronate, glycerin, and ceramides. [16,17]

Cell-communicating ingredients are any ingredients that can tell skin cells or other types of cells in skin to behave in a more healthy manner by producing "younger" cells. Over the years, because of sun damage, acne, age, and hormone fluctuations, skin cells and genes involved in cellular formation and repair become permanently damaged. The result is that the new cells being produced are now irregular, mutated, rough, defective, and older-acting cells, whereas before the damage they were healthy cells. [5,6]

Cell-communicating ingredients are substances that "communicate" with these defective cells, helping reverse the damage by helping the skin to produce healthier, younger cells. [5,6] In effect, the defective cells receive a message to stop making bad cells and start making better ones! It is an exciting area of skincare! The key players in this group are niacinamide, retinol, synthetic peptides, lecithin, and adenosine triphosphate. [5,14,18,19,20]

SKIN TYPE DETERMINES FORMULA

We know we're being painfully repetitive, but forgive us if we go over this one more time because it is so important. Once you know your skin type, you will have a clearer understanding of which product formulations and textures work best for you. If you have oily skin, you'll want to avoid overly emollient or greasy formulations at all costs. Conversely, if you have dry skin, you'll want formulations with a creamy, rich base. This is incredibly important to understand. So, while all skin types need antioxidants, skin-repairing ingredients, and cell-communicating ingredients, the texture of the products that contain those ingredients is determined by your skin type. It's fine to layer multiple products with the same texture in your routine, or, if you prefer, and if it's appropriate for your skin type, you can layer lighter-weight products under heavier, more emollient products.

WHAT INFLUENCES SKIN TYPE

Many people have no idea what their skin type is, which is completely understandable because skin type can be hard to pin down and because it can be a moving target. That's because almost anything can influence skin type—both external and internal elements can and do influence the way your skin looks and feels.

Things that affect your skin type that are generally beyond your control are:
» Hormones
» Skin disorders
» Genetic predisposition
» Medications (oral or topical)
» Exposure to pollution
» Climate (including seasonal changes)

Things that affect your skin type that you have some control over are:
» Diet
» Your skincare routine (using irritating products or products that are wrong for your skin type)
» Stress
» Unprotected/prolonged sun exposure or use of tanning beds

YOU MAY BE CAUSING A SKIN TYPE OR CONCERN

It probably isn't difficult to see how smoking, sun damage, diet, and genetics can negatively and dangerously affect your skin type and concerns. What many people don't realize is that the skincare products they use can also be a primary factor in exacerbating, or even creating, the very skin issues you are trying to resolve. In other words, what you do to your skin via your skincare routine may be causing or intensifying a skin type or skin concern you don't want!

You'll never know your actual skin type or get your skin concerns under control if you use products that contain ingredients that **create** the very problems you don't want.

If you're using products that contain irritants, you can create dry skin and still make your oily skin worse (think dry skin on top, oily underneath). Products with irritating ingredients also cause collagen and elastin to break down, damage skin's ability to heal, and make wrinkles worse. Alternatively, if you use overly-emollient or thick-textured products along with a drying cleanser, you can clog pores, prevent skin cells from exfoliating (which makes your skin look dull), and make your skin feel oily in some areas and dry in others. If you over-scrub, you can damage the barrier (surface), causing more wrinkles and dry skin.

Not surprisingly, the kinds of products you use make all the difference in the world when trying to reach your goal of having the best skin of your life now.

HOW TO DETERMINE YOUR SKIN TYPE

Once you've ruled out the controllable factors that can affect your skin type (for example, sun exposure, smoking) and eliminated problematic products (poor formulations, jar packaging, irritating ingredients) from your routine, you'll be able to more accurately determine your skin type.

A good thing to keep in mind is that almost everyone at some time or another has combination skin. That's because the center area of your face naturally has more oil glands, so you are more likely to be oily or have clogged pores in the "T-zone." Many people with dry skin often find their skin is less dry on the nose and center of the forehead than elsewhere. It's also typical for some areas of your face (the eye area, around the nose) to be more sensitive.

Before you get out your mirror and have a close look, it's best to wash your face with a gentle cleanser. Then, wait two hours to see what your skin does without additional products or makeup (you can apply a gentle toner after cleansing, if desired). You may see a combination of skin types—normal to dry in some areas, oily in others. It bears repeating that anyone's skin can have multiple "types," and that these types can change due to hormonal cycles, seasons, stress levels, and other factors.

HOW TO DETERMINE YOUR SKIN CONCERN(S)

In some ways this is the easiest section of the book because most of us are painfully aware of what our skin concerns happen to be. Most of us already know what wrinkles, breakouts, blackheads, sagging skin, or brown discolorations look like. That's the easy part. But there are some skin concerns that are far more difficult to identify, such as sebaceous hyperplasia (small whitish, crater-like bumps on skin), milia (small pearl-like bumps on skin), keratosis pilaris (tiny red rough bumps on the arms and legs), and rosacea (sensitive skin with flushing and redness) among others. We explain all of these in the next sections of the book.

The most important takeaway about skin concerns is that most people have multiple skin concerns at the same time. It is not unusual for someone to have rosacea, wrinkles, sun damage, brown discolorations, and patches of dryness. This is where skincare can get complicated because once you've identified your skin concerns, then you need to add the specialty treatment products that can address them. Your core skincare routine may be enough to handle some aspects of your skin concerns, but that all depends on how stubborn or deep the problems are. You are the only who can determine how targeted and precise a skincare routine you want and need.

There are specific treatment products, both prescription and non-prescription, targeted for the treatment of acne, rosacea or other types of redness, blackheads, very oily skin, advanced sun damage, wrinkles, eczema, hydration, skin discolorations, and so on. Those concerns, along with your basic skincare requirements, are explained in the following chapters—along with helpful tips on how to put a routine together, including the order of application.

BASIC SKINCARE REQUIREMENTS

This section presents a quick overview of the products you need to build a core or basic skincare routine. (We elaborate more on this topic in Chapter 4, *Which Skincare Products You Need and Which Ones to Avoid*.) In the following paragraphs, we list the products you would use every day to maintain your skin, to meet many of your skincare needs related to your skin type, and to address some of your skin concerns. Though this may sound like a sweeping comment, we believe strongly that everyone can benefit from following these steps, even teenagers. Although we know it's highly unlikely that any teenager will follow all these steps, starting them in the right direction with at least three would be a perfect beginning.

The basics are: Twice a day use a **gentle water-soluble cleanser** appropriate for your skin type; more emollient for dry skin, more of a lotion style for normal skin, and a gel or pearlized lotion with a bit of sudsing for oily/combination skin. You can start or follow with a makeup remover to be sure you've removed every last bit of makeup; you don't ever want to fall asleep in your makeup.

Next is a **toner**, and of course it must be one that contains no irritants of any kind. This step assures you that you are quickly giving back to skin the crucial substances we mentioned before, such as antioxidants, skin-repairing ingredients, and cell-communicating ingredients, in a lightweight sheer formula that's appropriate for your skin type; dry skin would have more emollients, normal skin would be a fluid without extra emollients, and oily/combination skin would have ingredients that are helpful to balance oily skin.

You then follow with an **exfoliant** in a formula appropriate for your skin type. We explain at length in the next chapter why an exfoliant is a basic item in any daily skincare routine.

A **serum** can be your next step to give your skin a concentrated dose of the brilliant ingredients skin is hungry for, including antioxidants, skin-repairing ingredients, and cell-communicating ingredients. This is a wonderful basic step that many overlook, but the benefit may be worth experiencing for yourself before you write this step off as being a waste of time.

It goes without saying, but we will say it anyway: During the day you must wear a **sunscreen** with SPF 30 or greater and you must experiment to find a texture of sunscreen that makes your skin happy. For someone with dry skin a creamier formula should be perfect, for someone with normal skin a lotion formula will be great, and if you have oily/combination skin, a matte-finish sunscreen would work best.

At night you need a moisturizer to feed your skin once again, with healthy amounts of antioxidants, skin-repairing ingredients, and cell-communicating ingredients. The texture of your moisturizer must be appropriate for your skin type. If you have oily/combination skin, a liquid, gel, or thin serum would be ideal; dry skin would need a rich emollient cream; and normal skin would do great with a lotion.

LAYERING SKINCARE PRODUCTS

The first building block for finally achieving the best skin of your life is a core skincare routine, as mentioned above. Those basic, and critical, steps—water-soluble cleanser, toner, exfoliant, SPF moisturizer during the day and moisturizer at night—are essential products for everyone. All of these core products must have a texture that is appropriate for your skin type and must contain the same indispensable ingredients for skin.

As we explained throughout the opening chapters, and it bears repeating, everyone needs antioxidants, skin-repairing ingredients, and cell-communicating ingredients. If you have dry skin, the texture of the products should be emollient creams and serums; if you have normal skin, they should be lightweight lotions and serums; if you have oily/combination skin, then gels, liquids, and thin serums are best. For some skin types and skin concerns, the basics might be all you need to have smooth, soft, and radiant skin. If your skin concerns are more complicated, or if you have more than one skin type on your face, then additional steps are vitally important—this is where layering skincare products becomes imperative.

Depending on your skin concerns (breakout-prone, blackheads, advanced sun damage, rosacea, among many others) and/or on your special skin type (seasonal changes to skin, more dry patches than typical for combination skin, super oily skin, extremely dry skin), you might want to consider layering one or several uniquely-formulated products with the products in your core skincare routine.

Layering involves supplementing your core routine with products usually referred to as specialized serums, essences, boosters, or medical treatments (over-the-counter as well as prescription), either every day or as needed. As you will see in the following chapters, we explain how you can add a specialized product or products to your core routine to address specific problems such as skin discolorations, extra moisturizing for dehydrated skin, more emollients for seasonal dryness, anti-acne products for breakouts, increased exfoliation for stubborn blackheads or advanced sun damage, and so on.

You can add these types of targeted, or focused, products at almost any point in your skincare routine, after cleansing and toning. Depending on the type of problems you are addressing, these targeted treatments can be used daily, every other day, once a week, or seasonally.

The most important thing to understand is that no single product can do it all when you have distinct and disparate skin concerns. It's possible that it may take only one extra product, but this depends entirely on the problems with which you are dealing. Layering is not a new concept in skincare, but given the new and advanced lightweight and highly compatible formulations that can truly make a marked difference in specific skin concerns, better skin awaits you once you understand how layering works and what products will produce the best results.

CHAPTER 4

Which Skincare Products You Need— and Which Ones to Avoid

CLEANSERS

No other aspect of skincare is quite as basic or as important as using a cleanser. Cleansing the face sets the stage for almost everything else that will take place on skin. A good cleanser removes excess oil, dirt, and makeup and helps exfoliate, leaving skin smooth and fresh without feeling greasy or dry.

If you don't cleanse your skin regularly or if you don't remove all your makeup, your skin will pay the price, with irritation, potential breakouts, dry patches, and puffy eyes being the cost.

Thorough cleansing is essential for every skin type, and it's equally critical—for every skin type—that the cleansing products be gentle. Over-cleansing or using cleansers that are too drying are major causes of skin problems, especially dryness, flaky patches, and redness.

On the other hand, using a cleanser that leaves a greasy film on the face or that doesn't clean well can lead to clogged pores and dull-looking skin, and prevent moisturizers from absorbing and doing their job. It is essential to get this step right, and that means thoroughly, but gently, cleansing your face.

Should you start with a makeup remover? Many people feel their cleansing routine should start with a makeup remover, such as a liquid, makeup wipes, or cleansing oil. Although these work well for some people (particularly if you wear a heavier makeup application), they are merely an option, not a requirement.

Regardless of the type of makeup remover you use, the action of wiping at the face, especially around the eyes, is a problem. Tugging on skin damages its elastin fibers, increasing the potential for sagging. The less you pull, the better your skin will hold up in the long run.

We recommend starting out by washing your face with a gentle water-soluble cleanser because it reduces the amount of pulling necessary (the water reduces friction) and because most, if not all, of your makeup is rinsed down the drain. Then, if you still need a makeup remover to remove the last traces, it will be only for touch-ups (such as along the hairline or lash line), causing minimal pulling.

As is true for many aspects of skincare, you should experiment to see what works best for your skin type and your own personal preferences—but do take care not to pull or tug on skin.

What about facial cleansing oils? As stated above, using a makeup remover, which includes facial cleansing oils, that needs to be wiped off has inherent problems because the wiping and pulling at your skin increases sagging by breaking down the elastin fibers in skin—that's just a physiological fact. If you see skin moving up or down, you're helping it to sag faster than it would normally. Gravity will take its eventual toll, but in the meantime you don't have to make matters worse by constantly pulling at your skin. The goal for facial skin is to move it as little as possible.

The term "facial cleansing oil" is a bit confusing because the category is not clear-cut. Some facial cleansing oils are "oils" in name only; they're actually more like emollient water-soluble cleansers that are meant to be rinsed off. These can be a great option if you have normal to very dry skin.

Traditional facial cleansing oils, meaning an actual oil or blend of oils, that are gently removed can be effective for many reasons. They dissolve makeup quickly and efficiently while feeling soothing and softer than a water-soluble cleanser.

If you have very dry, sensitive skin, the cleansing oil doesn't need to be rinsed off, although you may prefer to do so depending on how you want your skin to feel once you've applied everything else in your routine. If you have normal to oily, combination, or breakout-prone skin, you'll most likely want to wash this residue off your face. Regardless of how you choose to use a cleansing oil, the caveat is always to pull at your skin as little as possible.

There are lots of myths circulating about facial cleansing oils, from a variety of sources. We prefer facts to myths, and the fact is that facial cleansing oils are not miracles for skin, just another option that may or may not be helpful for you depending on your skin type and concerns.

The notion that cleansing oils can somehow unclog pores by some force of chemistry pulling blackheads out of the pore (we still don't understand the explanations we've seen as they defy science and physiology) is not supported by any research—or even reality, for that matter.

Keep in mind that many facial cleansing oil products also contain fragrant oils, which present a serious problem for skin. As we will repeatedly state throughout this book, fragrance, whether natural or synthetic, causes problems for skin. [5,6,10,11,12] Non-fragrant plant oils are the only ones you should ever consider putting on your face.

What about bar soap? We wish we could say bar soaps are great for skin as that would make choosing a cleanser so much easier and less expensive; regrettably, however, that's not the case. For many reasons it's best to never use bar soap on the face, and it's also helpful to avoid it from the neck down. This is particularly true if you have problems with dry skin or breakouts; however, there are significant issues with using most bar soaps or bar cleansers no matter what type of skin you have.

Many people with breakout-prone, combination, or oily skin believe that the tight sensation they feel after washing with soap means their face is really clean. The thinking is that the more squeaky-clean their face feels, the better their skin will be, yet just the opposite is true!

The feeling associated with being squeaky clean is most likely an indication skin is being irritated, dried-out, and stressed, which makes all skin problems worse. [21]

The major issue with bar soap is its high alkaline content (meaning it has a high pH). "The increase of the skin pH irritates the physiological protective 'acid mantle', changes the composition of the cutaneous bacterial flora and the activity of enzymes in the upper epidermis, which have an acid pH optimum." [22] That technical explanation basically presents the fact that the skin's normal pH is about 5.5, while most bar soaps have an alkaline pH between 8 and 10, which negatively impacts the surface of skin by causing irritation and increasing the presence of bacteria.

There's research showing that washing with a cleanser that has a pH of 7 or higher increases the presence of bacteria significantly when compared to using a cleanser with a pH of 5.5. [23,24] Water-soluble cleansers, unlike bar soaps, are typically formulated with a lower, and thus more desirable, pH, one more reason to use this type of cleanser instead of a bar soap.

There are specialty soaps with non-soap-sounding names you're likely wondering about. These products typically contain creams and emollients and appear to have none of the properties of regular soap, but they still present problems similar to soap. First, bar cleansers (technically they're not soap; they're sometimes called syndet bars, for the "synthetic detergent" cleansing agents they contain) often have a lower (less alkaline) pH, which means they can be somewhat less irritating to skin; but, they're still more irritating than gentle water-soluble cleansers, and gentle is vitally important to skin.

Second, the other problem all bar cleansers share is that the ingredients used to keep them (bar cleansers or soaps) in bar form can leave a pore-clogging film on skin.

Soaps that are marketed for oily or acne-prone skin often contain even harsher ingredients. Even bar soaps marketed for dry and sensitive skin, which often contain beneficial ingredients such as glycerin, petrolatum (mineral oil), or vegetable oil, that reduce the irritation potential and make your face feel somewhat less stiff after you rinse, present a problem—skin just doesn't need the ingredients that hold the soap in its bar shape. [25,26]

How do I choose a gentle cleanser? Generally, liquid or lotion-style cleansers are going to be more gentle than bar cleansers. Unfortunately, this is not always true because not all liquid and lotion cleansers are created equal. Not making things any easier, it's nearly impossible to choose a cleanser based on its ingredient label because the technical names of the ingredients are absurdly complicated and there are hundreds of options a formulator can use. In short, how to choose a cleanser is not an easy question to answer.

What we can say for certain is that the best cleansers, regardless of your skin type, should never leave your face dry, greasy, or tight. There's a fine line between a cleanser that cleans well but doesn't strip vital barrier substances from skin, and this is true for all skin types.

For those with normal to oily or breakout-prone skin, cleaning skin well or getting skin really clean is often misunderstood. Overzealous cleansing or wanting skin to be squeaky clean can mean skin is stripped and ripped (OK, that's a bit of an exaggeration, but you get our point), and that type of cleansing worsens oiliness, prolongs post-acne marks, hurts healing, and can cause a host of other problems.

In short, for everyone, if a cleanser makes your skin feel like it's not clean, then you need a stronger cleanser. If a cleanser makes your skin feel tight after rinsing, you need to find a more emollient cleanser. It will take some experimenting to find the best cleanser for your skin type.

Do I need a scrub or a Clarisonic device? Scrubs and Clarisonic (or other types of cleansing brushes, sonic or not) are certainly options as part of your daily cleansing routine. Both can provide extra cleansing, and scrubs also offer superficial manual exfoliation; for many reasons, however, scrubs aren't the best way to gently, evenly, and naturally exfoliate skin. The way skin exfoliates naturally is beyond what manual exfoliation can provide. Skin can't exfoliate as it should when you have sun damage, blackheads, breakouts, or oily/combination skin. If you have those issues, you need to resort to a more efficient type of exfoliation, which is what AHA and BHA exfoliants (discussed further in this chapter) do.

Scrubs have considerable limitations when compared to the numerous, truly impressive benefits of exfoliating skin with a leave-on exfoliant such as an AHA or BHA (but more about those in the next sections). Scrubs deal only with the very top, superficial layer of skin, while most of the unhealthy and built-up dead skin cells are deeper, and thus beyond the reach of a scrub.

The real benefit of scrubs and the Clarisonic, or other powered cleansing brushes, is to be sure you get your skin clean, but with the goal to always be sure you don't over-cleanse skin.

What is most problematic about many scrubs is that they have a rough, coarse, uneven texture that can cause skin damage by tearing into skin as it abrades away the surface. This causes tiny tears that damage skin's barrier. The result? Skin takes longer to heal, red marks from acne get worse, dryness intensifies, and skin tends to become more sensitive and reactive, among other problems.

If you do want to use a manual scrub, be sure it doesn't contain any abrasive ingredients, even if they are natural. If you're using the Clarisonic or a similar cleansing device, be sure you use it as directed, and consider using only the device's "sensitive" brush head option. The brushes on such devices should feel very soft and flexible, *never* stiff or wiry.

You also have the option of simply using a gentle washcloth with your daily cleanser, which works just as well to exfoliate the surface of skin as any cosmetic scrub you can buy (really!). As a bonus, washcloths are softer (thus more gentle), less expensive, and, of course, they don't contain pore-clogging ingredients, something oily, acne-prone skin doesn't need!

TONERS: DO YOU REALLY NEED ONE?

Toners have become a confusing category of skincare products. Because of misperceptions, many fashion magazines, dermatologists, and even cosmetics salespeople advise against using a toner, or they simply dismiss toners as an optional step. That's disappointing, because a well-formulated toner can provide truly amazing benefits for your skin.

Once you understand how toners work, and know what ingredients are bad for skin versus what ingredients to look for, you'll find a toner can be the perfect addition to your skincare routine for achieving a healthy, radiant glow!

Toners are meant to be used after cleansing. They were once recommended as a way to restore skin's pH balance after using a bar soap or bar cleanser because, as mentioned, those types of cleansers can raise skin's natural pH to a level that isn't good for your skin. However, with today's gentle, water-soluble cleansers, which are formulated at a pH of 5 to 7—water has a pH of around 7, depending on region—this has become a non-issue.

What we now know is that after cleansing, your skin needs a range of ingredients to restore and repair its surface. A liquid toner can instantly give skin a generous dose of these important substances in a way that a moisturizer can't (lotion and cream moisturizers work in a different manner than liquids). Plus, you can't give your skin too much of these important ingredients, which include antioxidants and skin-repairing substances such as glycerin, fatty acids, and ceramides.

The right toner can give your skin a healthy dose of what it needs to look younger, fresher, and smoother, right after cleansing and throughout the day, as well as provide a bit of extra cleansing just in case you missed some areas, such as around your hairline or jaw.

Toners for oily or breakout-prone skin: If you have oily or breakout-prone skin, you need to be especially careful when shopping for toners. Almost without exception, the toners that claim to be specifically for these skin types and concerns are a problem. That's because most toners for oily, breakout-prone skin contain irritants (such as alcohol, witch hazel, or menthol) that hurt your skin's healing process, make breakouts worse, delay healing, and, surprisingly, stimulate oil production at the base of the pore. [4,27,28,29] Using the wrong toner on oily, breakout-prone skin guarantees you'll see more oil, redness, and longer-lasting red marks, and possibly a dry, flaky surface with oily skin underneath.

The toners that are best for oily or breakout-prone skin are those with ingredients that help repair skin's surface, make skin feel smoother, reduce enlarged pores, and contain cell-communicating ingredients that help pores handle excess oil in a more efficient manner. For some skin types, especially during summer or in warmer climates, a well-formulated toner may be the only "moisturizer" your oily skin needs!

Toners for dry or sensitive skin: Those with dry or sensitive skin typically shy away from toners because of their astringent, drying reputation. After all, the last thing dry, sensitive skin needs are irritants that make it sting or become even drier or redder! But, the right toner for dry or sensitive skin can make a world of difference: You'll see less redness, less flaking, and your skin will feel soothed and comfortable.

If you're skeptical (and we can't say we blame you) give a well-formulated toner a try—we know you'll be pleasantly surprised with how fast your skin improves!

Toners for combination skin: If your skin is oily on your forehead, nose, and chin and dry to normal on your cheeks and jaw area, then you have classic combination skin. Using the wrong toner on combination skin will exaggerate the dry areas and make oily areas worse (this is doubly true if breakouts and clogged pores are present).

What's the solution? You need a gentle, alcohol-free toner with ingredients that help normalize your skin, so you'll see less dryness and reduced oiliness. With ongoing use as part of a complete skincare routine, you'll also see enlarged pores become smaller.

When shopping for toners it's critical that you consider only those that treat your skin to nothing but beneficial ingredients. There's never—never—a good reason to use a toner with irritants (especially fragrance—natural or synthetic, as it's a serious problem for skin, and witch hazel, which often shows up in these types of products), regardless of the "gentle" or "good for sensitive skin" claims on the label. Despite its frequent appearance, witch hazel can be a skin irritant. [30]

WHY LEAVE-ON EXFOLIANTS ARE SO IMPORTANT

If scrubs aren't an ideal option for exfoliation, what *should* you use? Without question, almost everyone can benefit from daily use of a well-formulated leave-on AHA (alpha hydroxy acid, such as glycolic and lactic acids) or BHA (beta hydroxy acid, also known as salicylic acid) exfoliant. These work far differently from a scrub or Clarisonic brush. A gentle leave-on exfoliant picks up the slack where natural exfoliation should be taking place but has become faulty. This type of exfoliation provides multiple benefits, including fighting signs of aging and alleviating uneven skin tone, dullness, and breakouts, so don't let the "acid" in the name of these amazing ingredients scare you.

Your skin naturally sheds millions of skin cells every day, but this shedding process can slow or stop due to sun damage, dry skin, oily skin, genetics, or various skin disorders that can cause a buildup of dead skin cells or affect how cells move through the pore lining. The not-too-pretty results are unmistakable: dull, dry, or flaky skin; clogged, enlarged pores; blackheads; white bumps (milia); wrinkles; loss of firmness; and uneven skin tone.

Adding a well-formulated exfoliant to your routine helps put everything in balance again. When you gently get rid of the buildup of skin cells, you can unclog pores, stop breakouts, smooth wrinkles, and even make dry, dull skin a thing of the past!

OK, so **what's the difference between AHA and BHA exfoliants?** When properly formulated, both AHAs and BHA are brilliant options for exfoliating the surface layers of skin. Both AHAs and BHA have a lot in common when it comes to improving hydration, reducing wrinkles, stimulating collagen production, and firming skin. Both can also reduce discolorations from sun damage and the visible marks left after a breakout is gone. But, each also has unique qualities you'll want to consider when deciding which one to use:

> » **AHAs are preferred for those whose chief concerns are sun damage and dry skin** because they exfoliate primarily on the top layers of skin. [31,32] They do not cut through oil so they are less compatible for those with oily/combination skin.

> » **BHA is preferred for oily, acne-prone skin and for treating blackheads, enlarged pores, and white bumps** because BHA can penetrate the oil that's clogging your pores, thus normalizing the lining of the misshapen pore that contributes to acne and clogs.[33,34]

> » **BHA has anti-inflammatory and antibacterial action.** [33] That's two more reasons to use a BHA exfoliant if you have acne or sensitive, reddened skin.

> » **BHA is preferred for those struggling with rosacea.** Not everyone with rosacea can tolerate an exfoliant; however, given the multiple benefits of BHA, it's wise to experiment with a BHA product to see how your skin responds. Due to the anti-inflammatory and antimicrobial properties of BHA, it's likely you'll see reduced redness and smoother, more even skin with fewer red bumps and fewer acne breakouts. [33] (The antimicrobial action also may benefit rosacea because there is some research suggesting that certain microbes on skin may be causing or contributing to the disorder.)

If your skin is sun damaged and you're also struggling with acne or clogged pores, add a BHA product to your routine. If you want to use an AHA and BHA at the same time, that is an option. Some people find they work well when applied at the same time; others have better results if they apply one in the morning and the other in the evening. You can also alternate days, applying AHA one day, BHA the next. It takes experimentation to see what works best for you, but, for most of us, using one or the other is usually enough to get and maintain positive results. You don't have to use both kinds, but there's no harm in trying both and seeing which you prefer.

Note: Those allergic to aspirin shouldn't use a BHA exfoliant because of aspirin's close relationship to BHA: BHA is salicylic acid, while aspirin is acetylsalicylic acid.

Tips on Getting the Most from Your AHA or BHA Exfoliant:
» Experiment with different strengths of AHA and BHA to see which concentration gives you the best results without any signs of irritation.
» You can apply an AHA or BHA product once or twice per day.
» You can apply either type of exfoliant in the eye area, but not on the eyelid or directly under the eye (along the lower lash line).
» Apply the AHA or BHA product after your face is cleansed and after your toner has dried.
» Once the AHA or BHA product has been absorbed, you can apply any other product in your routine, such as moisturizer, serum, eye cream, sunscreen, and/or foundation.
» If you're using a topical prescription product such as Renova, other retinoids, or any of the topical prescription products for rosacea or acne, apply the AHA or BHA exfoliant first, and then follow with your medications from lightest to heaviest texture. Some people will find their skin doesn't tolerate a topical retinoid along with a AHA or BHA, but it can provide brilliant results for others, so it's definitely worth seeing if this combination works for you.

It's important to understand that exfoliating with an AHA or BHA does not negatively affect how healthy skin cells are generated in the lower layers of the skin. That's because AHA and BHA ingredients do not penetrate that deep below the surface layers of skin or beyond the inside of the pore. Exfoliating these dead skin cells can improve collagen production, increase skin's ability to hold moisture, and allow pores to function normally! Contrary to myth, AHA and BHA exfoliants do not thin the skin. [35,36]

Wondering if you can just use a rinse-off scrub or a Clarisonic device instead of an AHA or BHA? We discussed this earlier in the chapter, but it bears repeating: The benefits of manual exfoliation are not even remotely the same as the benefits from a well-formulated, leave-on AHA (glycolic or lactic acid) or BHA (salicylic acid) exfoliant. These chemical physical-type exfoliants are best thought of as an extra-cleansing step (much like using a soft washcloth or Clarisonic brush) to boost the results from your cleanser.

SERUMS: WHY YOU REALLY SHOULD USE ONE

While it's true that every product in your routine should contain a skin-pleasing array of antioxidants and cell-communicating ingredients, you should have higher expectations for your serums. Why? Well-formulated serums differ from moisturizers in that they don't "make room" for the traditional emollients or thickeners found in moisturizers—these are the ingredients that give moisturizers their lotion or rich cream textures. Likewise, serums won't contain the sunscreen actives that a daytime moisturizer would. Instead, serums use that extra space to pack in other beneficial ingredients or even more antioxidants than any other product in your routine.

Serums won't replace your daytime or nighttime moisturizers, but they will boost your anti-aging results and overall skin health when used morning and evening. Exception: If you have oily skin (and thus don't need extra moisture), a well-formulated serum can work as a double-duty product that replaces your nighttime moisturizer. It can be the only moisturizer your skin needs at night!

Finding a good serum is akin to starting a long-term relationship—the real benefits come from sticking with your serum day in and day out. While you'll likely see some improvements right away (because the antioxidant-rich formula soothes redness and brightens skin), over the long term you'll see other signs of damage fade and your skin will look and feel healthier and firmer!

Look to serums that contain anti-aging ingredients that are proven effective based on a large number of independent, peer-reviewed studies. Such substances include potent, stable antioxidants, such as vitamin C, green tea/EGCG, grape, and resveratrol, and cell-communicating ingredients such as retinol and niacinamide.

There's no single "best" serum, so choose based on your skin type and concerns. No matter how well-formulated a serum is, if it isn't right for you or isn't a match for your skin type, you'll end up disliking the results, and you won't stick with it. For example, if you have oily or combination skin, look for a water-light serum that won't feel heavy or greasy. Alternatively, if you have dry skin, you'll likely love a serum packed with antioxidant-rich moisturizing plant oils! All others can choose a serum based on personal preference, and don't be afraid to rotate among two or three serums so you can enjoy the unique benefits each provides. Sensitive skin? Choose a serum's texture based on how oily or dry your skin is, and make sure it's loaded with anti-irritant ingredients like willow herb, sea whip, and licorice root among others.

Note: Well-formulated serums tend to be concentrated, and so also tend to cost more than moisturizers, even though serums typically offer a smaller amount of product than moisturizers.

When should you begin using a serum? It's common knowledge that eating a balanced diet and exercising keeps your body healthier and younger-acting as you age. With that in mind, does it make sense to wait until you're unhealthy and in your 50s or 60s to start a healthier lifestyle? Of course not! The same is true when it comes to anti-aging for your skin!

Start using serums loaded with these types of impressive ingredients before signs of damage occur (it's never too soon) and you'll be on track for a more even complexion and firmer, healthier skin as you age. Your skin never "gets used" to these types of ingredients, just like your body never "gets used" to eating healthy foods.

Of course, these ingredients will work even after skin damage starts showing up, but without question, sooner is better than later!

A MOISTURIZER BY ANY OTHER NAME...

Moisturizer. Wrinkle cream. Firming fluid. Anti-aging cream. However the cosmetics industry refers to them (and the name variations are endless), a moisturizer is supposed to improve skin's softness, smoothness, and ability to hold on to the vital substances it needs to look and act younger. Some moisturizers are brilliant at this, but a surprising number of them fall short—and this applies to a lot of the more expensive options.

The standard term for this skincare step is "moisturizer," but this step is not about giving skin moisture, and it isn't about applying a lotion or cream. In reality, not everyone needs a "moisturizer," but everyone needs to add antioxidants, skin-repairing ingredients, and cell-communicating ingredients to their skin every day. These types of ingredients are essential to maintain and achieve the skin you want by giving it the substances it needs to repair itself, create healthy skin cells, make healthy collagen, and (to the extent possible) repair damaged elastin and improve skin's immune response. [5,6,15,16,17] Regardless of the product's name or texture, choosing a product loaded with these elements is vital for making any skin function more normally and look as young and healthy as possible.

As long as a product in this general, large category of moisturizers is well-formulated and includes an array of those key ingredients, the only thing you need to think about is the texture, because aside from that the name on the product's label is irrelevant.

Among products that are well-formulated, the only thing that differentiates all the "moisturizers" and antiwrinkle or similar products from one another is their texture. If you have dry to very dry skin, you need a product that comes in a cream form; if you have normal to dry skin, a lotion will work well.

If you have normal to slightly dry skin or combination skin, a lightweight lotion or thin fluid is your best choice. If you have oily or breakout-prone skin, a gel or liquid toner is an excellent form, but you may also want to consider a mattifying serum (not to be confused with foundation primers, which typically do not have impressive formulas in terms of providing the types of ingredients outlined above).

What a Moisturizer *Shouldn't* Include

We listed above the types of ingredients a good moisturizer should include to heal and improve skin. But almost as important, is what a moisturizer should not contain. Many moisturizers, including those labeled for dry or sensitive skin, contain ingredients that can make the problem worse, or counteract the beneficial properties of their good ingredients. We're talking about alcohol (not the "good" fatty alcohols, but those such as denatured alcohol and isopropyl alcohol) and fragrance, including fragrant oils such as those from lavender, rose, lemon, and mint.

If any of these are included in the moisturizer you're considering, walk away! Many of these ingredients, especially the volatile plant oils (think lavender and citrus oils) are pitched as natural or organic solutions to skincare problems, but they cause irritation and inflammation—the last thing dry skin needs!

Packaging Matters!

Avoid any moisturizer packaged in a jar! As we explain in Chapter 14, *Common Beauty Questions Answered and Myths Debunked*, no matter how great a product's formula, jar packaging, and to a lesser extent clear packaging (i.e., it lets light in), is always a deal breaker. This type of packaging exposes the beneficial delicate ingredients to light and air, causing them to break down. Given the number and variety of products available today that come in air-reducing or airless packaging, why waste your money on products whose most beneficial ingredients will be gone (or at least be less effective) shortly after the first use?

EYE CREAMS

Eye creams are certainly an option if it's a well-formulated product, meaning it contains ingredients that are helpful to skin around the eyes and if it omits ingredients that can be problematic. We know this sounds like a really basic idea, a no-brainer, but there are lots of eye creams that contain ingredients that aren't suitable for the eye area, or for anywhere on the face.

A serious concern about eye creams is that most of the ones labeled as being for daytime use don't contain sun protection, which would make them pro-aging, not anti-aging (if you aren't wearing them under a sunscreen). Sun damage is one of the major causes of wrinkles and sagging around the eye area, so this area needs sun protection as much as the face does.

Speaking of sunscreens, we strongly recommend using only mineral-based sunscreen formulas in the eye area. In this case, "mineral" means they contain titanium dioxide and/or zinc oxide as the only active ingredients. Both of these active ingredients are gentle on skin and provide broad-spectrum sun protection. It's not that synthetic sunscreen ingredients aren't effective; they just aren't as gentle and non-irritating as mineral sunscreen ingredients. This is true whether the product is labeled as an eye cream or not.

All of the marketing hype you've heard about how eye creams are specially formulated for the sensitive, thin skin around the eyes, that they get rid of puffy eyes, dark circles, and lift or tighten sagging skin is often not true. There are a few ingredients that can be considered special for the eye area, but, for the most part, the same essential ingredients that benefit the face benefit the eye area, too. A great facial moisturizer can absolutely be used around the eye area, which is why we maintain that not everyone needs an eye cream (or eye gel or eye serum).

The exception to this is when the skin around your eyes is different from the skin on your face. For example, if the skin around your eyes is drier than the skin on your face, you'll need to use a more emollient moisturizer around the eyes.

This is especially true if your skin is oily. The gel or liquid moisturizing formula that would work great on the face for those with oily or combination skin would probably not be enough for the eye area. But again, it doesn't have to be labeled "eye cream," but if it helps you to use a special product for this area, then as long as it's a great product we couldn't be happier.

We discuss eye creams and concerns like puffy eyes and dark circles in Chapter 14, *Common Beauty Questions Answered and Myths Debunked.*

MOISTURIZERS WITH SPF: THE CORNERSTONE!

It's OK to be obsessive about some things, like eating healthy, flossing your teeth, driving safely, and using sunscreen every day. That last item, daily application of a moisturizer with sunscreen, should absolutely be on your list. Your dedication to this step means you'll have the last laugh when it comes to laugh lines and other signs we associate with aging—which are overwhelmingly about sun damage.

Without a doubt, **sunscreen is the #1 antiwrinkle, anti-sagging, and anti-brown spot product you can use.** Unprotected UV exposure is the #1 cause of virtually every sign of aging. We refer to sunscreen as the cornerstone of a skincare routine because without it, nothing else you do to improve the health and appearance of your skin will have much impact; UV damage without protection literally destroys skin, slowly and surely. [8,9,37]

See Chapter 6, *Sun Damage and Sunscreen Questions Answered*, for key details on this most critical product in your daily skincare routine.

TARGETED TREATMENTS: FOR SPECIFIC CONCERNS

At some point, most people's skin will have a need for one or more products we refer to as targeted treatments. As the name states, these specialized treatments target a specific skin concern, such as breakouts, dark spots, wrinkles, stubborn bumps, redness, and so on.

For example, those who struggle with acne will likely benefit from a targeted acne treatment that contains the topical disinfectant ingredient benzoyl peroxide. Those with brown spots will likely benefit from a targeted treatment that contains ingredients like hydroquinone, niacinamide, or high concentrations of vitamin C. Very dry skin can benefit from targeted treatments that are a blend of facial oils, either used alone or mixed with a moisturizer.

If you're using multiple treatment products over the same area, which one you apply first comes down to texture (go from thin to thick) and personal preference. The good news is you don't need to worry about the ingredients in different treatments interfering with one another; almost without exception, you can layer such products or use them as needed, morning and/or evening, depending on your concerns.

Targeted treatments also include topical prescription products, such as retinoids like tretinoin (Renova) for wrinkles or Finacea (azelaic acid) for rosacea.

FACIAL MASKS AND THEIR PLACE IN YOUR ROUTINE

Despite their enduring popularity around the world, we've never been big fans of facial masks. It's not that masks are a problem (at least not when they're well-formulated, but many aren't) or that they can't be helpful. It's because what you do to take care of your skin daily matters far more than any mask you might apply once or twice per week, however indulgent or special it may seem.

In East Asian cultures, many use masks once daily. Although masks may not be all that helpful if you use them only once a week, if you're willing to use them more often, they can provide greater benefit—but it's even more critical that they be well-formulated. Most important, masks must work in harmony with your skincare routine. For example, if everything in your routine is gentle and well-formulated, but the mask contains irritating or problematic ingredients, it's merely undermining what the rest of your skincare routine is doing to help you get (and keep) the best skin of your life.

There are two main types of masks: those that moisturize and hydrate (best for normal to dry skin) and those that absorb oil and help dislodge superficial blackheads, leaving skin smooth and matte (best for those with oily or combination skin). Those with truly normal skin (a rarity!) who want to use a mask should err on the side of a more emollient mask rather than an oil-absorbing one. If you have combination skin (dry and oily areas), consider using two masks: a moisturizing formula in the dry areas and an absorbent mask in the oily areas.

Whether you use a mask or not, know that, despite claims to the contrary, they're not essential. Peel-off or sheet masks, masks that change color or feel warm as they dry, or special eye-area "cooling" masks can be fun ways to pamper yourself, so if that floats your boat, go for it—just make sure the masks you're considering don't contain problematic ingredients like denatured alcohol, menthol, witch hazel, fragrant plant oils, or other known skin irritants. Even if you apply something only infrequently, the emphasis should always be on being gentle and not exposing your skin to damaging ingredients.

How often and how to apply a mask are a matter of personal preference and the usage instructions specific to each facial mask. Generally, a mask is applied to clean skin, then rinsed or massaged in, to be followed by the rest of your morning or evening skincare routine. It is perfectly fine to leave moisturizing masks on overnight; clay or peel-off masks, however, should always be rinsed or removed after 10–15 minutes because leaving them on longer increases the risk of skin feeling unusually dry and tight. Eye-area masks may be left on or massaged into skin after a certain period of time, based on the product's usage instructions.

CHAPTER 5

How to Put Together the Perfect Skincare Routine

SKINCARE ROUTINES THAT PROVIDE RESULTS

We promised the best skin of your life in this book's title, and here's the secret: The only way to have beautiful skin—and keep it that way—is to start (and never stray from) applying a state-of-the-art skincare routine based on what unbiased, scientific research shows works for your skin! There's really no other possible way to finally have the skin you've always wanted. Focusing on the claims for the product, on suspicious before-and-after photos, or on fictional marketing about a new miracle ingredient or miracle product will hurt your skin and waste your money time after time. If you've been at this skin thing for a while, aren't you tired of that crazy merry-go-round? We've all gotten to that point—it's what inspires us to find out what works and what doesn't—and why!

With a wiser outlook in mind, the next step is to understand what kinds of products work together, how they benefit your skin, and the order in which to use them. The information we present in the table that follows is an easy-to-follow guideline to help you put together your own skincare routine or to custom-select products based on what works best for you and your specific skin concerns, step by step.

We explain the purpose of each type of product, why you need it, and what results you can expect, whether you prefer a basic or more advanced routine. Keep in mind that if you have multiple skincare concerns, you may need to add more than one treatment or targeted treatment product. We wish we could tell you there's one skincare product that can do it all, but it just isn't possible. Addressing a variety of skincare concerns requires more than one bottle or tube, no matter the product's claims or cost.

A note on targeted treatments: You may be able to merely add one targeted treatment product to your daily routine, or you might need to alternate its use with other treatment products. If your routine is complex and involves several products (including topical prescription products), you might need to experiment to discover which method and what frequency of application works best for you. Now let's go over the products and steps to get you started!

THE PRODUCTS YOU NEED (AND WHY)

CLEANSER
(STEP 1)

What is this for?	A gentle, water-soluble, soap-free cleanser removes debris, oil, and makeup.
Why do I need this?	Rinsing with water is not enough to clean your face. When your face is clean, it allows the other products you use to work even better, morning and evening.
What results will I see?	**With a well-formulated cleanser, your skin will look and act healthier, feel smoother, and be ready to receive maximum benefits from your other products.**

TONER
(STEP 2)

What is this for?	A well-formulated toner smoothes, softens, and calms skin, while removing the last traces of makeup. It also adds vital skin-repairing ingredients after cleansing.
Why do I need this?	Toners with skin-repairing ingredients hydrate and replenish the skin's surface immediately after cleansing. They also help reduce redness and dry patches.

What results will I see?	With a well-formulated toner, your skin will feel softer and look smoother, and redness will be reduced. Those with oily skin will see smaller pores.
	Daily use will give your skin what it needs to function in a younger, healthier way.

AHA OR BHA EXFOLIANT
(STEP 3)

What is this for?	A leave-on AHA or BHA exfoliant gently removes built-up dead skin cells, revealing new skin.
	AHAs exfoliate the surface of skin and bind moisture; BHA exfoliates the surface of skin and inside the pores as it reduces redness.
Why do I need this?	Sun damage causes the surface of the skin to become abnormally thick. Acne and oily skin complicate this further. Exfoliating eliminates this buildup, which otherwise would cause clogged pores, uneven skin tone, dullness, and deeper wrinkles.
What results will I see?	**Overnight your skin will look radiant, smoother, and younger (really)!**
	Daily exfoliation with a well-formulated AHA or BHA exfoliant will unclog pores, reduce redness, blackheads,* and breakouts, diminish wrinkles, build collagen, and improve uneven skin tone. *BHA is best for blackheads.*

ACNE TREATMENT
(STEP 4, IF NEEDED)

What is this for?

After exfoliating with an AHA or BHA exfoliant, an acne treatment with benzoyl peroxide kills acne-causing bacteria and helps reduce redness.

Why do I need this?

When acne is your concern, research shows that topical treatment with benzoyl peroxide is an essential step for achieving clear skin.

What results will I see?

With consistent use of a well-formulated, non-drying acne treatment, you'll see fewer breakouts and a reduction in large, red, swollen blemishes. **Your acne will be reduced, possibly eliminated.**

SKIN-LIGHTENING TREATMENT
(STEP 4, IF NEEDED; STEP 5, IF YOU'RE USING AN ACNE TREATMENT)

What is this for?

Used at least once daily, skin lighteners gradually reduce, and in some cases eliminate, brown spots and discolorations from sun damage or hormonal influences.

Why do I need this?

Using a skin-lightening product reduces the over-production of melanin, the skin pigment that causes brown spots and discolorations.

What results will I see?

After 8–12 weeks of daily use, you'll see discolorations fade or even disappear completely. **Your skin tone will be more even and radiant.** Ongoing use is needed to maintain results.

SERUM
(STEP 4, IF YOU'RE NOT USING AN ACNE TREATMENT OR SKIN LIGHTENER; OTHERWISE, THOSE GO ON FIRST)

What is this for?

Applied morning and evening, serums filled with antioxidants and other anti-aging ingredients protect your skin from environmental damage, including sun damage* and pollution. *When used with a sunscreen.*

Why do I need this?

Well-formulated serums with antioxidants improve your skin in numerous ways, from reducing redness to stimulating healthy collagen production for firmer skin and fewer wrinkles.

What results will I see?

Immediately, your skin will feel smoother and look radiant. **With twice-daily use, signs of damage will fade and your skin will look and behave healthier and younger.**

ANTI-AGING/ ANTIWRINKLE MOISTURIZER WITH SUNSCREEN
(THE LAST STEP IN YOUR MORNING ROUTINE)

What is this for?

This essential morning step keeps your skin shielded from sun damage. It must have an SPF 30 or higher rating, and offer broad-spectrum protection.

Why do I need this?

Moisturizers with SPF and antioxidants are essential to protect your skin from sun exposure, which is the #1 cause of wrinkles, brown spots, and other signs of aging.

What results will I see?

Protecting your skin from further sun damage allows it to generate younger, healthier skin cells. This is the critical step to having radiant skin. **You'll see fewer signs of aging!**

ANTI-AGING/ ANTIWRINKLE MOISTURIZER
(THE LAST STEP IN YOUR EVENING ROUTINE)

What is this for?   All skin types will benefit from a well-formulated moisturizer that contains the types of ingredients research has shown help your skin look healthier and younger.

Why do I need this?   Used daily, moisturizers (cream, lotion, gel, or liquid texture; choose based on your skin type) improve your skin's healthy functioning and keep it feeling smooth and soft. You can also use them around the eye area.

What results will I see?   When you use the right moisturizer for your skin type, you'll see smoother, radiant skin that's hydrated and healthier. **Dry, dull, or flaky skin will be replaced by skin that looks and acts younger!**

TARGETED TREATMENTS
(WHEN AND HOW OFTEN TO APPLY DEPENDS ON THE PRODUCT)

What is this for?   These are optional extras you can add, depending on your personal skincare concerns. Examples include facial masks, eye creams, and boosters.

Why do I need this?   These products may be needed as an extra step to hydrate skin, absorb excess oil, reduce redness, or treat a special need or occasional skin concern.

What results will I see?   Results depend on the targeted product you choose and may include oil absorption, plumping of wrinkles, extra moisture, etc.

EXAMPLES OF A.M. AND P.M. SKINCARE ROUTINES

Depending on your needs, your skincare routine can include only the basics (what we call the Essential routine) or can be more complex (what we refer to as an Advanced routine). The following step-by-step Essential routines (for morning and evening) cover the types of products everyone should use and the order in which to use them every day. These steps apply regardless of your skin type, whether oily, dry, normal, or combination.

The textures of each type of product will vary based on your skin type and preferences (lotion instead of cream, gel instead of foam), but the fundamentals and the order of application remain the same.

The ingredients that everyone's skin needs can be found in products with a wide variety of textures within each category (step) of product in your skincare routine. In Chapter 12, *How to Treat Special Skin Problems*, we detail additional products and steps you can use to treat special skin concerns stemming from disorders like rosacea or brown spots from sun damage.

ESSENTIAL ROUTINE: MORNING

» Cleanser
» AHA or BHA Exfoliant
» Moisturizer with sunscreen rated SPF 30 or greater

ESSENTIAL ROUTINE: EVENING

» Cleanser
» AHA or BHA Exfoliant
» Moisturizer without sunscreen (sun protection isn't needed at night)

If you have multiple concerns, an Advanced routine is the best way to go. It includes targeted treatments you can add to your Essential routine to treat your personal skincare concerns, such as acne, red marks, wrinkles, sun damage, brown spots, or rosacea.

Which to choose? Here's an example: If your sole concern is dry skin, you'll do fine using the Essential routine; however, if you have dry skin and wrinkles or oily skin and wrinkles *and* breakouts, you'll want to use an Advanced routine for best results. An Advanced routine includes more products and takes a bit more time, but each product plays an important, critical role in achieving the skin you want to see! Once you get the hang of it, an Advanced routine, although more involved, becomes second nature and takes only a few extra minutes.

An Advanced routine includes a toner as your second step, morning and evening. If you've never used a well-formulated toner before, prepare to be amazed by the results! You can add targeted treatments if/when needed.

ADVANCED ROUTINE: MORNING

» Cleanser
» Toner
» AHA or BHA Exfoliant
» Treatment (such as a serum or eye cream or both; for daytime the eye-area product should provide sun protection)
» Moisturizer with sunscreen
» *Optional:* Targeted treatment (applied as needed before sunscreen)

ADVANCED ROUTINE: EVENING

» Cleanser
» Toner
» AHA or BHA Exfoliant
» Treatment (such as a serum or eye cream)
» Moisturizer without sunscreen
» *Optional:* Targeted treatment, as needed, applied before or after your Step 3 treatment product.

MIXING AND MATCHING PRODUCTS

You may have been told that adding products from different brands will make the other products you're using ineffective, or they won't work as well as they could, or that you MUST use products from one brand or else your skin won't improve, or the products will no longer be guaranteed "or your money back." None of this is true in the least.

Not only is it perfectly OK to mix and match products from different brands (especially prescription products, depending on your skincare needs), but sometimes doing so is essential if you want to get the best results possible! Think of all the other areas in life where we successfully mix things up—food, for one! Who buys all of their food from only one brand, or eats at only one restaurant?

What really counts are the formulas, and whether or not those are appropriate for your skin type and your skin concerns. As long as you're consistently using products that are well-formulated and suitable for your skin type and concern, you should see positive results. However, **keep your expectations realistic:** No topical product will work like Botox, and no spot treatment will completely erase a stubborn pimple or deep wrinkle overnight. If your goal is clear, smooth, radiant, healthy, and younger-looking skin, then you can absolutely achieve that with daily use of brilliantly-formulated products, no matter the line or brand.

DO DIFFERENT SKIN COLORS OR ETHNICITIES NEED DIFFERENT SKINCARE PRODUCTS?

It might surprise you to learn that whether your heritage is European, Asian, or anywhere else in the world, you do not require special skincare products based on your skin's color or your ethnic background. Why not? Because **skin color is not a skin type**! None of the research on the differences between ethnicities indicates that skin color has anything to do with the skincare products you need.

Darker skin tones have some physiological differences from lighter skin tones, but those differences don't impact what products you should be using. Think of it like your diet: Regardless of our ethnic background and skin color, we all need the same nutritious foods (ones that supply antioxidants, fatty acids, protein, vitamins, and so on) to be healthy. The exact same concept applies to skin. Skin is the body's largest organ, and everyone's skin needs the same ingredients to address dry skin, acne, wrinkles, sun damage, uneven skin tone, oily skin, rosacea, sensitive skin, and so on. All of these problems affect every color of skin.

Everyone's skin also needs the same basic care—gentle cleansing, sun protection, and state-of-the-art products for the specific skin type. It is also important to avoid problematic ingredients, such as alcohol, menthol, peppermint, eucalyptus, lemon, lime, and natural or synthetic fragrances, because exposure to irritants always will worsen any condition on any color of skin. [2,5,7]

Research shows that the only significant difference between African-American skin and Caucasian skin is the amount, size, and distribution of melanin (the cells that produce our skin's pigment). [38] Excess melanin, for example, accounts for the darkened or ashen appearance of darker skin when it's irritated or sun damaged, whereas the same irritation and damage would cause lighter skin to appear pink, red, or, if more melanin is present or stimulated, mottled tan.

Although the extra melanin is good news for those with darker skin tones, it doesn't mean damage from unprotected sun exposure isn't happening. Uneven skin tone, wrinkles, and slower healing time (particularly for scars) is primarily a result of sun damage. Even though it takes longer and more intense sun exposure for visible damage to occur on darker skin, sun damage is always greater on skin that's chronically exposed to sun than on skin that's properly protected. [8,9]

By now you can tell that many beauty myths drive us over the edge—this is one more to add to our list. Simply put, as far as biology and physiology are concerned, regardless of your ethnic, racial, or cultural background, you do NOT need special skincare products. Let go of this idea—in most cases, it won't help (and could actually hurt) your skin.

You've probably heard or read that Asian skin is more sensitive and, therefore, needs products that don't contain irritating ingredients. Even if that were true, no one in the world, whether Asian or not, needs products with irritating ingredients. Everyone needs beneficial ingredients that are gentle on skin, and everyone should be treating their skin gently. Using irritating, overly fragranced products is detrimental, no matter who you are.

Whether you have normal, oily, combination, or dry skin or your skincare concerns involve sun damage, wrinkles, breakouts, large pores, uneven skin tone, rosacea, sagging skin, and on and on, there's no research showing that different skincare formulas are needed based on your race or heritage. The ingredients that benefit skin and the ingredients that are a problem for skin are global. Aligning your skincare routine to a specific brand that wants you to believe this myth would do your skin a disservice.

DO THE NECK AND CHEST NEED SPECIAL PRODUCTS?

Wrinkles, crepey skin, and brown or ashen discolorations show up sooner on areas that haven't been shielded from the sun. This is especially true for the neck and chest because we tend to neglect those areas far more than our face, leaving them exposed to the sun and the damage it causes. That's why, for women, skincare really needs to start at your boobs! What we mean by that is that the products you use on your face can and, in fact, should also be used on your neck and chest!

Cosmetics counters are packed with endless creams and treatments targeting the neck and chest (often labeled as for the "décolletage"). The truth is that buying a separate neck, chest, or décolleté cream or treatment is a complete waste of money. These "specialized" products are rarely well-formulated, rarely contain sunscreen, and almost always are overpriced given what they contain. Most important, they're completely unnecessary because the products you use for your face (provided they're well-formulated) will work beauti-fully on your neck and chest, too.

There's no research showing that the neck and chest need ingredients or formulations different from those you use on the face. In fact, copious research makes it absolutely clear that what it takes to keep skin anywhere on your body acting and looking young requires the same brilliant ingredients. Gentle cleansing, products loaded with antioxidants, skin-repairing ingredients, and cell-communicating ingredients, along with dedicated use of a well-formulat-ed broad-spectrum sunscreen work for your face, neck, chest, and décolletage.

It's important to point out that the neck is a bit of a different issue, not in terms of what products you use, but in what happens to the neck as we age. For certain, the neck will show the same signs of aging as the face, but usually not as quickly because the neck typically is shielded from the sun by our heads. Regardless of how slowly the sun damage may show up, if you neglect your neck it will suffer the same woes as any other part of your body that you don't protect from the sun.

What's frustrating about the neck is that it tends to sag faster than other parts of the face. This is to some extent about skincare (or lack thereof), but it's also because of gravity and physiology.

Skin on the face and chest are well supported by bone, while the front of the neck has no supporting bone structure (only the back of the neck does, but not all that much given the size and shape of the neck's vertebrae). The elaborate network of neck muscles don't provide much support. This means that the neck and its fat pads can be affected by the pull of gravity sooner than other parts of your body and face. [39, 40]

Regrettably, despite the claims and gibberish you've probably heard, there are no special skincare ingredients that will help tighten a sagging neck—the same products that help firm skin for the face work for the neck; it's that sim-ple. But (you knew this was coming, didn't you?), there is a point of no return where age-related sagging can be fixed only with surgery, not skincare.

WHY SKIN REACTS BADLY TO PRODUCTS

Sometimes, using a new product or a new mix of products can cause skin to have a negative reaction—even if the products are well-formulated. Such reactions are usually perplexing because it's hard to determine exactly what's happening and why. Even more frustrating, it isn't always clear what to do about it, especially when you hoped the product would work as promised. You may wonder if you did something wrong, or if the product itself is faulty.

There are five primary reasons why skin reacts negatively to a new product, a new skincare routine, or even to products you've used for months or years.

» **The product was poorly formulated** with ingredients that can irritate your skin, such as alcohol, fragrance, or fragrant plant extracts. The reaction can happen immediately or it can develop over time; sometimes, when several fragranced products are used, the skin reaches a critical tipping point and suddenly reacts, often strongly. [2,5,7]

» Often **an allergy to a specific ingredient or combination of ingredients** in the formula is to blame. This has nothing to do with the quality of the product; rather, it's a personal reaction to an ingredient or a mix of ingredients. It's like being allergic to cats, an unpleasant fact for some, but not the fault of the cat, nor does it mean cats are bad.

» **Using the wrong products for your skin type**; for example, using oil-absorbing products when dry, flaky skin is the problem or using overly emollient products when oily skin, large pores, and breakouts are the problem.

» **Using too many "active" products at one time**. With anti-aging or anti-acne products, some people think that if a little is good, then more (or more often) must be better. So, they use three types of exfoliants at the same time twice daily, followed by a high-strength vitamin C serum, a prescription retinoid, and then a prescription skin-lightening product. For some, this combination may work at first, but it can quickly backfire, causing skin to become overly sensitive or reactive when it was normal before. This reaction can be even worse if you're also getting professional peels or aggressive facials involving lots of massage, steaming, and extractions.

» Some people have **skin that's just more reactive and sensitive to cosmetics**, no matter the ingredients. For them, the more products they use, the greater the risk of a reaction, especially if the products contain fragrance or fragrant plants. If that describes you, the worst thing you can do for your skin is to hop frequently from product line to product line, hoping *something* will stop this skin misery merry-go-round.

WHAT TO DO

First, be certain the products you used don't contain problematic ingredients that are known to cause irritation. Using only well-formulated products (preferably without fragrance, because fragrance is a common allergen for everyone) is essential. [5,6,10,11,12]

Next, be certain the products are a good match for your skin type. Oil-absorbing or matte-finish ingredients will be a disaster on dry skin, while emollient, thick moisturizers will be a problem for someone with oily skin or when applied over the oily areas of combination skin.

In situations where highly reactive skin is a primary concern, be cautious about products with active ingredients; don't use too many of them or use all of them at the same time. It's OK to alternate application of such products; anti-aging and anti-acne isn't an all-or-nothing deal.

After investigating the ingredients and the types of products being used, consider the combination and frequency of the products you're applying. Although sunscreen, skin lighteners with hydroquinone, AHA or BHA exfoliants, anti-acne treatments, and anti-aging products with ingredients like retinol can have remarkable benefits, they can also cause reactions for some, especially when used together in your everyday skincare routine.

In such a scenario, a starting point would be to change the sunscreen to one that contains only the mineral active ingredients titanium dioxide and/ or zinc oxide, which have minimal risk of causing a reaction. These mineral actives also are super-gentle, making them good for use around the eyes and on reddened skin.

Another test would be to reduce the frequency of use. Rather than using every product in your routine twice per day, alternate them, apply one in the morning and the other in the evening.

It can also be helpful to alternate days. For example, instead of using a retinol-based product or a prescription anti-acne treatment every day, try applying these every other day and see how your skin reacts. If reducing the frequency doesn't improve matters, then stop using the most suspect product (or products) and see how your skin reacts.

Keep a notebook handy so you can record how your skin progresses. Briefly jot down the pros and cons, and what you did differently. Yes, it does take a bit of time, but you can refer back to it later to help you better handle a future reaction.

Although active ingredients or problematic ingredients are typical causes of skin reactions, even basic skincare products like cleansers, toners, or moisturizers can trigger negative skin reactions. In such cases, it usually starts when you introduce a new product into an existing skincare routine or when you begin using a new group of products.

If the reaction is mild, it might be helpful to stop using one of the products and see what happens. If that doesn't help, stop using another one of the new products and see what happens after a day or two. If *that* doesn't resolve the problem, then go back to the previous routine that didn't cause your skin to react. Sadly, when you reach this point, the hunt for products that won't cause a reaction starts anew—unless you want to keep using your former products, assuming they're well-formulated.

USING PRESCRIPTION PRODUCTS WITH YOUR SKINCARE ROUTINE

There are many reasons why you may want, or need, to add topical prescription products to your regular skincare routine. For example, if you have stubborn acne, prescription-only medications such as topical antibiotics like BenzaClin or topical retinoids like Differin or Retin-A can make a world of difference.

For wrinkles, Renova, the prescription-strength form of retinol, can be extremely beneficial. Topical medications for rosacea, including MetroCream, Atralin, and Finacea; cortisone creams for eczema; medications such as Calcipotriene for treating psoriasis; or topical acne medications like Tazorac are often the only way to keep these irksome skin disorders under control.

There's a great deal of research about how topical prescription products work to help different skin disorders and about their potential side effects. Surprisingly, there's minimal to no information on how you're supposed to incorporate topical prescription products into your daily skincare routine. After all, you still must clean your face, use a skin-healing toner, protect with an effective sunscreen, apply moisturizers or serums appropriate for your skin type, and, for most people, exfoliate ... but how are you supposed to do that and apply prescription products? How does it all work together? *Can* it work together?

Sadly, there isn't any agreement among dermatologists as to what non-prescription skincare products you're supposed to use with your topical prescription-only medications or about the order in which to apply them. Frustrating, huh? Even more shocking is the lack of consensus or suggestions about how to avoid some of the most typical reactions from prescription medications, such as redness, irritation, dryness, and inflammation.

We have pored through massive amounts of research to uncover tips on how you can assemble the most ideal skincare routine for your skin type and concerns—and how to incorporate topical prescription medications into that routine. The goal is to use these topical products consistently because none of them are cures. If your skincare routine causes irritation and inflammation, dryness, or additional problems, you'll not be able to get the best results or (in many cases) continue to use these helpful medications.

Step 1: Use only gentle water-soluble cleansers. Regardless of the medications you apply, everyone first needs to use a gentle water-soluble cleanser appropriate for their skin type. If the cleanser isn't gentle, it will cause irritation and dryness, which will only be exacerbated by the medication(s) you apply afterward.

Do not use abrasive scrubs with any topical prescription medications. Most scrub particles create tiny micro-tears on the skin's surface, which will aggravate the skin condition you have and increase the irritation from the medications you're applying. If you want a bit of extra cleansing, use a washcloth with a gentle water-soluble cleanser.

Caution: Think twice before using a prescription topical product and a cleansing brush like the Clarisonic. This combination can prove too irritating, especially if you're also using products like exfoliants, skin lighteners, and serums with retinol.

Step 2: Use a great toner. Most toners are loaded with irritating plant extracts such as witch hazel along with alcohol and fragrance—in one word: Ouch! On the other hand, toners loaded with beneficial skin-repairing ingredients can create the optimal environment on your skin for the medication(s) you'll be applying.

Step 3: Use an AHA or BHA exfoliant. Most people's skin reaps incredible benefits from exfoliation. This is true even if used in combination with most topical prescription medications.

Tip: There's a risk of irritation from exfoliants, so you need to start slowly, initially applying a lower concentration exfoliant once (morning or evening) every three days to see how your skin does, and then increasing the frequency and/or concentration based on how your skin responds. If you experience irritation, and it continues, cut back on the frequency, reduce the concentration, or stop altogether.

Step 4: Apply a serum filled with antioxidants, barrier-repair substances, and other beneficial ingredients. These kinds of ingredients are compatible with almost any topical prescription product.

Note: Many people ask us about using an over-the-counter retinol product, such as a serum, plus a prescription retinoid like Renova. It's fine to use both; generally, you should apply the over-the-counter retinol product first, followed by your prescription retinoid. Do you need both? No, but some people see greater benefit from the combination, or they simply like to alternate a stronger and weaker retinol product. As with any active ingredient, pay attention to how your skin responds and adjust your routine accordingly. **Doubling up on retinol products** is too much for some people's skin—more isn't necessarily better, and you never want to tip the scale in favor of irritation.

Step 5: Apply your prescription product. This is the best place in your routine to apply your prescription product, especially if it has a cream or lotion texture. If it's a liquid, apply it after Step 3.

Step 6—DAYTIME: Never forget to apply a moisturizing, broad-spectrum sunscreen rated SPF 30 or greater every day. Protecting your skin from the sun not only prevents signs of aging, but also helps repair skin and helps heal many skin disorders by reducing the underlying inflammation. So, unless your physician says otherwise (which may be the case for those with severe psoriasis), always apply sunscreen.

Step 6—NIGHTTIME: Apply a skin-repairing moisturizer and/or serum every night. Moisturizers and serums work effectively with almost any topical prescription; choose one or both based on your skin type and personal preferences, and apply it around the eyes, too. You can add a separate eye cream if needed.

If you're also using **targeted treatment** products, apply these either before your daytime or nighttime moisturizer or, if spot-treating, dab the product on top of your moisturizer, after having already applied your prescription product.

A lot of experts suggest you **mix your topical prescription medication with your moisturizer** to minimize the risk of dryness or irritation. That's an option, but it's unlikely to make a big difference; applying your prescription product first and then applying your moisturizer or serum afterward essentially does the same thing. (However, with regard to mixing products, you shouldn't mix any skincare product with a sunscreen, because diluting a sunscreen with a serum, moisturizer, or prescription product decreases the sunscreen's effectiveness.) Sunscreen should always be the last step in your skincare routine, regardless of the prescription product.

If you're experiencing bothersome side effects, talk to your physician about cutting back on how frequently you apply the topical medication, but keep in mind that if you cut back too much you won't get any benefit. If you're using your prescription product less than three times per week, and it still causes irritation, you should talk with your physician about using a different medication or trying a lower dose, which your skin may tolerate better.

In our research and personal experience, we've noted that there are doctors who recommend prescription and over-the-counter products and usage steps that don't seem to make sense, at least to us, and likely not to you, either—we hear from a lot of people who are dissatisfied with their doctor's advice. Despite these issues, you must follow your doctor's recommendations—or get a second opinion from another medical doctor or pharmacist.

CHAPTER 6

Sun Damage and Sunscreen Questions Answered

SUN DAMAGE IS NEVER PRETTY

Sun protection is so important it has its own chapter and merits us repeating as often as we can: Daily exposure to UV light without protection, even for a minute, is the single worst thing you can do to your skin. Research has made it clear that repeated, unprotected sun exposure, getting sunburned, or repeatedly getting tan causes DNA damage that triggers skin cells to mutate. [8,9,37] Over the years and in the absence of sun protection and sun-smart behavior, these mutations often turn into skin cancers.

Even if you're lucky enough to avoid skin cancer, years of unprotected sun exposure or, worse, deliberate tanning either from the sun or a tanning bed, puts your skin on the fast track to aging. You'll see wrinkles, sagging, brown spots, texture changes, large or misshapen pores, and reduced skin healing (including from acne breakouts) far sooner than those who are diligent about protecting their skin from UV light. [7,41,42]

We emphasize "UV light" because, although the sun emits other wavelengths of light as well, UV light is what really causes sun damage to skin, even on cloudy or overcast days. In other words, sun damage isn't only a threat when the sun is shining; it's a threat whenever and wherever you see daylight. And the damage starts happening the first minute your skin sees daylight! [43,44] That research shocked even us. Protecting skin every day of the year, rain, snow, or shine is critically important if your goal is to have healthy, young-looking skin for as long as possible.

The problem is that the topic of sunscreens and all the details surrounding their use has become a confusing mess of incomplete or misleading information—which is what this chapter aims to sort out!

HOW AND WHEN YOU APPLY SUNSCREEN IS IMPORTANT!

Using a daytime moisturizer with sunscreen and knowing how to apply it is a complicated, confusing, and controversial issue, and we certainly can understand if you're wondering what to do. This is especially true about the recommendation to reapply sunscreen every two hours—no matter what! This seems ridiculously inconvenient, to say the least. If you're wearing makeup, are you supposed to wash it all off, reapply sunscreen, and then redo your makeup every two hours throughout the day? Who has time for all that?! We straighten that out below.

There's no question that wearing sunscreen daily, 365 days a year, minimizes signs of premature aging. Whether you decide to be sun smart is up to you; we know lots of you still feel that a summer or vacation tan is a must or that getting "just a little tan" is fine, but please at least consider the information below because, and we're not exaggerating, your skin's life depends on it.

The following research-supported facts will help you make sense of sunscreen, so you can get the best protection from the sun's harmful rays:

» "SPF," which stands for **S**un **P**rotection **F**actor, is an indicator of the length of time that your skin can be exposed to sunlight without turning pink (meaning your skin will start burning) when wearing an SPF-rated product.

» Although using a product rated SPF 15 is acceptable, the latest research suggests that higher SPF ratings are far more desirable because they provide better protection. [45,46] Look for sunscreens rated SPF 30 or greater, and/or consider layering SPF products for enhanced anti-aging protection.

» The two types of UV rays that damage skin are UVA and UVB. UVA rays are far more damaging because they're present all day long, year-round, and penetrate deeper into the skin than the shorter wavelength UVB rays. UVB rays are present with visible sunlight and can cause sunburn, while UVA rays promote tanning. UVB rays are strongest in sunny climates and between the hours of 10:00 A.M. and 2:00 P.M. UVA rays maintain a consistent intensity during daylight hours, throughout the entire year. [9,47]

» Sunscreens labeled as providing "broad-spectrum" protection should protect your skin from both UVA and UVB rays. [9,47]

» All sunscreens with an SPF rating provide reliable UVB protection, as there are numerous UVB filters approved for use in sun-protection products. The best active ingredients for reliable UVA protection are titanium dioxide, zinc oxide, avobenzone, ecamsule (Mexoryl SX), and Tinosorb (which may be listed as methylene bis-benzotriazolyl tetramethylbutylphenol). [9,47]

» You must apply sunscreen liberally to obtain the benefit of the SPF number on the label. Unfortunately, most people don't apply sunscreen liberally and that is detrimental for their skin. This common mistake might lead you to believe that the sunscreen you applied isn't effective. [9,47]

What about the recommendation you often see about reapplying sunscreen every two hours even if you're not swimming or sweating? That's a great question, with a somewhat complicated answer—but hang in there and we know you'll get it.

Does the sunscreen you apply in the morning still work in the late afternoon, following a day at the office or at school? The answer is yes, depending on how much time you spend outdoors because the sunscreen actives break down in response to direct exposure to daylight, not in response to the passage of time during a single day. [9,47]

On an average day (if you're in an office or otherwise indoors), your morning application of sunscreen is still going to provide sufficient UV protection on your way home, assuming you applied a liberal amount of an SPF 30 (or greater) in the morning.

If you spend the majority of your day outdoors, then the recommendation is to reapply every two hours, especially if you're perspiring or swimming. This recommendation to reapply every two hours is based on the following.

» Most people don't apply sunscreen liberally, and if you don't you won't get the SPF protection rating shown on the label. If you're one of those people who does not apply sunscreen liberally, then the apply-every-two-hours guideline makes sense, however impractical it may seem. The thinking goes like this: If you aren't good about applying sunscreen liberally, then reapplying every two hours after direct daylight exposure will add up to liberal application because of the extra layers of sunscreen you're putting on. [8,9]

» **How much to apply:** There are many measurements given to help you figure out how much sunscreen to use, but in reality how much to use depends completely on the size of the area you're covering. What we like to suggest is to smooth a layer of sunscreen over the skin that will be exposed to the sun so you can see it and then gently smooth it into skin and let it absorb. And, yes, we understand that it may feel a bit unpleasant until it is absorbed, but the protection it affords is worth this temporary feeling. Don't forget your chest, arms, and hands (or any other areas of exposed skin)!

» **How often to apply:** We know this one is repetitious, but we're on a mission to ensure the best skin of your life starts now, and this is the first rule to make sure that happens. Aside from everyday use (no exceptions), a single application each morning with a product rated SPF 30 or greater will keep you protected for a normal workday (indoors), a walk to lunch, and the drive home. If you spend more than three or four hours in direct sunlight during the day, it's a good idea to reapply your sunscreen—and, yes, that means redoing your makeup, which is why we advise touching up with a pressed powder rated SPF 15 or greater.

» If you sweat profusely (think outdoor exercise or what can happen on a really humid day) or if you wash or sanitize your hands, swim, or get wet, you must reapply your sunscreen regardless of the SPF number on the product. If the sunscreen is labeled "very water resistant," you get about 80 minutes of protection while perspiring or swimming. If the label states "water-resistant," you get only about 40 minutes of protection if you get wet. [48] But don't forget, even if you use those types of sunscreens, you'll be rubbing them off when toweling dry, so in that scenario, be sure to reapply.

As you've seen, the rules for applying and reapplying sunscreen if you're getting wet or sweating are entirely different from the rules if you stay dry and spend only limited time outside.

It's also critical to understand that being inside doesn't mean your skin is protected from sun exposure. If you're sitting next to a window, it's highly unlikely you'll get sunburned because almost all windows protect you from UVB rays, the rays that cause burning. However, unless the window has special UVA shielding, your skin will NOT be protected from the sun's UVA rays because these rays penetrate windows. [49] This is one of the factors you must take into consideration when deciding how often to reapply your sunscreen, or be sure you're wearing sunscreens with higher SPF. You can also consider the following:

» Find out if the windows filter both UVB and UVA rays.
» Use blinds to control the amount of daylight that enters your work space.
» Add a UV-filtering film to your office window; these films are sold in most major hardware stores and are easy to apply.

COMMON SUNSCREEN QUESTIONS, ANSWERED!

What does "liberal" application really mean? As we mentioned above, there are varying measurements given to help you figure out how much sunscreen to apply. The standard often cited by dermatologists is to use an ounce of sunscreen (what would fill a standard shot glass) for head-to-toe coverage.[8,50] But, although well-meaning, this is just an impractical and some-what illogical guideline.

The shot glass rule would apply only if you're a thin, petite person wearing minimal clothing, such as a bathing suit for the beach or a tank top and shorts. If you're a tall, heavyset person wearing minimal clothing, a shot glass amount literally won't cover it. The total surface area exposed is what matters and a shot glass may or may not be enough. Following our rule of applying a layer of sunscreen you can see and then smoothing it over skin to let it absorb should work well.

Keep in mind that the more skin that's covered by opaque clothing with a tight weave that doesn't let sunlight through, the less sunscreen you need to apply because the clothing also provides protection. Don't count on your clothing alone, however, especially for long days outside; for that, look to spe-cial sunscreen clothing companies, such as the Sun Precautions and Coolibar brands, which sell their products online and in some sporting goods stores.

Another option we recommend for achieving liberal application on your face is to layer sunscreens. For example, apply an amount of your daytime moisturizer with SPF 30 or greater that feels comfortable, and then follow it with a foundation rated SPF 15 or greater and set that with a pressed powder that provides additional sun protection. Voilà, you get great sun protection without skin feeling too slick or heavy from a liberal application of sunscreen.

Keep in mind that layering sunscreens is not additive; for example, apply-ing an SPF 15 and an SPF 30 doesn't net an SPF 45. However, adding sun-screen ingredients by layering different SPF-rated products absolutely helps boost protection, just how much more isn't exact. Applying more sunscreen ingredients to your skin is how chemists formulate sunscreens to achieve higher SPF ratings—they add more active sunscreen ingredients! Now that's sun-smart behavior!

When should you apply sunscreen? Every day, as the last step in your skin-care routine. The vast majority of medical experts and skin researchers agree: **Sunscreen is always, always, the final step in your skincare routine.** [47,51] Any skincare product applied over a sunscreen dilutes the sunscreen, reducing its effectiveness to some degree. So, if you apply a moisturizer or a serum over your sunscreen, the amount of protection you get is reduced, and that's a se-rious problem.

With the exception of a small minority of naysayers, the above guidelines are universally agreed on as the correct way to use sunscreens. Forgoing this important step is a disservice to the health and appearance of your skin, but, of course, this is your decision to make.

Do you need moisturizer AND sunscreen during the day? Typically, no. That's because most sunscreens are formulated in a moisturizing base. Plus, the best ones also contain other beneficial ingredients, so most people can skip applying "regular" moisturizer during the day—your sunscreen product should provide enough moisture, so there's no need to layer moisturizer underneath. Instead, consider applying an antioxidant-rich serum before your sunscreen or a booster (sometimes labeled "essence") to increase skin's environmental defenses. Research has demonstrated that sunscreens work better and provide even more benefit when paired with an abundant amount and variety of antioxidants. [13,14]

We're occasionally asked if it's necessary to use a "regular sunscreen" on top of a daytime moisturizer with SPF. A sunscreen is a sunscreen; whether labeled a "daytime moisturizer" or a "sunscreen," it will provide you with the same UV protection benefits as long as it is rated SPF 30 or greater and contains active ingredients that, singly or together, provide broad-spectrum protection.

The primary difference between a daytime moisturizer with an SPF rating and a larger-sized product labeled a sunscreen is that the daytime moisturizer with sunscreen typically also contains larger amounts of other beneficial ingredients (that is, antioxidants and cell-communicating ingredients) than a "regular" sunscreen formula. Thus, a facial moisturizer with SPF should pack a greater anti-aging punch than that giant bottle of sunscreen you keep in your beach bag, even though their SPF ratings are identical. But, if all you're after is protection from UV light, then a regular sunscreen can also be applied to the face, and, of course, doing so saves money, too.

What about the recommendation to wait after application before venturing outside? Synthetic sunscreen actives (common examples include avobenzone, octinoxate, and oxybenzone) should really be applied 20 minutes before exposing your skin to daylight because they need time to "get situated" in the uppermost layers of skin before they can provide optimal protection. [9,52]

On the other hand, the mineral sunscreen actives—titanium dioxide and zinc oxide—provide immediate sun protection, so it's not necessary to wait if your sunscreen contains them. [9,52] That's why we recommend using a mineral sunscreen for your hands when you're outdoors, and always reapplying after washing or sanitizing them.

We're occasionally asked whether it's OK to use makeup that contains mineral sunscreen actives on top of a sunscreen that contains synthetic sunscreen actives. This is fine—the manner in which today's sunscreen actives are encapsulated, coated, and stabilized makes this a worry-free way to apply your makeup and sunscreen formulas. In fact, many sun-care experts recommend layering like this to get maximum protection!

What about applying foundation (one that doesn't contain sunscreen) over the sunscreen you've just applied? As mentioned above, this will dilute the sunscreen and reduce its effectiveness somewhat, but there are steps you can take to minimize this effect:

» Wait 3–5 minutes for the sunscreen to set before applying the foundation.
» Make sure you apply in smooth, downward motions; do not use a rubbing or back-and-forth motion or apply the foundation with a damp sponge.
» Do not use excess pressure, regardless of the application tool you prefer.
» Use a dry (not damp) foundation sponge or brush rather than your fingers.

If you're not the sort to wait, opt for a foundation or tinted moisturizer rated SPF 15 or greater (and in this case greater is better), of which there are plenty in all price ranges. Secondary to that, you may also set your foundation with a pressed powder rated SPF 15 or greater.

You may have read that you can't rely on your foundation or tinted moisturizer with sunscreen rated SPF 30 or greater as your sole source of sun protection. We disagree with that strongly! There's no research showing that a foundation or tinted moisturizer (or BB or CC cream either) with sunscreen is a problem as long as you stick to the same rules for all sunscreen application. In this case, the primary consideration should be how much coverage you want from these products. If you don't apply foundation, tinted moisturizer, or BB or CC cream with SPF 30 or greater liberally, you won't get the amount of sun protection stated on the label. So, if you're someone who likes a very sheer light application, then you shouldn't rely on these alone for sun protection. But, if you like a more generous application then you'll be covered quite well. Don't forget, you'll still need a sunscreen for your neck, as applying makeup there can result in higher dry-cleaning bills!

While foundations, tinted moisturizers, and BB and CC creams can be applied generously to achieve great sun protection, we feel that is unlikely in the case of loose or pressed powders that contain sunscreen. The kind of liberal application you would need to get the best protection would create a caked-on look that most people would find unacceptable (and we think would look fairly strange). Loose and pressed powders with sunscreen are best for the layering approach of wearing sunscreen, as we mentioned above.

Can you mix a tinted moisturizer or foundation that doesn't contain sunscreen with the mineral sunscreen you use to counteract the white cast

it can cause? We don't recommend it. Diluting a sunscreen is never a good idea for this critical step of skincare. Just apply your mineral-based sunscreen first, let it absorb, and then you apply your foundation in a light layer to eliminate the white cast. Or, you can add just a drop or two (literally) of a liquid bronzer or specialty makeup product like Cover FX Custom Cover Drops to your mineral sunscreen to offset the white cast. In this case, the tiny amount of product added is unlikely to have a negative effect on the mineral sunscreen's ability to protect your skin.

What does the PA++ designation mean? As if the whole SPF situation weren't confusing enough, along comes the PA rating system! The letters PA followed by plus signs (PA++, PA+++) on a sunscreen product label are a rating system developed in Japan. Although interesting, this system has its drawbacks. The PA system concerns only UVA protection; PA++ indicates moderate UVA protection and PA+++ indicates high UVA protection. Some regulatory experts argue that this type of rating isn't reliable because it looks only at UVA radiation, and UV rays from natural sunlight are a mix of UVA and UVB, each of which damages skin in different ways. [51]

The testing for the PA ratings differs from the UV critical wavelength testing, which is what's used to determine the UVA protection of sunscreens made in the United States and in European Union (EU) nations. The U.S. and EU method is considered more reliable because the subjects are exposed to the UV light (both UVA and UVB) they will encounter in real-world settings; that is, the sunscreen's UV protection ability is measured against this type of real-world exposure. [51]

The other issue is that the PA ratings of a product are established based on what's known as "persistent pigment darkening" (PPD). As mentioned previously, UVA rays are the ones that cause tanning; so, if exposed to UVA, your skin will become browner or darker, but that's not true for everyone. In the actual testing to determine the PA rating, even on people who have the same skin tone before UVA exposure, the color their skin turns after UVA exposure is routinely inconsistent; some skin gets darker, some not as dark. These variations make this type of testing inconsistent and unreliable in the long run. [51]

Whether the sunscreen you're considering uses the PA rating system or not (and it's definitely not essential nor a mark of a superior product), a well-formulated sunscreen will provide broad-spectrum protection and, as with any sunscreen, must be applied liberally and reapplied as needed to maintain protection.

Does sunscreen cause cancer? No, and there's no research proving otherwise. We're shocked how some people overlook the huge amount of research showing that regular use of sunscreen actually prevents cancer, prevents premature aging of skin, reduces brown spots, improves wrinkles, and helps skin heal. We discuss this issue in detail in Chapter 14, *Common Beauty Questions Answered and Myths Debunked!*

Bottom line: While understanding sunscreen isn't necessarily easy, if you remember to liberally apply a broad-spectrum SPF 30 sunscreen daily as the last step of your skincare routine that is a great start. After that, the next step is to be sure you use a water-resistant sunscreen if you'll be swimming or sweating and to reapply it every 40 to 80 minutes (which is determined by whether it is water-resistant or very water-resistant) when sweating or swimming. You also need to reapply regular sunscreen after every few consecutive hours of direct daylight exposure and anytime you towel off.

When we say the best skin of your life starts here, this is how it begins—with daily, diligent sun protection, your skin will look and act younger. You'll also reduce the risk and presence of brown spots, degree of sagging skin, formation of deep wrinkles, and impairment of skin's healing. Most important, it will reduce your risk of skin cancer!

RECOMMENDED SUNSCREENS:

Following is a list of sunscreens with different textures that we're particularly fond of. All provide broad-spectrum protection and also include other beneficial ingredients like antioxidants. In addition, the brands mentioned tend to produce consistently good SPF products, whether they are facial moisturizers with sun protection or "regular" sunscreens for the body.

» Alba Botanica Very Emollient Mineral Sunscreen Protection, Fragrance Free SPF 30 ($11.49)
» Clinique Sun Broad Spectrum SPF 30 or SPF 50 Body Cream ($23)
» KINeSYS SPF 30 Alcohol-Free Sunscreen with Mango ($18.99)
» MD SolarSciences Mineral Crème Broad Spectrum SPF 50 UVA-UVB Sunscreen ($30)
» Olay Regenerist Regenerating Lotion with Sunscreen Broad Spectrum SPF 50 ($25)
» Replenix Sheer Physical Sunscreen Cream SPF 50 ($29)
» Paula's Choice Resist Super-Light Daily Wrinkle Defense SPF 30 ($32)
» Paula's Choice Resist Youth Extending Daily Fluid SPF 50 ($32)
» Paula's Choice Sunscreen Spray Broad Spectrum SPF 43 ($25)
» Yes to Cucumbers Natural Sunscreen SPF 30 Stick ($8.99)

CHAPTER 7

Stop Acne and Breakouts (No Matter Your Age)

UNDERSTANDING ACNE

Acne is one of the most troublesome and common skincare problems for people around the world and, emotionally, one of the most embarrassing skin disorders. Although most often associated with teenagers and the onset of puberty, the truth is that you can suffer from acne at any age. Even if you never had it when you were younger, acne can still occur.

Most of us are familiar with acne to some degree, even if we don't know the specifics of what makes it acne and not some other skin problem. Acne's textbook definition describes it as a skin disorder occurring when hair follicles (every pore on your face is actually part of a follicle) become plugged with dead skin cells and oil that causes skin to become inflamed, erupting as a white fluid-filled sac. [27]

That mixture of oil and dead cells allows the bacteria responsible for acne, *Propionibacterium acnes (P. acnes)*, to flourish inside the follicle instead of remaining on the skin's surface, where it normally resides without causing too much trouble. [27]

These bacteria feast on the follicle's contents (gross, huh?), which starts a domino effect that leads to the production of inflammatory chemicals and enzymes. This process then triggers the immune system to send white blood cells to combat the bacteria—a call for help that leads to further inflammation.

Acne is, first and foremost, an inflammatory disorder, so it's important to remember that when treating it! Anything and everything you can do to reduce inflammation will help acne and the red marks it leaves behind heal faster. The reverse is true as well: Irritation will make inflammation worse and, therefore, cause more breakouts! [3,4]

The last stage in the development of acne is when the wall of the plugged follicle breaks down, spilling everything inside to nearby skin, causing inflammation that leads to the formation of a pimple. [27] Exactly what triggers this process, how fast a pimple develops, and why some pores are affected instead of others remains unknown.

Acne can show up on many areas of the body, including the face, neck, chest, back, shoulders, and arms. When a typical pimple (also called a pustule) forms, it can be one of several types of breakouts, as described below. [53]

Comedones: Comedones are considered non-inflammatory precursors to acne, but these lesions are not acne. In other words, comedones are evidence that conditions are present that could lead to acne breakouts. Comedones come in two forms, whiteheads (sometimes referred to as "closed comedones") and blackheads (sometimes referred to as "open comedones" because you can see the pore opening).

When too much oil is produced in the pore it can mix with dead skin cells and cellular debris, causing it to get stuck and form a "plug." This plug pushes to the surface and, if it's covered by skin, it appears as a slightly raised, whitish, firm bump called a whitehead. These are not pimples.

If these plugs come to the surface and are not covered by skin, they are exposed to the air, which causes the plugs in the pore to oxidize, resulting in a black spot referred to as a blackhead. That dark spot is not dirt showing beneath the surface of the skin!

Papules: These are small, raised bumps that indicate inflammation is occurring in the hair follicles. Papules are unsightly, but typically not painful or sore.

Pustules: Larger than papules, these red, tender bumps have white pus at their tips and are a sign of more advanced, deeper inflammation. They can be painful.

Nodules: One of the most painful forms of acne, these bumps remain below the surface of the skin and are large and solid. They develop when buildup occurs deep within the hair follicles that are severely clogged.

Cysts: These are markedly painful, swollen, pus-filled lumps that form beneath the skin. They present increased risk of scarring due to their depth and collagen-destroying potential. These are also the type of breakout least likely to respond to topical treatments, especially traditional over-the-counter acne products.

Sebaceous filaments: If you look closely at the tip of your nose, you might see tiny dots that resemble blackheads. These marks may be blackheads if they are quite dark, but the dark "dot" you see when you look very closely is also the tip of the columnar structures that fill your pores. They're known as sebaceous filaments, naturally occurring hair-like formations that channel the flow of oil along the lining of the pore in which they lie. [54] It's a natural part of skin's follicle (pore) structure that everyone has, but if your skin is oily or if your pores are large and prone to becoming clogged, you're more likely to notice it. Removing these filaments manually is possible, but they return shortly, and truth be told, chances are no one besides you and your magnifying mirror notice them anyway. Nevertheless, if sebaceous filaments bother you, regular use of a BHA exfoliant can potentially make them less of a noticeable concern.

WHY DOES ACNE HAPPEN?

You might be wondering: Who gets acne? It's estimated that 80% of *all* people between the ages of 11 and 30 will have acne breakouts at some point during this period of their lives, and it's quite common for many women to have breakouts well into their 40s, 50s, and 60s. [53]

Believe it or not, as long as people have been struggling with acne and even though hundreds of studies have been done, the exact cause remains unknown. Researchers have narrowed it down to a group of several related factors. [27]

» **Hormonal activity.** Androgens (male hormones) increase in both boys and girls at the onset of puberty, causing the body's sebaceous (oil) glands to enlarge and produce more oil. Oil production can also increase during pregnancy, or with starting or stopping oral contraceptives. In women, it decreases during menopause. [55]

» **Medications.** Medicines that contain or stimulate androgens, corticosteroids, and/or lithium can play a role in the development of acne.

» **Heredity.** Researchers believe that good old genetics could have a hand in whether or not a person gets acne. [56] Thus, if your parents suffered from breakouts, you're at greater risk of suffering from them, too.

In addition to the actual causes of acne, there are other factors that can make acne worse if you're already prone to breakouts, such as those below. [27]

» **Hormonal changes** that occur in girls or women two to seven days before the beginning of their menstrual cycle. It's no surprise to women around the world that breakouts are quite typical during your period.

» Breakouts and oily skin can also plague women going through **perimenopause** (the beginning phase of menopause that normally begins after a woman turns 40) and during menopause. What happens is that estrogen levels (estrogen is the "female" hormone) drop, but the androgen levels (the male hormone that women also have) remain constant. [55] Androgens are a primary trigger of acne and when you have more of them in your body without the estrogen to balance it, your skin can start acting like you have a teenager's skin, and not in a good way. The extra androgens cause the oil glands to produce more oil, and a stickier oil to boot, that can clog pores. There's also the issue of older women having excess skin cells due to accumulated sun damage which can also lead to clogged pores.

» **Sensitizing reactions** to makeup, irritating skincare ingredients, specific foods (rarely), allergies, or medicines. Sometimes such reactions aren't true acne, but rather what's known as "irritant contact dermatitis." The red bumps seen with this type of reaction can resemble acne and tend to happen quickly, while true acne develops over a longer period of time. [27,57]

» **Inflammation** caused by conditions inside the pore or by outside influences, such as using products that contain irritating ingredients, trying to "dry" up a pimple, or over-scrubbing. Squeezing pimples doesn't increase the incidence of acne, but when done incorrectly, it can further inflame the breakout, potentially push the contents deeper into the pore lining, and generally keep it around longer. [27]

» **Allergic reactions** to foods such as milk and milk products, gluten, nuts, or fish can cause acne in some people, but there's research showing that this may not be true. Nonetheless, if you want to see if certain foods are acne triggers for you, it's easy enough to experiment to see how your skin reacts if you eliminate one or more of these from your diet for several weeks. [27]

We touched on this above but to elaborate a bit before moving on to the next section: Acne and its typical partners-in-crime whiteheads and blackheads aren't the result of dirty skin. The black dots that comprise the tip of blackheads aren't dirt; dead skin cells and oxidized oil make these plugs appear dark. You cannot wash or scrub acne, whiteheads, or blackheads away, so please ignore all products making such claims. In truth, finally getting your acne under control is far more involved than that.

GETTING ACNE UNDER CONTROL IS THE SAME FOR EVERYONE

Although there really isn't a cure for acne, there's a lot you can do to greatly reduce the problem and get it under control. No matter what else you do, the most important thing to remember about acne is that it's an inflammatory disorder, which means anything you can do to reduce or avoid inflammation is going to help keep breakouts, the swelling, and the telltale redness at bay.

We describe below key steps you can take to make sure acne doesn't stick around for long.

Keep skin clean, but don't overdo it. Clean skin is a good thing because washing removes the excess oil and dead skin cells that contribute to clogged pores and create conditions ripe for acne to occur. However, washing too often, especially if you use harsh cleansers or scrubs, will lead to irritation and chronic inflammation. (Remember, anything that causes inflammation will increase acne conditions in your skin.) The best way to go is to wash your skin twice a day (once in the morning, once at night) with a gentle, water-soluble cleanser. We can't stress the "gentle" part enough!

Also stay away from bar soaps and bar cleansers—they can leave a film or residue on your skin, which in turn can clog pores and reduce the effectiveness of any anti-acne products you apply after cleansing. [58]

Avoid skincare and makeup products that can cause irritation. Irritation = inflammation, and that's bad news! Unfortunately, many skincare and makeup products, including many claiming to treat acne, contain irritating, drying ingredients. Don't use products that contain SD or denatured alcohol because it dries out skin and actually can lead to increased oil production. [3,4,53]

Also on the "do not use" list are mint (including menthol and peppermint), witch hazel, eucalyptus, or citrus ingredients, as they will wreak havoc on your skin—yet these ingredients show up in a shocking number of products claiming to help acne.

Be sure to remove all your makeup before going to bed. Sleeping with makeup on will prevent skin from exfoliating and also block pores, which increases the conditions that promote acne. If you wear heavy makeup or just want to feel extra clean (without causing inflammation), it can help to use a Clarisonic brush or a washcloth with your gentle water-soluble cleanser. After you've rinsed your face, follow with a gentle toner that contains anti-inflammatory ingredients or a gentle makeup remover to be sure every last trace of makeup is gone before your head hits the pillow.

Avoid overly emollient or thick moisturizers. These types of products not only make oily skin feel more oily and greasy, but also can block pores and even absorb into pores, adding to the clog that's already there or creating a new one. No matter how you look at it, these types of products are usually a problem for someone struggling with breakouts and oily skin.

Exceptions to this are the small percentage of the population who have acne, clog-prone skin and dry skin with little to just-visible pores. This confusing skin type is not easy to treat. More emollient moisturizers may be necessary to deal with the dryness, but they can also clog pores. The best way to deal with this is to follow our skincare routine suggestions and then experiment to find the lightest lotion moisturizer that will take care of your dry skin and not trigger more breakouts. Layering two or three thin-textured hydrating products (for example, a water-based serum layered with a lotion moisturizer) may be necessary.

Does wearing makeup cause acne? Not for most people. Foundations are designed to stay on the top of skin; they don't absorb into the pore and cause problems like thick, emollient moisturizers can. But what can cause acne is not getting all of your makeup off at night. So don't blame your breakouts on the makeup you're wearing, blame it on being a bit too tired at night to follow your skincare routine.

Use lighter hair-care products. If your hairstyle is such that your hair touches your forehead or the sides of your face, traces of the products you use to style your hair will also end up on your skin. Therefore, if you have acne-prone skin, you should avoid thick, waxy hairstyling products along the hairline because they can clog pores and lead to breakouts. Conditioners can also trigger acne breakouts, so avoid getting these on your face. If you have neck or back acne, try rinsing the conditioner in a way that prevents those areas from coming into contact with it.

Protect yourself from the sun. You might have heard that a good dose of sunlight can "clear up" acne breakouts, but there's no research indicating that sun exposure clears up acne. Sun damage is yet another form of inflammation, and inflammation is necessary to avoid. [4,27] If you're concerned that the emollient texture of your sun-protection products might cause breakouts, look for lightweight options. See the end of Chapter 9, *Managing Oily Skin*, for a list of some of our favorite lightweight, matte-finish sunscreens.

We realize that this is a lot of information to digest all at once, but preventing (or at least reducing) acne once you know what to use and what not to use can be surprisingly simple. We hope the information in this book will make your decision process far easier.

ACNE MYTHS: A REALITY CHECK

Regarding acne, there's no shortage of advice and there are all sorts of theories as to what works and why. Among them are the following myths that turn up all the time, no matter how many times they've been debunked.

MYTH: You can dry up blemishes. Water is the only thing you can "dry up," and a pimple has nothing to do with skin being wet. Drying up the water and other moisture-binding substances in skin actually hurts its ability to heal and fight inflammation, which *encourages* bacterial proliferation. [3,4,53] Absorbing oil that's on the skin's surface or in the pore is radically different from "drying up" skin with harsh ingredients such as SD or denatured alcohol, sulfur, camphor, and witch hazel.

MYTH: Acne is caused by not cleaning your skin well enough. This mistaken belief often leads to over-cleaning or scrubbing of the face with soaps and strong detergent cleansers, which only increases the risk of irritation, inflammation, and dryness, while doing nothing to prevent pimples. [53]

MYTH: You can spot-treat acne. Although you can greatly reduce the redness and swelling of a breakout with a salicylic acid (BHA)–based product or with a benzoyl peroxide disinfectant (both explained below), that doesn't help prevent other breakouts from popping up on other parts of your face. Dealing with only the pimples and pustules you see means you're ignoring those that are in the process of forming. [27,34]

As you may have guessed, spot-treating leads to a never-ending cycle of chasing acne around your face. Spot-treating tends to be most useful for those whose breakouts are consistently infrequent and localized (for example, always on the chin, nowhere else), rather than for those who experience them more frequently and/or randomly all over the face.

MYTH: If it tingles or feels cooling, it must be working. Ingredients that make your skin tingle, such as menthol, peppermint, eucalyptus, and lemon, show up in countless anti-acne products, yet there's no research showing they have any benefit for acne or oily skin.

In fact, these ingredients irritate and inflame skin, only making matters worse! Irritating skin triggers stress-sensing nerve endings at the base of the pore, which in turn stimulate oil production. [4] That cooling sensation, however nice, has no ability to reduce acne.

MTYH: Eating chocolate or greasy food causes acne. Although it's absolutely true that eating healthy food and an overall anti-inflammatory diet is good for your skin and your overall well-being, specifically eating chocolate or greasy food isn't going to give you acne. [53] If that were true, then everyone who ate either of these things would have acne, and that's simply not the case! On the other hand, diets high in sugar, dairy products, gluten, nuts, and fish may worsen acne for some people. [59,60,61,62,63]

MYTH: You can scrub acne, whiteheads, and blackheads away. It can help to use a gentle scrub as an extra cleansing step, but it won't change acne conditions in skin. None of these problems are about skin being dirty or needing a "deep" cleansing.

In terms of blackheads, gentle scrubbing can remove only the top portion of the problem, kind of like mowing over a weed rather than pulling it out of the soil, roots and all. That's why, within a day, if not within hours, of scrubbing blackheads, the dark dots are again lining your nose and cheeks. [64] The same concept applies to blackhead-removing pore strips, and the adhesives on these strips can be quite irritating. Depending on the scrub and how you use it, you most likely will be inflaming your skin, making matters worse!

MYTH: "Non-comedogenic" products won't cause breakouts. You've no doubt seen the term "non-comedogenic" dozens of times—you may even look for it when shopping for makeup, in the belief that a product with this claim won't clog pores or cause acne. Unfortunately, non-comedogenic is a totally unhelpful claim; the term was coined under test conditions that are not even remotely applicable to how you, or anyone else for that matter, use beauty products.

How did the non-comedogenic myth get started? It stems from a 1979 study published in the *British Journal of Dermatology*. [65] This study examined the potential of various ingredients (cocoa butter, for example) to clog pores and lead to the formation of comedones (a fancy word for blackheads and whiteheads). This potential was determined by applying a pure amount of an ingredient to the skin on a rabbit's ear.

Here's the kicker: Each ingredient was layered *five times* per application over a period of two weeks, without cleansing the skin at any time. [65] Can you imagine? This methodology easily dispels the entire notion of these tests relating in any way to how skincare products or makeup are actually formulated (it's the rare skincare product that contains only one ingredient) and to how people really use them.

What really determines whether an ingredient in a makeup (or skincare) product is likely to trigger a breakout is how *much* of an ingredient is present in the formula. A tiny amount of an ingredient, even mineral oil or a thickening agent, in your moisturizer, blush, foundation, or concealer is not going to cause or exacerbate a breakout. By the way, the researcher largely credited for developing the concept of comedogenic, Albert Kligman, said as much in his 1972 study, "Acne Cosmetica":

"It is not necessary to exclude constituents which might be comedogenic in a pure state. **The concentration of such substances is exceedingly important**. To exile such materials as lanolin, petroleum hydrocarbons, fatty alcohols, and vegetable oils from cosmetics would be irrational. What is ultimately important is the comedogenicity of the finished product." [66]

Like most of the beauty advice from the 1970s (for example, when we used baby oil to increase the effects of the sun to get a deeper tan while sunbathing), it's time to retire the whole concept of "non-comedogenic." It's just not helpful, and how many of us have bought products claiming they won't cause breakouts—yet we broke out anyway?

WHAT TO AVOID

OK, so we know that no one can say with certainty whether or not a product will or won't exacerbate a breakout if you're already prone to acne. What we can do is make your search easier by helping you identify the biggest culprits—namely irritating ingredients and products with thick, waxy textures. If you start experimenting by eliminating these from your skincare routine, we're sure you'll see important changes for the better.

Avoiding products that contain irritating ingredients is critical for everyone, but especially for those who have oily, acne-prone skin, because inflammation can worsen breakouts and oiliness.

The tricky part about irritation is that research has demonstrated that you don't always need to see or feel irritation or inflammation for your skin to suffer damage.[2] Just because you don't see redness on the surface doesn't mean that damage isn't taking place underneath the surface, silently hurting the skin in a variety of different ways. This fact explains why some people can use irritant-laden, anti-acne products, yet not suffer obvious signs of irritation.

It's also important to understand that the effect of inflammation on skin is cumulative, and repeated exposure to irritants contributes to a weakened skin barrier, slower healing (including of red marks from acne), and a dull, uneven complexion. [67]

If that weren't enough, inflammation in the skin plays a major role in increased breakouts and making oily skin *oilier*. [28,29] It's really, really important to avoid alcohol-based or fragrance-loaded skincare and makeup products.

As discussed above, it's also helpful to avoid any product with a thick, heavy, or creamy texture, such as some moisturizers and makeup products. If you're acne-prone, **thick or solid makeup products** such as stick, pancake, cream, or cream-to-powder compact foundations and concealers should be on your "must avoid" list—or at least avoid using them on areas where you're prone to breaking out. The problems with these kinds of products are that they're harder to remove from skin and because the heavier waxes they contain can become stuck inside the pore lining, creating a clog.

The same goes for bronzers or blushes in stick, cream, or cream-to-powder forms. The types of ingredients that keep these products in a solid form are iffy for use by those with breakout-prone skin.

OVER-THE-COUNTER ACNE TREATMENTS THAT WORK

When you're battling acne breakouts, the key is to look for ingredients that are proven to combat acne effectively, yet *gently*. The two best over-the-counter acne-fighting ingredients, as demonstrated by peer-reviewed medical and scientific research, are salicylic acid (also known as beta hydroxy acid or BHA) and benzoyl peroxide. [33,68] Research has shown that these two ingredients are as beneficial, if not more so, as prescription-only acne medications for mild to moderate acne.

Salicylic Acid: Also known as beta hydroxy acid (BHA), salicylic acid is an amazing multifunctional ingredient that treats acne in several ways. It not only has potent anti-inflammatory properties, but also exfoliates to remove the buildup of dead skin cells on the surface of the skin as well as inside the pore. Salicylic acid also has mild antibacterial properties. [33,34]

Because salicylic acid is a derivative of aspirin (both are salicylates; aspirin's technical name is acetylsalicylic acid), it also has some of aspirin's anti-inflammatory properties. That means it reduces inflammation, redness, and swelling, helping skin heal. [33] This in turn helps prevent scarring, while also decreasing the chance of further breakouts. Salicylic acid's antimicrobial properties also help kill the bacteria that cause acne. [69] Together, these properties make salicylic acid an MVP in the game of you versus your acne—a game we want you to win!

For salicylic acid formulas to be effective, they must have a concentration of at least 0.5%, although 1% to 2% is far more effective; plus, the formula's pH is a critical factor, with a pH of 3 to 4 being optimal. [70] Surprisingly to us, many salicylic acid products for acne don't meet these requirements, so they don't work well, if at all, on acne and clogged pores.

In addition, the product must not contain any irritating ingredients because such ingredients cause inflammation as we've stated so many times (because it's so important), potentially delaying healing and increasing oil production deep within the pore, keeping you on an endless cycle of clear skin–more acne, clear skin–more acne…Fortunately, well-formulated salicylic acid products do exist, and you'll find them from Paula's Choice and from other brands recommended at the end of this chapter.

Benzoyl peroxide is considered the most effective over-the-counter choice for a topical antibacterial agent in the treatment of acne. It penetrates into the pore and kills acne-causing bacteria, thus reducing inflammation. It does present a risk of irritation, but the risk is low compared with the benefits, and unlike antibiotics used to treat acne, it doesn't have the potential to create bacterial resistance. [33]

The concentration of benzoyl peroxide in products usually ranges from 2.5% to 10%. A 2.5% benzoyl peroxide concentration is far less irritating than a 10% concentration (not irritating skin is always the goal), and it can be just as effective. If your skin doesn't respond to the 2.5% concentration within a week or so of daily use, try a 5% concentration. [33]

Generally speaking, if your acne doesn't respond to a 5% concentration of benzoyl peroxide, then the next step is to consider topical prescription options (such as a topical antibiotic mixed with smaller concentrations of benzoyl peroxide) before trying a product with 10% benzoyl peroxide. Concentrations of benzoyl peroxide over 5% have been shown to tip the scale in favor of irritation, causing dry, flaky, and inflamed skin. Not surprisingly, this causes more problems than it helps. [71]

Note: Research shows that combining benzoyl peroxide with topical antibiotics reduces the risk of the bacteria developing resistance to the antibiotic, which means the antibiotic will be effective over a longer period of time. [72] This combination also has been shown to reduce inflammation, making it a good ingredient in some prescription options for stubborn breakouts that aren't responding to over-the-counter treatments such as benzoyl peroxide and salicylic acid. There are numerous topical prescription products that contain benzoyl peroxide + an antibiotic. Your dermatologist can help you determine which one is best for you.

Important note: When you're struggling with acne, you must be consistent with your anti-acne treatments. For many, breakouts are an ongoing problem, not a "one and done"–type deal. Ongoing, consistent use of anti-acne treatments is required to maintain the results and to keep new breakouts from forming. Daily adherence to a treatment routine is essential for success!

WHEN OTC ACNE TREATMENTS AREN'T ENOUGH

Some cases of stubborn acne just won't go away with over-the-counter medications alone, no matter how well-formulated they are. Instead of spending more money on product after product, if you notice your acne isn't improving after several weeks of being consistent with your skincare routine, it's time to see a dermatologist.

A dermatologist has numerous topical and oral prescription options to treat acne, from retinoids like tretinoin or Differin® to antibiotics and oral vitamin A (isotretinoin, formerly sold under the brand name Accutane). Each has its share of pros and cons, which you should discuss with your doctor. Following is an overview that will help you understand the options your doctor may suggest.

Important reminder: Using prescription-only products for your acne doesn't change the basic skincare routine you need to follow. Bar soaps, harsh cleansers, abrasive scrubs, and products that contain irritating ingredients or overly waxy products will still harm your skin and increase the likelihood of your skin not being able to tolerate these prescription treatments.

Prescription topical antibiotics are an option if you haven't gotten good results using over-the-counter treatments containing salicylic acid and benzoyl peroxide.

There are several topical antibiotics to consider; the main ones to discuss with your dermatologist are **erythromycin**, **clindamycin**, **minocycline**, and **tetracycline**. These can be used alone, but a good deal of research indicates that you can derive greater benefit without some of the side effects by combining one of these antibiotics in lower doses with benzoyl peroxide to create a far more potent and effective treatment.

Dapsone is a topical disinfectant gel available by prescription in 5% strength. The brand name for this anti-acne drug is Aczone. A recent study involving 347 adolescents and 434 adult women showed dapsone 5% gel used twice daily was effective in reducing inflammatory and noninflammatory acne lesions in both adolescent and adult women, but was even more effective for adult women. [73]

Retinoids, such as prescription tretinoin (Retin-A, Avita, Atralin, and generics) and other vitamin A derivatives, such as tazarotene (Tazorac®, Avage®) and adapalene (Differin®), can play a significant role in an anti-acne treatment routine. [74]

Retinoid is the name of the general category for any and all forms of vitamin A. Prescription retinoid options are viable treatments for breakouts because they change the way skin cells are formed in the layers of skin as well as in the pore, improving how skin cells shed while unclogging pores, thereby significantly reducing inflammatory lesions. Retinoids also have anti-inflammatory action, making them even more compelling.

Topical tretinoin and many antibacterial agents have complementary actions, and they work well together, but applying both at the same time increases the chance of side effects such as dryness, redness, and/or peeling. If you experience side effects, it's best to use the two separately, applying the antibacterial product in the morning and the prescription retinoid (be it tretinoin or another type) at night. Benzoyl peroxide does not deactivate newer formulations of tretinoin as it did in the past. [75]

Azelaic acid is believed to work against acne-causing bacteria in concentrations of 15%–20%, and it may also pack an anti-inflammatory punch. [76] Azelaic acid was approved for the treatment of acne in the United States in 2002, and also is prescribed to manage the symptoms of rosacea (some of which are similar to those of acne). It's definitely on the A-list of prescription options for treating acne—no pun intended. (Azelaic acid is not a prescription treatment in most Asian countries.)

Stay the course! For any topical acne treatment to work, whether prescription or over-the-counter, consistency is vital. Unfortunately, because almost all topical options can be hard on skin (at least at first), it's even more important to follow our suggestions for gentle skincare. Too often, skincare recommendations, even from dermatologists, include using products with irritating, drying ingredients that cause damage and inflammation. This means you'll struggle with being able to use acne-fighting treatments successfully. Please don't make the mistake of reverting to an outdated, problematic way of caring for acne- or breakout-prone skin. The research is clear that irritation makes acne worse, but a lot of salespeople, aestheticians, and physicians ignore or aren't familiar with this—but now you are!

Oral antibiotics can be extremely effective in controlling acne, but they also pose a risk of serious side effects that you must consider. Oral antibiotics do indeed kill the bad bacteria, but they also kill the good bacteria in the body. Thus, ongoing use can lead to chronic vaginal yeast infections as well as stomach problems. In addition, the acne-causing bacteria can become immune or resistant to the oral antibiotic. [77] That means if you've been taking an oral antibiotic to treat your acne for longer than six months, it can, and almost always does, become ineffective against the acne, although the negative side effects—killing good bacteria and causing stomach and other problems—could continue.

However, some research has shown that taking low doses ("sub-microbial" or subclinical doses) to fight acne is moderating the concern about bacterial resistance and adaptation. [68] Taking such low doses of oral antibiotics over the long term can improve acne, while minimizing, if not completely eliminating, the problem of the bacteria becoming resistant. It seems that lower doses of oral antibiotics have anti-inflammatory benefits instead of antibacterial benefits, but they still can kill acne-causing bacteria. That doesn't mean you won't suffer from possible systemic effects, though; so, whether you opt for regular or low-dose oral antibiotics, be sure to discuss the pros and cons with your dermatologist.

Birth control pills (some types) have been shown to reduce acne lesions and oil production, in part by decreasing androgens (male hormones), which are largely responsible for causing acne.

Birth control pills are a combination of different synthetic estrogens and progestins (female hormones). Some progestins can increase the amount of androgens in the body, while others block the production of androgens. Because androgens stimulate oil production, blocking androgens for those prone to breakouts and oily skin is a good thing.

As a result, some of the birth control pills that block androgens have been approved by the Food and Drug Administration (FDA) and other regulatory organizations for the treatment of acne. These include Ortho Tri-Cyclen (active ingredient: norgestimate/ethinyl estradiol), YAZ (active ingredient: drospirenone/ethinyl estradioland), Estrostep Fe (active ingredient: norethindrone/ethinyl estradiol). Diane-35 (chemical name: ethinyl estradiol cyproterone acetate) has been approved for such use in Canada.

Keep in mind that there are risks associated with taking any type of birth control pill (especially if you smoke), and you should discuss these matters with your doctor. [78] Birth control pills also should not be the sole therapy for acne; think of them as a partner product for use with a skincare routine designed to reduce acne.

ALTERNATIVE ACNE TREATMENTS

The world of alternative acne treatments is wide and varied. It includes options that are easily obtained at the drugstore, some that you can find at your local health supplement retailer, and even options in your grocery store, particularly if you frequent natural markets. We describe some of these options below.

Tea tree oil has some interesting, though minor, research demonstrating that it's an effective antimicrobial agent, although it's not without its drawbacks. In a study comparing tea tree oil with benzoyl peroxide, it was found that a 5% concentration of tea tree oil has an efficacy similar to that of 5% benzoyl peroxide. [33] That sounds as if the two are equally effective, but in the world of skincare it doesn't work that way. It turns out there aren't any skincare products that contain 5% tea tree oil. The highest concentration of tea tree oil we've ever seen in a cosmetic product is less than 0.5%, which likely makes it ineffective for treating acne. [33] "Pure" tea tree oil is typically only a 3% concentration diluted in a carrier oil, so even that isn't strong enough, despite the "100% tea tree oil" statement you might see on the label.

Niacinamide and nicotinic acid are derivatives of vitamin B3. There are a handful of studies showing they can be helpful for improving the appearance of acne, which most likely is the result of their anti-inflammatory and barrier-restoring properties. [79,80] When included as part of an anti-acne skincare routine, these B vitamin ingredients can be part of a powerful combination of products and ingredients to combat the series of events taking place in the skin that lead to acne. Niacinamide has anti-aging benefits as well, so it's a brilliant solution for those struggling with wrinkles as well as acne. [79,80]

Prebiotics and probiotics are microorganisms that occur naturally in the body and are present in many of the foods we eat, such as yogurt. Although they can be helpful when consumed, the research on prebiotics and probiotics related to topical application and their effect on acne is non-existent, so any benefit remains theoretical, although there has been at least one study that indicates they may have potential. [81] There's no harm in trying this option, via foods and/or supplements. As far as skincare products, we just haven't seen any that would be able to keep the prebiotics and probiotics stable or contain enough to provide any meaningful benefit.

Fatty acids are an interesting group of ingredients that can have an effect on breakouts, but exactly what that effect is, either positive or negative, isn't clear; far more research is needed. [82,83] There are only a few studies showing how fatty acids may improve matters but none are conclusive in the least.

Fatty acids, such as lauric, oleic, and palmitic acids, can have an antibacterial effect on *P. acnes*. However, their stability is an issue: A product that contains a fatty acid must be carefully formulated to ensure the fatty acid can exert its antibacterial action before it breaks down. If these fatty acids are present in skincare products that are packaged in a jar, chances are good they'll break down before they can really help your skin, because air exposure causes these fatty acids to turn rancid.

Sulfur can have some benefit as a disinfectant for breakouts. [33] However, compared with other options, it's an overly strong ingredient for skin, potentially causing more irritation than needed to fight acne-causing bacteria. For this reason, using sulfur to manage acne has largely fallen out of favor, so it's actually hard to find sulfur-based acne products, which in the long run is best for most people's skin. Nonetheless, when all else has failed, this may be an option to consider.

Diet can have both a positive and negative effect on acne. Reactions to certain foods can cause acne, while other foods may help reduce the frequency of occurrence. [63] Reactions to foods such as dairy products (mostly due to naturally-occurring hormones in dairy) or excess sugar intake can have varying degrees of influence on acne breakouts, depending on the individual. [59,60,61,62] Identifying which, if any, are true for you can lead to a significant and relatively rapid improvement in your skin. It takes experimentation to see what's true for your acne. Links to dietary factors such as shellfish, gluten, or peanuts are anecdotal, and haven't yet been demonstrated in research, but if you're wondering if this is true for you it's easy enough to experiment by eliminating one or all of these to see how your skin reacts. [84]

What theoretically can be great for skin is a diet high in foods known to have anti-inflammatory properties, such as antioxidants and beneficial fatty acids like omega-3 and omega-6. These can potentially fight acne from the inside out by reducing the inflammation present in the pore. Whole grains, fresh fruits and vegetables, and other healthy foods just might help your acne, too!

DO I HAVE TO BREAK OUT BEFORE MY SKIN GETS BETTER?

When starting a new skincare routine or product for acne, the age-old question is: Does your skin have to get worse before it gets better? In other words, does your skin have to go through a period of "adjustment" or "purging" and suffer through more breakouts first before you see positive results? The answer is no, that shouldn't happen from using new products. For many of you, however, that is exactly what you have experienced. You start a new product and begin breaking out like crazy! There are a few primary reasons why you may break out after starting a new product, as described below.

First: You would have broken out anyway. When you have acne-prone skin, especially women, acne can occur at specific times of the month or just randomly even if you haven't started a new skincare routine. What that means is that you might have started using new products when your skin was going to flare up anyway. The only way to find out if this is what's happening for you is to wait it out, keep using the product, and see if your skin starts getting better after about two to three weeks. If your skin doesn't get better after that time, then it's probably the products that are the problem, not you.

Second: Perhaps the anti-acne product(s) are just poorly formulated. If the products contain irritating ingredients, such as alcohol, mint, eucalyptus, witch hazel, lemon, lime, and/or fragrance (either natural extracts—especially "essential" oils—or synthetic ingredients), they will inflame skin and trigger breakouts. This reaction can happen immediately, especially if you are using more than one problematic product, or it can happen over time. Either way, you know that your skin is supposed to be getting better and that you should have seen significant improvement after two to three weeks. In this scenario, the products are the problem, not you.

Third: Your skincare routine is the problem. If your current skincare routine includes harsh scrubs, toners, or serums with irritating ingredients, then adding anti-acne products with active ingredients, even if they are brilliantly formulated, can be hard on your skin. In this case, it's the combination of a poor skincare routine plus anti-acne products that cause an irritant reaction that triggers immediate breakouts.

What about BHA—can it make skin purge? The answer is: Maybe ... for some people. Occasionally, first-time BHA users report experiencing a "purging phase," where they actually have more breakouts initially. Because BHA is oil-soluble, it exfoliates not only on the surface of skin, but also inside the pore lining. That kind of exfoliation can trigger a mass exodus of inflammatory substances and oil that, under certain conditions, can lead to more breakouts. Another possibility is that a concentrated BHA formula can bring to the surface pimples that were already brewing before you started using the product. It sounds counter-intuitive, but it can happen for some people. Our recommendation? Give your BHA exfoliant a couple weeks of consistent use before deciding whether or not it's working for you.

The bottom line: Unfortunately, it isn't always easy to tell why you are breaking out after starting a new anti-acne routine, but your skin should show some signs of improvement after about two to three weeks. Following our recommendations on how to choose the best over-the-counter anti-acne treatments can help, but when all else fails, see a dermatologist for prescription options.

HOW TO TREAT RED MARKS AND ACNE SCARS

Acne is enough of an issue on its own, so we openly admit it's not fair that long after a breakout has healed you're left with pink, red, or brown marks where the breakout once was. There are skincare steps you can take to prevent these marks (to the extent possible) and, more important, help them go away faster than they would on their own.

A common point of confusion is the difference between an actual acne scar and a post-breakout red mark or discoloration. Some people who ask us about solutions for acne scars are actually referring to the superficial pink, red, or brown marks from a breakout, which will heal over time; others are referring to a genuine acne scar that looks like a dent or depression in the skin. These actual scars are a result of deep, large pimples or from not letting acne breakouts heal by constantly picking at them.

A mild to moderate breakout often leaves a red, pink, or brown discoloration, which eventually fades over time. Although people often refer to such marks as acne scars, they are **post-inflammatory hyperpigmentation marks**, which appear as your body heals. Luckily, such marks are not really scars at all, and it's rare for them to be associated with permanently damaged skin. [85] That means there are steps you can take to speed up their healing and return to clear, even-toned skin!

A true acne scar results when there's damage to the deeper layers of your skin (that is, the skin below what you see on the surface) that has broken down the skin's support structure. Moderate to severe acne can damage these deeper layers of skin, causing the permanent breakdown of collagen and elastin. This leaves you with an actual indented, semi-circular, or jagged "ice pick" scar. Physical scarring of skin cannot be improved without the aid of medical or cosmetic corrective procedures. [86]

A quick note: If you have the bad habit of picking at a pimple—don't! Picking can further damage your skin and turn a pimple or white bump into a permanent scar, which otherwise could have been merely a red mark that diminished over time.

OK, now that we've defined the difference between a post-breakout discoloration and an acne scar, let's talk about what works and what doesn't for each!

Skin-lightening or skin-whitening treatments don't work on red marks because these products contain ingredients meant to reduce melanin production (melanin is responsible for giving color to your skin). Although they can reduce the appearance of brownish discolorations caused mostly by sun damage, they won't help fade post-acne marks because these red marks are not related to melanin production. The one exception is for those with darker skin tones whose post-acne marks are brownish in color from the skin's pigment, melanin, which in darker skin tones is more involved in skin's immune response to acne. In those cases, hydroquinone and other melanin-inhibiting ingredients are an option for fading their appearance. [85,86]

At-home treatments, such as rubbing lemon juice or other citrus fruits on your face won't work, either. They can't exfoliate skin properly and their acidic juices are potent skin irritants that actually can prolong the healing process. Don't fall for that one! There are no solutions in the kitchen for this skin issue.

Following are tips to help you achieve your skincare goals of fading post-acne discolorations and treating the underlying causes that lead to breakouts, and they work for any skin tone or ethnicity.

Use only well-formulated, gentle skincare products. It's tempting to try abrasive scrubs and all manner of irritating treatments in a desperate effort to get rid of acne discolorations, but irritation only causes more harm, which impedes your skin's ability to heal itself. [3,4,87]

Use a leave-on AHA or BHA exfoliant daily. The benefits of a well-formulated leave-on AHA or BHA (especially BHA) product can be truly impressive in helping to heal red marks. Both AHA and BHA increase cell turnover in the upper layers of skin to remove unwanted, built-up skin cells that prevent new healthy skin cells from coming to the surface normally. BHA's inherent anti-inflammatory properties mean it can reduce redness.

Use a broad-spectrum SPF 30 product every day, without exception. Unprotected exposure to UV light (which will get to your skin whether it's sunny or cloudy) hurts your skin's ability to heal, which means the red marks from acne will stick around longer. Protecting your skin from UV exposure every day is critical to fading discolorations, plus it keeps your skin healthier-looking longer! [7,9]

Use products loaded with antioxidants and cell-communicating ingredients. These two categories of beneficial ingredients defend your skin by helping it heal while also "communicating" with your cells to speed up their ability to repair damage. [88] The result is reduced inflammation and a shorter healing time for your discolorations. Using a toner, serum, and/or moisturizer formulated with a variety of these ingredients is the best way to reap their skin-repairing benefits. The cell-communicating ingredients niacinamide and retinol are particularly beneficial in the fight to fade your post-acne annoyances.

Consider professional help. Research shows that difficult or stubborn post-inflammatory red pigmentation responds well to a series of intense pulsed light (IPL) treatments. [85,86] Those with deeper skin tones, speak with your dermatologist about alternatives to IPL, as it can have the reverse effect on dark complexions. Another option is prescription tretinoin (Retin-A, Renova) and/or a monthly BHA or AHA peel performed by a cosmetic dermatologist. [85,86] These options should be considered only after the other choices we listed here didn't work for you (but do give them at least a few weeks of daily use to work before giving up).

For true acne scars (the pitted, indented kind), treatment options aren't as easy. Due to the extensive damage to and the loss of skin-supporting collagen, no skincare product can reverse their appearance. Injected dermal fillers can plump up the indentations, and you can combine dermal fillers with AHA or BHA peels or a series of fractional laser treatments (Fraxel) to achieve the best results. [85,86] This approach isn't cheap, but can produce truly remarkable results on scarring that seemed beyond help.

Dermabrasion is another option, but there's a much greater risk of damage to your skin than with laser treatments or high-strength AHA or BHA peels. The results aren't as impressive either, yet the risks are greater. [85,86] The medical options described above have advantages and disadvantages, so it's important to discuss them with your dermatologist.

HOW TO POP AND TREAT A BREAKOUT

Using a great skincare routine is vital to reducing or even preventing breakouts, but what you do with that pimple you see in the mirror is important, because it can determine how long you have to live with its memory.

You've probably read or heard people say to never pop a pimple, but we strongly disagree with that recommendation. Almost all of us are going to pop a pimple anyway because who wants to sit with that white swollen lesion sitting on their face all day?

Thankfully, it turns out that popping a pimple *correctly* can reduce inflammation, reduce the likelihood of scarring, and speed up healing time. And, of course, it gets rid of the way-too-obvious skin-distorting white bump— but only if you do it right!

Doing it right is key—you absolutely must not over-squeeze, pick, puncture, or do anything else that can cause serious scabs or you'll end up with a leftover mark that can take forever to go away or result in a permanent scar. It's easy to go too far, so proceed with caution!

Learning when and how to extract the contents of a pimple or other type of raised breakout properly is essential. You'll know the offending breakouts are ready when you see a white head. As long as you can see an obvious head, and you're certain you're not dealing with cystic or nodular acne (deep, red swollen bumps far below the skin's surface), you can use the following steps to remove the contents, which "deflates" the bump. Here's what to do:

» Buy a comedone extractor. Many beauty stores (like Sephora and ULTA) carry them, as does Paula's Choice.

» Cleanse your face with a gentle water-soluble cleanser first. Do NOT use very cold or very hot water (that will inflame the breakout and hurt skin's ability to heal).

» With the cleanser, lightly massage the skin with a soft, wet washcloth to remove dead skin cells—this makes extracting the pimple easier—but don't over-scrub.

» Dry your skin gently. Do not use the comedone extractor or squeeze when your skin is wet because it's more vulnerable to tearing and creating a scab, which can cause scarring.

» Center the comedone extractor's opening over the pimple. Then gently (and we mean *gently*), and with very little pressure (and we mean very little pressure), push the comedone extractor down on the whitehead and move it across the bump. That should release the contents.

» You may have to repeat this one or two more times, but that's all you want to do, as you can easily damage the skin and exacerbate the breakout.

» Remember to be gentle; the goal is to remove the white head without creating a scab or damaging the surrounding skin (scabs are not any better to look at than a pimple).

After your gentle extraction, follow up with a 2.5% or 5% benzoyl peroxide product and/or a 1% or 2% salicylic acid (BHA) product. Both salicylic acid and benzoyl peroxide can help by reducing inflammation and disinfecting, and will definitely help prevent further breakouts. [33]

RECOMMENDED OTC ACNE TREATMENTS:

The products listed below are suitable for all skin types struggling with breakouts. They should be used as part of a gentle daily skincare routine that includes cleansing, sun protection, moisturizing, and other steps needed for your skin type and concerns.

» Ambi Even and Clear Spot Treatment with 5% Benzoyl Peroxide ($5.99)

» Avon Clearskin Professional Acne Mark Treatment (salicylic acid, $11)

» Clinique Acne Solutions Emergency Gel-Lotion (benzoyl peroxide, $17)

» Kate Somerville Anti Bac Clearing Lotion (benzoyl peroxide, $39)

» La Roche-Posay Effaclar K Daily Renovating Anti-Relapse Salicylic Acid Acne Treatment ($31)

» Paula's Choice Clear anti-acne products (complete routines, $12–$29)

» Paula's Choice Clinical 1% Retinol Treatment ($55)

» Paula's Choice Resist Weekly Retexturizing Foaming Treatment 4% BHA ($35)

» philosophy clear days ahead oil-free salicylic acid acne treatment and moisturizer (BHA; $39)

» ProActiv Clarifying Night Cream (BHA; $28.75)

» ProActiv+ Pore Targeting Treatment (benzoyl peroxide; $42)

CHAPTER 8

Anti-Aging (From the Outside In and Inside Out)

HOW YOUR SKIN AGES AND WRINKLES

Before you spend another dime on products claiming to get rid of wrinkles and firm your skin, it's crucial to know what causes the signs of aging to show and to know how skincare products can either help or make matters worse. Just hoping the next product you buy will finally be the answer is a gamble for skin that can waste your time and money.

Dark spots, wrinkles, sagging skin, and other signs of aging are caused by a variety of factors, some of which can be treated by skincare products, while others cannot. The primary factors are as follows:

» **Sun damage**, meaning repeated exposure to the deadly, carcinogenic, aging rays of the sun or tanning beds. This cumulative damage destroys collagen and elastin, and causes DNA damage that leads to abnormal skin cells that cannot behave like young skin. Sun (daylight) damage is the major cause of wrinkling, uneven skin tone, and brown spots. This is known as extrinsic aging. [5,6,7]

» **Genetic factors**, such as skin color, affect how your skin handles sun damage. If you have inherited a darker skin tone, then you'll be less vulnerable to the sun's impact on your skin—but not immune. [5,6,7]

» **Chronological aging**—every year we get a little older and those added years negatively affect our skin, just as they do the rest of our body. This is known as intrinsic aging. [5,6,7]

» **Hormone loss for women** during menopause changes the texture and elasticity of skin. The most common sign? Skin becomes crepey, thinner, and doesn't bounce back when pinched. Breakouts and large pores that give skin an orange-peel texture may also be issues. [5,6,7]

» **Fat and bone depletion** occurs as you age. Your skin is supported by both fat and bone, so as some of that support is lost, skin begins to sag—there's simply less scaffolding to keep it in place, especially as gravity takes its inevitable toll! [5,6,7]

» **Muscle and fat pad movement** determine what areas begin to show signs of aging first; the parts of your face you use the most wrinkle the fastest and deepest. Plus, facial muscles become lax over time, causing further sagging. This, coupled with the random movement and gradual depletion of fat pads in the face, also contributes to sagging and a sunken, hollowed appearance of what was once plump. [89]

» **Disruption of skin's protective barrier,** from unprotected sun exposure or from irritating ingredients, decreases vital substances in the skin (such as ceramides, antioxidants, hyaluronic acid, and lecithin), leaving your skin more vulnerable to damage by the sun, smoke, air (oxygen), and pollution. [5,6,7]

With this information, you can get a better handle on what you can realistically expect from skincare products to make the biggest difference in your skin. And you'll more easily be able to spot cosmetics claims that are beyond the capability of even the best (or most expensive) skincare products.

CAN ANTIWRINKLE PRODUCTS HELP?

The answer is yes, antiwrinkle products absolutely can help, but only if you use the right products in a consistent, synergistic skincare routine. For many people, the results can be miraculous, or at least as close to a miracle as you can get without medical treatments such as lasers, Botox, dermal fillers, or cosmetic surgery.

Achieving such results is never about any one product or one ingredient (however much it's hyped), just like a healthy diet isn't about eating only one food or one nutrient. Skin is far more complicated than any one ingredient or one product can address. The fundamental ways to fight aging require a combination of the following types of ingredients, which should always make an appearance in your skincare routine!

ANTIOXIDANTS

Without question, topically applied antioxidants are essential for skin, and the more included in your skincare products, the better. [5,6,7] There are a wide variety of antioxidants, including different forms of vitamins A, C, and E, superoxide dismutase, beta carotene, glutathione, selenium, green tea, soy extract, grape extract, pomegranate extract, and dozens of others. Antioxidants help your skin by:

» Reducing or preventing some of the daily free-radical damage and inflammation that destroy skin's ability to heal, to remain healthy, and to stay firm over time. [5,6,7]
» Boosting the effectiveness of sunscreens and helping skin resist environmental assaults. [13,14]
» Helping skin heal and produce healthy collagen. [5,6,15]

Important note: As powerful as antioxidants are, they're also delicate! Therefore, as we state throughout this book, they must be protected from exposure to air and light to remain effective in a skincare product. When antioxidants are packaged in a jar, they're exposed to air the second the jar is opened, causing them to deteriorate. [5,6,15] Likewise, an antioxidant-rich product housed in clear packaging that exposes the formula to UV light will lose its potency, so it's imperative to seek opaque packaging. Keeping antioxidants as potent as possible before they contact your skin is critically important.

SKIN-IDENTICAL/SKIN-REPAIRING INGREDIENTS

Healthy young skin naturally contains skin-identical (repairing) ingredients in abundance—these help keep the skin smooth, retain moisture, protect itself from the environment, fight infection, and repair its outer and inner barrier structure. [16,17] When skin's barrier is maintained, it can go about repairing some of the damage that leads to the telltale signs of aging. Used regularly, these ingredients will make signs of aging and skin sensitivity (how reactive it is) less apparent.

Skin-identical ingredients range from ceramides to lecithin, glycerin, fatty acids, polysaccharides, hyaluronic acid, sodium hyaluronate, sodium PCA, collagen, elastin, proteins, amino acids, cholesterol, glycosaminoglycans, triglycerides, and many more. Skin-identical ingredients are critical to skin health, and (especially) if you have dry skin or the skin disorder rosacea, you should look for them in abundance in your moisturizers, toners, and serums.

CELL-COMMUNICATING INGREDIENTS

Factors such as sun damage, age, and hormone fluctuations damage skin cells—subsequently, those damaged cells regenerate irregular, mutated, rough, and defective cells. [5,6] These "defective" cells are responsible for all manner of skin concerns—from wrinkles and uneven texture to irritation and more. As these damaged cells reproduce more copies of themselves, the health and appearance of your skin suffers. [5,6] Essentially, skin can get to a point where you have more damaged irregular cells than healthy cells—and you'll see this degradation in the mirror!

Cell-communicating ingredients are substances that "communicate" with the defective cells, helping reverse the damage by signaling the skin to produce healthier, younger cells. [5,6] The defective cells receive a message to stop making bad cells and start making better ones! It's an exciting, fascinating area of skincare! The key players in this group include niacinamide, retinol, synthetic peptides, lecithin, ceramides, and adenosine triphosphate. [5,14,18,19,20]

SUNSCREEN

Unprotected exposure to UV light, i.e., daylight (and UV light is there whether the sun is shining or not), ages skin and causes skin cancer—in fact, UV exposure is one of the most potent natural carcinogens around! [8,9] About 80% of what we think of as aging is caused by unprotected UV exposure. [37] This damage begins within the first minute of skin's exposure to daylight. [43,44]

Other than sun-smart behavior, using a daily sunscreen is vital—even on days when the sun isn't shining, as UV damage occurs on cloudy days, too![8,9] See Chapter 6, *Sun Damage and Sunscreen Questions Answered*, for the full scoop on this critical topic.

Note: The only real difference between a daytime moisturizer and a nighttime moisturizer should be that the daytime moisturizer contains sunscreen. A product labeled day cream or day lotion that doesn't provide sun protection is an invitation to more wrinkles and other unwanted signs of aging! Also, research has demonstrated that beneficial antioxidants added to a sunscreen boost its ability to defend your skin against the damaging effects of UV exposure. [13,14] Don't bother with sun protection products that omit antioxidants; you won't be getting your money's worth!

LEAVE-ON EXFOLIANTS

One major aspect of skin aging and sun damage is that the outer layers of skin become thick and rough, while the inner layers become thin and collagen breaks down. [32,36] Alpha hydroxy acids (AHA) such as glycolic and lactic acids, and beta hydroxy acid (BHA, also called salicylic acid) each have unique properties to address these concerns.

When these types of exfoliating products are well-formulated, they gently exfoliate the surface layers of skin, providing a smoother, less wrinkled appearance. Both AHAs and BHA also reduce skin discolorations and can aid your skin in producing collagen to increase the support in the lower layers of skin:

» Both BHA and AHAs help create smoother and firmer skin.
» Both BHA and AHAs can reduce or eliminate dry, flaky skin.
» BHA can noticeably reduce the size of enlarged pores.
» BHA can reduce blackheads, white bumps, acne, and large pores. [32,36]

For more on the benefits of AHA and BHA exfoliants, see Chapter 4, *Which Skincare Products You Need—and Which Ones to Avoid*.

If the products you use contain a combination of the beneficial ingredients listed above (and come in opaque, air-restrictive packaging), then you're doing exactly what research indicates you can do to fight the signs of aging with skincare products. The result? You'll help your skin look and act younger and keep it that way for as long as possible. It's never too late to get the best skin of your life!

DO FIRMING AND LIFTING CREAMS REALLY WORK?

The truth is: While you can help create healthier, firmer skin, the results aren't going to replace a cosmetic procedure—this is a fine line of distinction that's often (OK, endlessly) exploited by the majority of cosmetics companies churning out treatments with "works like Botox" or all manner of "lifting" or "re-contouring" claims. We're asked time and time again, "but what about *this* product," or "what about *that* new cream I read about in _____ magazine?"

Reality check: No matter what tempting claims or blatantly retouched before-and-after photos you see in advertisements, no firming or tightening products can provide results even remotely similar to what you can get from procedures such as dermal fillers, lasers, and cosmetic surgery. If a product could work that way, it certainly wouldn't be for sale over-the-counter, it would be available only with a prescription (with good reason), and only then after a great deal of safety and efficacy testing.

Knowing the truth about how skin elasticity works and what can and can't affect its structure is the only way to be sure that what you buy can actually make a difference. Wasting money on products that don't work is never pretty!

» **Elastin** is the support fiber in the body that allows skin to "bounce" back into place. Think of elastin like the springs in a mattress and the stuffing between the springs as **collagen**, along with other elements of the body, such as fat, cartilage, muscle, and so on. When elastin is damaged and pulled to the breaking point, skin begins to sag; just like when mattress springs get old and damaged, the mattress begins to sag and can't bounce back to its original form. [5,6]

» During development in the womb and in early childhood, the skin makes lots of elastin; **older skin, on the other hand, makes almost none**, even with medical procedures—and definitely not with skincare products (though some ingredients can play a role in repairing damaged elastin). [20]

» **Sun damage and age degrade elastin**, and cause faulty repair mechanisms in the skin, resulting in crepey, paper-like skin. Skin gradually loses its ability to maintain elastin. [7,41,42]

» **Stretching and pulling at the skin also breaks down elastin**. As much as possible, avoid pulling at the skin, especially around your eyes. This constant tugging stretches the elastin in your skin; just like a rubber band, eventually it will not snap back to its original shape. It can actually stretch to the point where it becomes brittle and weak or breaks; in fact, that's what stretch marks are, broken bands of elastin! [42,90]

» The collagen and/or elastin in skincare products **cannot fuse with the collagen and elastin in your skin** to help rebuild or reinforce those structures. The molecular sizes of both collagen and elastin are too large (WAY too large!) to penetrate the skin's surface. [91]

Some products claim that the collagen or elastin they include has been "bioengineered" so it's small enough to be absorbed into the skin. As helpful as that sounds, it's completely useless. No matter how small these ingredients are engineered to become, they still will not fuse with the collagen and elastin in your skin. Claims to the contrary are not supported by independent, peer-reviewed research.

Even if there were some remote possibility that the collagen and elastin in skincare products could reinforce those elements in your skin, how would the collagen and elastin you applied all over your face know which collagen and elastin to attach to in your skin, and which to leave alone so the wrong parts of your face don't start puffing out or becoming lumpy?

Many times when you buy a product claiming to tighten sagging skin, its effects, if any, are due to high amounts of ingredients such as film-forming agents. Just like the name states, film-forming agents form a film on the skin, and, as they set, they can make the skin "feel" tighter—think of the sensation when hairspray (which uses film-forming ingredients to create hold) is sprayed onto skin.

The "tightening" effect of products that contains a high amount of film-forming ingredients is temporary and you won't see a noticeable lifting of sagging skin. However, the sensation is often enough to convince users that the product is working, and we want so desperately to believe that it really will lift skin. Skin "feeling" tighter is not the same as making a real change for the better in the tone or laxity of your skin. However, with the right products (and, yes, this must include sun protection), you can create healthier, younger-looking skin. That won't give you Botox- or surgery-like results, but the difference healthier skin can make is absolutely dramatic in and of itself! Here's the game plan:

» **Helping skin build more collagen is the key.** Although collagen doesn't help crepey skin bounce back, it does help support the skin so that sagging is less apparent—you can help your skin stimulate collagen production with skincare products that supply potent antioxidants and skin-repairing ingredients. [5,6] Good news: Healthy, protected skin LOVES making collagen and will continue to do so in a controlled manner.

» **Sunscreen rated SPF 30 or greater is non-negotiable.** Because sun damage destroys collagen and elastin, daily sun protection is critical. [7,41] Don't forget your neck and chest, or those areas will age prematurely as well!

» **Daily use of an AHA or BHA exfoliant** can really help. Along with exfoliating for smoother skin, there's also a good amount of research showing these ingredients lead to building more collagen and, to some extent, because of how they exfoliate skin, can make skin feel and appear firmer. [31,32] Hey, we'll take all we can get, right?

» **Vitamin A, also called retinol, applied topically, can improve the shape of the elastin** your skin still has; there's even a small amount of research showing it can build elastin—it definitely can build more collagen. [19,92] Applying a retinol product every night can help a lot, and the same is true for prescription retinoids such as Renova or generic tretinoin. If your skin can tolerate a retinoid, use it!

» **Medical procedures—lasers and other light or ultrasound therapies—** such as Fraxel and Ultherapy® have impressive skin-firming results and can also improve crepey skin by reshaping and reforming collagen (sadly, not elastin)! Rather than spending money on expensive lifting creams and facials that don't—and won't—work, set those funds aside and in a few months you can save enough to afford these types of skin-changing treatments from a dermatologist.

» **After doing all these things, natural aging can still cause your skin to sag and that's where cosmetic surgery plays a role.** Various types of face-lifts can make a dramatic difference without making you look "pulled too tight." When artful surgery is combined with a brilliant skincare routine, the results can be nothing short of show-stopping! See Chapter 13, *Botox, Fillers, Lasers, and Surgery*, for full details.

DRINKING COLLAGEN?

What about drinking collagen? Can it shore up damaged collagen from the inside out? The collagen-drinking trend is big business, especially in parts of Asia and in the United Kingdom, but it's not one we recommend, regardless of where you live. Here's what happens: When you drink collagen (and the commercial preparations usually contain fish collagen), the body's digestive system breaks it down just like it does any other protein, so it can't reach your skin as intact collagen.

There's no scientific research proving that drinking collagen can affect one wrinkle, spot, or pore on your face, although drinking fluids that don't dehydrate the body—that means not too much alcohol or too much coffee—will have a positive impact on anyone's skin.

DRINKING HYALURONIC ACID?

Hyaluronic acid is a substance in our skin that is abundant in the epidermis (skin's uppermost layers) when we're young, but diminishes with the passage of time. [20] This ingredient has been modified in laboratories to be used as dermal fillers (an example would be the Juvéderm brand) to plump out wrinkles and restore lost facial volume that occur with age. It also has impressive properties for skin, including hydration, wound healing, and skin repair, because it is so naturally compatible with skin. [93] This has made hyaluronic acid a very popular skincare ingredient. Often the claims about it are overblown, but the attention it gets isn't without merit.

Another use for hyaluronic acid in medicine is to inject a form of it into arthritic or injured joints, especially knees, as a fluid to cushion the painful area. All of these varied uses and the fact that it's a natural component of the body has led some to believe that drinking the stuff might be a way to prevent dryness, maintain hydration from the inside out, and improve aching bones. It turns out there's a small amount of research suggesting this may be valid and better for the skin than for the body. While the research is limited, most of it performed on animals or in petri dishes, what may be true is that when you drink hyaluronic acid it does congregate in the skin and improve hydration. [94]

Just to be clear, applying hyaluronic acid topically or drinking the stuff won't work like the injectable hyaluronic acid–based fillers doctors use to plump out wrinkles and restore lost volume to an aging face. The diffuse benefit in skin isn't the same as targeted injections benefiting deep wrinkles and folds. It will definitely help skin a great deal, but it won't replace in any way what medical cosmetic corrective procedures provide.

RETINOL: THE ANTI-AGING (AND ANTI-ACNE) HERO

There are dozens and dozens of remarkable "heroic" skincare ingredients, but in some ways retinol stands out from the rest. Retinol is another name for the entire vitamin A molecule, and vitamin A—in all its forms—works as a cell-communicating ingredient.

By "cell-communicating," we mean retinol can actually tell a skin cell to behave, and even to look like a more normal, healthy, younger skin cell. When you have sun-damaged or breakout-prone skin (and many people have both, especially in their 30s, 40s, 50s, and beyond), this communication is incredibly beneficial because improved skin-cell health means an improvement in the condition of sun-damaged and breakout-prone skin—even pore size can be improved with retinol! [95]

The term "retinol" is used most often to refer to the non-prescription version that you can find in many products, with varying strengths—you'll see this ingredient referred to by name on a product's label.

When dermatologists talk about "prescription retinol" or "retinoids," they're referring to various forms of vitamin A that appear only in prescription medications due to their potency. The technical names for the prescription forms of retinol are typically tretinoin (found in Renova or Retin-A), adapalene (found in Differin®), and tazarotene (found in Tazorac®).

In the world of skincare products, retinol stands alone because it can function similarly, and some researchers say identically, to the prescription versions. [95,96] Generally, pure retinol is considered more effective than retinol derivatives, but retinyl palmitate (a natural substance found in skin) and retinaldehyde are acceptable and helpful in skincare formulations.

Why does the pure retinol found in the cosmetics world work like the prescription versions? It's because once it absorbs into the skin, enzymes break it down into the active form (all-trans retinoic acid) that's found in prescription vitamin A products in ingredients like tretinoin. [19,95]

So how do you choose? Keep the following facts in mind to help you determine **which form is best for your needs:**

» Prescription-strength forms of retinol are technically "stronger" and work faster. The retinol found in non-prescription products is a lower concentration (under 0.5%), and takes longer to have an effect, but, in the end, it works the same. [96,97] However, 1% retinol is considered identical in action to most prescription-only forms. [96,98]

» Prescription-strength forms of vitamin A/retinol (tretinoin) present a greater risk of irritation, as do higher concentrations of retinol (1% or higher). [98,95] For some people, the irritation side effects never go away, and they just cannot use it; for others, the results are amazing, often occurring within the first week and improving day after day.

» Cosmetic retinol (that is, not the prescription strength) has a far lower risk of causing irritation, but because it still breaks down in your skin to become the active prescription form (tretinoin), it can also be irritating for some. [95]

» It takes experimenting to see what frequency of application works best for you; many find that using retinol 2–3 times per week works great, while others can use it every day, morning or evening. It's fine to use a retinol product during the day if you're also protecting your skin with sunscreen.

» Aside from using lower strength retinol products or alternating days of application, adapting part of your skincare routine can reduce the potential irritation from retinol. We have found that applying a non-fragranced, non-greasy, plant oil–based booster/treatment before or after the retinol product (or you can mix them together) can make a huge difference. You can also experiment with applying a moisturizer and serum first and then applying the retinol product. All this may be worth the trouble because of the impressive benefits retinol can deliver.

A common misperception about retinol is that it exfoliates your skin. That is not true: Vitamin A/retinol, in any of its forms, does NOT do the same thing as AHAs or BHA. Vitamin A/retinol, whether in an over-the-counter or prescription product, is a cell-communicating ingredient **that works from the deeper layers up**, helping skin cells make healthier, younger cells and enhancing the production and proliferation of new skin cells. [19,95,99]

This confusion about thinking retinol exfoliates might be because retinol, in both over-the-counter and prescription products, can cause flaking, which you see on the surface. [95] Because of this side effect, people assume it's also exfoliating their skin. **Flaking skin is not exfoliation**. As described above, AHAs and BHA are exfoliants because they help skin shed naturally, and skin's natural, healthy exfoliation never includes seeing flakes or dryness. You never see healthy skin cells being shed. Instead, you just see a smooth, renewed skin surface and a healthy glow. That's the goal when it comes to exfoliation. Retinol works in a completely different manner; it's only the potential irritation it causes that results in flaking skin.

For the best anti-aging, antiwrinkle benefit, it is ideal to use both an exfoliant and a vitamin A/retinol product. If you've heard that you can't use retinol along with vitamin C (or with AHA and BHA exfoliants) because the ingredients deactivate one another, don't believe it; this isn't accurate in the least and there's no research supporting it. Below we explain the reasons why you absolutely can and should consider using both, depending on your skin-care concerns.

Important note: Whether you choose an over-the-counter or prescription retinol product, daily use of a well-formulated sunscreen rated SPF 30+ is critical! Even the most effective, research-proven anti-aging ingredients won't work like you want them to if you're not diligent about sun protection. After all, it was sun damage that created most of the problems you're now using the anti-aging products to improve!

For best results, you should use any form of vitamin A/retinol **with other anti-aging products containing rejuvenating ingredients** such as antioxidants, skin-repairing ingredients, and cell-communicating ingredients. [100,101] Despite retinol's superstar status, treating signs of aging is far more complex than any one ingredient—however good it may be—can address!

FIVE RETINOL MYTHS BUSTED!

Given retinol's popularity and benefits, we're often asked about the claim that AHA and BHA exfoliants "deactivate" or reduce the effectiveness of retinol. We've also read similar cautionary statements in beauty magazines that retinol works better without AHA or BHA exfoliants—or that, gasp, it shouldn't ever be paired with vitamin C, lest your skin face certain doom.

If smoother, younger-looking skin is your goal, what should you do given all this misinformation? The confusion ends here—as always, we turn to the research to bring you the myth-busting facts.

Myth #1: You can't use retinol with an AHA or BHA exfoliant. False! No research anywhere (we repeat, anywhere) demonstrates or concludes that AHA or BHA exfoliants deactivate retinol or make it any less effective when used in the same skincare routine—even if these ingredients are applied at the same time.

In fact, whenever we see a comment or recommendation about not using retinol with AHA or BHA exfoliants, the statement is never supported by research that demonstrates such an incompatibility. It's one of those falsehoods that gets repeated so often that people (even dermatologists) tend to believe it rather than question it. After all, doctors are supposed to have our best interests at heart, right?

It turns out that the claim of retinol not working with AHA or BHA exfoliants involves a misunderstanding about how skincare ingredients work together, and how each affects the structure of the skin. We discuss how wrong this claim is in our next myth....

Myth #2: The pH of AHA and BHA exfoliants reduces retinol's effectiveness. The confusion about using retinol with AHA or BHA products has to do with concern over the exfoliant's acidity lowering the skin's pH, and by doing so (as the claim goes), disrupting the retinol's ability to work its anti-aging, skin-smoothing magic.

The reasoning behind this claim is that if the pH of skin is below 5.5 to 6 (which is typical), an enzyme in your skin won't be able to convert the retinol into retinoic acid (a form of vitamin A), which is the active form of retinol. This is all based on the assumption that these acidic exfoliant ingredients lower the pH of skin, thus destabilizing the retinol and/or deactivating the enzyme in skin that converts retinol to its prescription strength. But, that's not what happens.

Just like most skincare rumors, this one sprang from a misunderstanding about the research. Only one study mentions the pH range and skin enzyme issue described above. However, that 1990 study was performed on a blend of animal and human proteins, and the pH relationship issue developed only when a fatty acid by-product was added to the mix; in other words, it was not on normal human proteins and not on healthy, intact skin. [102]

To further demonstrate how misguided the assumption of retinol's incompatibility with AHAs or BHA is, the study in question clearly stated, "no clear optimal pH range was seen when the assay was run without fatty acid by-product."

In the end, this single study was used only to compare how animal and human skin metabolize the form of vitamin A naturally present in skin, not about how **topical** vitamin A benefits (or functions in) skin. The study's conclusions were not intended to be used to make decisions about skincare.

In short, low-pH products do not prevent retinol in any way from converting into its active form when applied to skin. Retinol even remains stable in low-pH formulations.

It's worth noting that no research has replicated the pH limitations of the 1990 study. Yet, despite the lack of follow-up supporting research and the reams of other research concerning retinol, that study is still cited (solely) to support the inaccurate claim that retinol cannot be used with AHAs, BHA, or, as you'll see in myth #5, with vitamin C.

Myth #3: Retinol works better without AHA or BHA exfoliants. You may be surprised to find out that research has shown just the opposite to be true and that retinol, when combined with exfoliants like AHAs, helps fade hyperpigmentation in skin and improve the results you get from both ingredients on the skin. [103,104]

Extensive research has shown that retinol works when applied to skin regardless of these other factors.

Myth #4: You can't use retinol during the daytime. Research has shown that retinol works well under SPF-rated products to protect skin from UV light, and that vitamins A, C, and E, even when in combination, also remain stable and effective under an SPF-rated product. [101,105]

Research also has shown that a vitamin A and E combination remains stable under UV exposure plus sunscreen, and so does pure vitamin A when used alone. [106,107] That's excellent proof of retinol's stability when paired with a sunscreen.

Antioxidants plus sunscreen are a formidable defense against wrinkles, uneven skin tone, loss of firmness, and brown spots. Vitamin A also is an antioxidant and cell-communicating ingredient, another reason why it is such a special, unique ingredient. For best results, be sure to apply antioxidant-rich skincare products morning and evening.

Myth #5: You shouldn't combine retinol with vitamin C. Vitamin C (ascorbic acid and its derivatives) is another ingredient often cited as a problem when combined with retinol. As with the AHA and BHA myth, this one is also based on the pH/acidity issue because most forms of vitamin C, especially the pure form (ascorbic acid), are naturally acidic.

Here are the facts: Vitamin C (depending on the form) requires a low pH to remain stable. We know that retinol works in an acidic environment, as mentioned above, and that skin's pH is naturally acidic. So, from what the research has shown us, using vitamin C+ retinol makes sense.

So why would you want to use both vitamin C and retinol? Research has shown that a combination of vitamins in cosmetics is the way to achieve the best results, including the combination of vitamins A, C, and E. [100] In a double-whammy myth-buster, not only did retinol prove to be effective when paired with vitamin C, but also the two worked beautifully to defend skin against free radicals when applied under a sunscreen! [101] That wouldn't be the case if retinol made vitamin C ineffective, or vice versa.

Vitamin C actually helps retinol work better because it fights the free radicals that can destabilize the retinol as it penetrates into skin; thus, it increases retinol's anti-aging benefits!

Vitamin C also has its own impressive benefits for skin. Research has shown it can lighten skin discolorations, reduce inflammation, help skin heal, and build collagen. Vitamin C is another superhero skincare ingredient. [108]

One other point: Vitamin C is found naturally in the skin, so it's there whether you apply it topically or not (although your skin loses its vitamin C content over time due to sun damage, which is why applying it topically is so important). Given that vitamin C is always present in skin, it clearly doesn't block or interfere with the benefit of any brilliant skincare products you apply to your face, including retinol.

VITAMIN C: ANOTHER ANTI-AGING HERO

We repeatedly state that there's no single ingredient that's best for skin—just like there's no single food that is best for your diet—but there are a few standouts and vitamin C is one of them.

Over 20 years ago, a Duke University scholar published a groundbreaking paper that showed how a form of vitamin C called L-ascorbic acid reduced UVB damage when applied to the backs of hairless pigs. [109] This evidence suggested that photodamage or "sun spots" could be repaired with topical use of vitamin C. As you might expect, that was big news for anyone concerned with signs of aging!

That original paper preceded an impressive and conclusive body of research that has since proven the benefits, stability issues, and usage requirements for vitamin C. Further research (*lots* of research) continued to show vitamin C's positive effect on skin, and a bona fide, legitimate skincare craze was born!

As widely used as vitamin C is in cosmetics now, it can get confusing because there are many forms, each with its own name and formulated in varying amounts to guarantee effectiveness. Here's what you need to know:

» The forms of vitamin C that are proven most stable and effective are: ascorbic acid, L-ascorbic acid, ascorbyl palmitate, sodium ascorbyl phosphate, retinyl ascorbate, tetrahexyldecyl ascorbate, and magnesium ascorbyl phosphate. [110,111,112,113,114]

» Regardless of marketing hype, there's no single "best" form of topically applied vitamin C.

» Vitamin C is also a powerhouse when mixed with other antioxidants, or when used alone in higher concentrations, such as 15% or 20% or greater, amounts that can be great for treating extra-stubborn concerns. [115,116]

» All antioxidants, including vitamin C, are vulnerable to deterioration in the presence of air and light. [117] If a product containing antioxidants does not come in opaque or light-protected packaging that also reduces or eliminates air exposure, *don't buy it!*

A well-formulated, stably-packaged product with vitamin C can do all of this for skin:

» Protect skin cells and the skin's support structure from UV-related damage.
» Improve the appearance of sun-damaged skin.
» Strengthen the skin's barrier response.
» Reduce inflammation.
» Promote collagen production via stimulation of fibroblasts (cells that make collagen).
» Enhance the effectiveness of peels and microdermabrasion treatments.
» Lessen hyperpigmentation (when used at concentrations of 3% or greater).
» Boost the effectiveness of sunscreen actives. [5,110,117,118]

From its humble beginnings atop the backs of hairless pigs to the countless studies since, vitamin C has definitely been shown to be a powerful antioxidant—one that should be on your short list if you're dealing with wrinkles, uneven skin tone, loss of firmness, brown spots, and redness and red marks from breakouts (because of its anti-inflammatory properties).

PEPTIDES FOR SKIN

Simply put, peptides are proteins composed of long or short chains of amino acids, which are the building blocks of proteins. Peptides may be natural or synthetic; most peptides included in skincare products and cosmetics are synthetic because lab engineering these ingredients gives chemists greater control over their stability and effectiveness in skincare products—one more example of the natural route not always being what's best for your skin!

In terms of the fuss over peptides, although there are intriguing reasons to consider them, the hype is mostly about the cosmetics industry's perpetuation that there's one magic ingredient or group of ingredients that's, finally, at long last, the anti-aging answer. It's simply not true. There's no single solution for all the signs of aging—we admit it would be great if it were really that simple—and it certainly makes for good marketing copy to play up the peptide du jour.

Here's what you need to know (and we keep repeating it because this is one marketing ploy that always wastes money and cheats your skin): Just like there isn't one healthy food to eat or supplement to take, there isn't one best, does-it-all ingredient or group of ingredients for your skin. Skin is the most complex organ of the human body, so as you can imagine, its needs cannot possibly come down to what a single peptide or blend of peptides can provide.

Although peptides aren't miracle workers, they are good ingredients to see in skincare products, though we still have much to learn about how to maximize their skincare benefits.

Most peptides function as moisture-binding agents and almost all of them have theoretical cell-communicating ability to help skin repair itself and produce healthier cells, potentially even healthier collagen. [18,92] Those are exciting benefits, so long as you don't rely on peptides alone. Peptides are naturally present throughout our bodies, but even then their action is dependent on several other factors, which is why they don't work all by themselves. [119]

No peptide works like Botox or dermal fillers to reduce wrinkles. Peptides are definitely not the topical answer for those who fear the needle! The research aiming to prove otherwise typically comes from the company that's selling the peptide or peptide blend to cosmetics companies eager to make such claims. More often than not, the concentration used in the company-funded study is much greater than what's present in skincare products, so the benefit simply cannot be realized—yet the claim can still be made (tricky, huh?).

Some wonder if a specific group of peptides—copper peptides (also known as copper gluconate)—are finally the anti-aging answer everyone's been looking for. The synthesis of the skin's chief support substances—collagen and elastin—is in part related to the presence of copper in the body. [120] There's also research showing copper can be effective for wound healing. [121] But so far, there's not much research demonstrating that copper bound with peptides has antiwrinkle or skin-smoothing benefits, and certainly no independent research.

What's more, the studies that do exist rarely, if ever, compare the allegedly wonderful results of copper peptides with the results of other, more established ingredients. Wouldn't you like to know if another ingredient (like vitamin C or retinol) performed even better than copper peptides? We sure would!

We've also received many questions about whether or not it's OK to use copper peptides with vitamin C, AHAs, or BHA because of the interaction between copper (a metal) and ascorbic acid. Copper peptides are amino acids and do not have the same properties in skin as the copper metal found in nature, so that's one concern you needn't think about! You can cross that off your list of skincare worries.

THE ANTI-AGING DIET

Similar to how eating the right kinds of foods can ward off disease and maintain a healthy body, a well-rounded diet can help keep skin looking younger, longer. Combined with a good skincare routine and being sun smart, a skin-friendly diet plays a significant role in achieving the best skin of your life!

INFLAMMATION FROM THE INSIDE OUT

In much the same way irritating skincare products and sun damage cause inflammation, eating unhealthy, processed foods can cause chronic inflammation in the body—which eventually shows up on skin. [1,5,15]

Chronic inflammation floods the body with stress hormones, destroys healthy collagen, limits cell renewal, slows your body's ability to heal itself, and may even trigger acne. [122] Many of the foods people eat on a regular basis worsen chronic inflammation, especially when paired with other unhealthy lifestyle choices such as unprotected sun exposure, smoking, being sedentary, and not getting enough sleep. That's why using great skincare products is only part of the long-term formula for younger-looking skin.

Perhaps the most tempting, yet pro-aging and possibly pro-acne, food to avoid is sugar. Here's why sugar isn't as sweet as you think!

AGEs: THE BITTER SIDE OF SWEET!

Sugar in the body triggers a process known as glycation, which is a chemical reaction that occurs when the sugar you eat interacts in a not-so-friendly way with your body's lipids and proteins. This reaction forms advanced glycation end-products (AGEs), which are destructive, inflammation-producing molecules that contribute to disease and increase free-radical damage, wrinkles, sagging, and, theoretically, acne (acne is an inflammatory skin disorder). [123]

Routinely consuming an excess of sugary sweets causes the rate of glycation to increase, speeding up the "AGE-ing" process. This includes sugary sodas and even fruit juices (whole fruit is preferred because the juices—yes, even the pricey ones juice companies sell—are mostly sugar and water).

CUTTING OUT AGEs AND CHRONIC INFLAMMATION

Eating the right foods and minimizing how much you eat of those that trigger inflammation and AGEs is an anti-aging MUST. In addition, a nutrient-rich diet helps reduce the risk of multiple diseases and other chronic health issues. Research has demonstrated that the following foods are the worst of the inflammation-promoting and AGEing offenders:

» **Sugar**, especially refined sugars such as high-fructose corn syrup, but any sugar (including honey and, yes, even agave nectar) causes the formation of AGEs.

» **Trans-fat** (any oil listed as "partially hydrogenated" qualifies), which includes margarine and most shortenings.
» **Processed or cured meats**, including bacon, which contains nitrites and nitrates, which are an acute source of inflammation.
» **Red meat**, choose the leanest cuts and avoid grilling with charcoal, or cooking it until it's dark brown or black, which increases AGEs and other harmful chemicals.
» **Highly processed foods**, which include most of the items on the menu at fast-food restaurants and lots of the pre-packaged meals and snack foods in grocery stores. Essentially, anything in the midsection of the grocery store likely isn't great for improving your midsection—or your skin!
» **White flour**, which is the source of simple carbohydrates present in most baked goods, no matter how fresh. **Wheat flour** is just as bad; white flour is simply bleached wheat flour.
» **Desserts such as cakes, pastries**, and, yes, even that breakfast bran muffin, are often loaded with sugar, and many of them are made from white flour. [124,125,126,127,128]
» Too much salt in your diet can also leave skin looking the worse for wear, including puffy, tired-looking eyes because of the water retention it causes. (This is not the kind of water retention that improves skin hydration.)

YOUR ANTI-AGING GROCERY LIST

Anti-aging foods are far from flavorless or boring! They've been shown to reduce inflammation and the glycation process inside the body. The next time you're jotting down your grocery list, be sure to add these anti-inflammatory, appearance-boosting foods, and do your best to leave the processed cheese doodles and sugared drinks on the shelf (we won't begrudge you the occasional cupcake).

» **Green, black, and red teas.**
» **Deeply colored berries**, such as blueberries, blackberries, and raspberries.
» **Deeply colored vegetables**, especially leafy greens and cruciferous vegetables, such as red cabbage.
» **Red, green, yellow, and orange bell peppers**, and all types of hot peppers.
» **Salmon and other cold-water, oily fish rich in omega-3 fatty acids**; choose wild-caught rather than farm-raised.
» **Walnuts** are considered the superman of nuts, but **most nuts have health benefits**, so buy the nuts you like the best. Choose raw if available, as too much processing can reduce the nutrient value of nuts.
» **Grape seed, walnut, rice bran, and canola oils**.

» **Whole grains** not only supply vitamins and antioxidants, but also boost your fiber intake, which reduces inflammation.
» **Spices such as basil, cardamom, cumin, curry, garlic, ginger, oregano, tamarind, and turmeric**—but be sure to use them often, as spices can deteriorate quickly, losing their nutritional punch.
» **Flax, sunflower, and pumpkin seeds**.
» **Coffee**, but most of us should limit consumption, especially if you have high blood pressure or other health concerns. Check with your doctor to determine what amount is best for you. [125,128]

An anti-inflammatory diet is one of the more beautiful things you can do for your health and your skin. Routinely eating the right foods can lead to the production of healthier skin cells, reduce dry skin, create a more radiant complexion, reduce the number of breakouts and wrinkles, and give your skin greater resiliency, so you look younger, longer. This dietary approach, combined with state-of-the-art skincare, really can give you the best skin of your life!

RECOMMENDED ANTI-AGING TARGETED TREATMENTS:

The innovative products listed below are those you may want to add to your regular anti-aging skincare routine (which MUST include a daily sun-protection product) to address special or more stubborn concerns like deep wrinkles or more pronounced brown spots. These products are suitable for all skin types:
» Algenist Targeted Deep Wrinkle Minimizer ($45)
» BeautiControl Regeneration Tight, Firm & Fill Eye Firming Serum ($45)
» Clinique Superdefense Age Defense Eye Cream Broad Spectrum SPF 20 ($41)
» Dr. Dennis Gross Skincare Hydration Super Serum Clinical Concentrate Booster ($68)
» Jan Marini Age Intervention Retinol Plus ($75)
» Mary Kay Timewise Repair Volu-Fill Deep Wrinkle Filler ($45)
» Murad Time Release Retinol Concentrate for Deep Wrinkles ($65)
» Olay ProX Even Skin Tone Spot Fading Treatment ($39.99-$44.99)
» Paula's Choice Clinical 1% Retinol Treatment ($55)
» Paula's Choice Resist C15 Super Booster ($48)
» Paula's Choice Resist Hyaluronic Acid Booster ($45)

CHAPTER 9

Managing Oily Skin

GET SHINE UNDER CONTROL

Oily skin is almost always the result of genetically determined changes in hormone concentrations in your body, which makes it difficult, if not impossible, to control oily skin topically. The hormones responsible for oil production in skin are androgens—male hormones—and they are naturally present in both men and women. [129,130,131] When the androgens create a balanced and healthy amount of oil (sebum), it has incredible benefits for your skin, such as preventing dryness, preserving the skin's healthy microflora, and maintaining hydration. [132,133] If too little oil is produced by the oil gland, it can be a problem; likewise, if too much oil is produced, you end up with a host of skin woes! So, when the oil gland produces just the right amount of oil, it does wonderful things for skin.

If there is too much oil, you end up struggling with oily skin, blackheads, and acne, and the pores become larger to accommodate the excess oil production. Androgens can also cause the pore lining to thicken, which prevents the oil from flowing through and getting out of the pore, and that can lead to blackheads, white bumps, and the conditions that cause acne breakouts. [27,64]

Not sure if you have oily skin? It's recognizable by a few classic characteristics:

» Your face is shiny only an hour or two after cleansing, and usually appears greasy by midday.

» Your makeup seems to "slide" off or disappear shortly after you apply it.

» The shiniest parts of your face have blackheads, white bumps, or acne.

» Your pores are visibly enlarged, especially on your nose, chin, and forehead.

The first step in caring for oily skin is to take a critical look at your current skincare routine.

Products that make your skin tingle (such as menthol, mint, eucalyptus, and lemon) or that contain SD or denatured alcohol may feel like they are helping your oily skin, but they're actually making matters worse. When your skin tingles, it means it's being irritated, and **irritating or drying ingredients** can actually trigger more oil to be produced in the oil gland. [4,27,28,29] This is a very important fact to keep in mind because lots of products loaded with irritating ingredients, especially alcohol, claim to be for oily skin and breakouts. Note that fatty alcohols in skincare (examples are cetyl, stearyl, and cetearyl alcohols) are not the bad kind of alcohols; they are not drying or irritating to skin.

Products that are overly thick and emollient can also make your oily skin worse because they add more oily, waxy ingredients to skin, which someone with oily skin doesn't need more of.

Any products that are thick and heavy, such as bar cleansers, stick foundations, thick, greasy concealers, or rich, emollient moisturizers or balms, are likely to clog pores. These types of products deposit ingredients that mix with your skin's abundance of oil, upping the grease factor. They can also be absorbed into pores and get stuck, adding to the problem in the pore lining.

Instead of using these kinds of products, use only liquid, serum, or gel formulations for both skincare and makeup. The excess oil your skin produces will take care of the rest in terms of extra moisture!

The following essential skincare guidelines will help you take control of your skin so you'll see less oil, smaller pores, and fewer breakouts. For further details on each step, see Chapter 5, *How to Put Together the Perfect Skincare Routine*.

Cleanse

Use a gentle, water-soluble cleanser twice daily. [58] Ideally, the cleanser should rinse without leaving a hint of residue or leaving skin irritated, tight, or dry. It should also be fragrance-free (fragrance is always irritating, whether it's natural or synthetic). Avoid cleansers with menthol; its cooling tingle isn't doing your oily skin any favors! Remember, irritation can trigger more oil production directly inside the pore.

Tone

An irritant-free toner (free of alcohol, witch hazel, and fragrance) that's loaded with ingredients such as antioxidants, barrier-repair ingredients to help healing, and cell-communicating ingredients to improve pore size is an important step for oily skin. Toners that contain these ingredients can help skin heal, minimize large pores, reduce inflammation, and remove the last traces of dead skin cells or makeup that can lead to clogged pores. Irritant-free is vitally important. We can't state this enough because irritation can trigger more oil production directly inside the pore. [3,4,53]

Exfoliate

Exfoliation is one of the most important skincare steps for oily skin. Oily skin tends to have an extra-thick layer of built-up dead skin cells on the surface, along with a thickened pore lining. Exfoliating skin's surface and inside the pore lining is the best way to remove that buildup, reduce clogged pores and white bumps, and at the same time make skin feel smoother.

The best exfoliating ingredient for oily skin is salicylic acid (BHA). Salicylic acid is oil soluble, so it exfoliates not only the surface of your skin but also inside the pore. This action improves pore function, allowing oil to flow easily to the surface, so it doesn't get backed up and clog the pore. In addition, regular use of a BHA exfoliant will help fade red marks from past breakouts. [33,64]

Another benefit of salicylic acid is that it has anti-inflammatory properties, so it reduces redness and irritation, which helps slow oil production. [33]

A.M. Sun Protection

Even if you have oily skin, a sunscreen is essential for preventing wrinkles and reducing red marks.[9,134] If you've avoided sunscreens because the ones you've tried felt too greasy or too occlusive, or you were afraid they'd make you break out, we provide product recommendations at the end of this chapter that will change your impression of sunscreens for good.

P.M. Hydration

At night, nix the heavy creams and choose a lightweight liquid, gel, or serum that doesn't contain pore-clogging, thickening ingredients. Liquids, gels, and serums can provide just enough hydration while treating your skin to the essential ingredients that all skin types need to function in a normal, healthy manner, improving healing and reducing inflammation: antioxidants, cell-communicating ingredients, and skin-repairing substances. [5,15]

Absorb Excess Oil

Even with our recommendations, when you have oily skin there are limitations to what skincare products can do. This means you'll probably still need to use oil-absorbing products during the day. These are products that contain ingredients such as clays (and it doesn't have to be a special clay, despite the claims made about miracle versions from volcanoes or rare earth (meaning dirt), silica (which is exceptionally absorbent), various powders, and starches such as aluminum starch.

This is an optional step, but many with oily skin find it helpful. A good trick for nixing excess oil during the day? Blot with oil-blotting papers, and follow with a light dusting of pressed powder with SPF. (**Bonus:** You're adding to your sun protection!)

RECOMMENDED PRODUCTS FOR OILY SKIN:

Cleansers
» Kiehl's Ultra Facial Cleanser, for All Skin Types ($19.50)
» Neutrogena Naturals Purifying Facial Cleanser ($7.49)
» Paula's Choice Skin Balancing Oil-Reducing Cleanser ($17)

Toners
» Clinique Even Better Essence Lotion Combination to Oily ($42.50)
» derma e Soothing Toner with Anti-Aging Pycnogenol ($15.50)
» Paula's Choice Skin Balancing Pore-Reducing Toner ($20)

BHA Exfoliants
» Paula's Choice Resist Daily Pore-Refining Treatment 2% BHA ($30)
» Paula's Choice Resist Weekly Retexturizing Foaming 4% BHA ($35)
» Smashbox Photo Finish More Than Primer Blemish Control ($42)

Daytime Moisturizers with SPF
» Coola Face SPF 30 Cucumber Matte Finish ($36)
» Paula's Choice Resist Super-Light Daily Wrinkle Defense SPF 30 ($32)
» philosophy miracle worker spf 50 miraculous anti-aging fluid ($60)

Nighttime Moisturizers
» md formulations Moisture Defense Antioxidant Hydrating Gel ($45)
» Olay Regenerist Micro-Sculpting Serum Fragrance Free ($23.99)
» Paula's Choice Resist Anti-Aging Clear Skin Hydrator ($32)

Oil-Absorbing Products
» e.l.f. Essential Shine Eraser ($1)
» Hourglass Cosmetics Veil Mineral Primer Oil Free SPF 15 ($52)
» Paula's Choice Shine Stopper Instant Matte Finish ($23)

CHAPTER 10

Healing Dry Skin

HOW TO CARE FOR DRY SKIN

Are you on a perpetual search for a good moisturizer to alleviate dry skin? Although there are some great moisturizers out there, many fall short. In fact, we're constantly surprised at how many contain ingredients that can absolutely make dry skin worse! Knowing what to look for in a moisturizer, as well as what factors actually caused the skin to become dry in the first place, is incredibly helpful in finding relief for your itchy, uncomfortable, tight-feeling skin.

As odd as it sounds, dry skin isn't about a lack of water in skin. Studies comparing the water content of dry skin with the water content of normal or oily skin show there is no significant difference between them. In fact, healthy skin is only 10% to 30% water.

Adding more water to dry skin is not necessarily a good thing! If anything, too much moisture, such as from soaking in a bathtub, is bad for skin. Excess water disrupts skin's outer layers, making it dry, flaky, dehydrated, and crepey. [135,136] The primary reason your skin becomes dry is because its outer layers become impaired; that is, it loses its ability to maintain normal moisture levels. For the most part, this is due to sun damage, and, to some extent, the use of skincare products that contain irritating or drying ingredients. [16,17,137]

Have you ever noticed that the parts of your body that don't have sun damage (the parts that are not routinely exposed to daylight) are rarely, if ever, dry? Just look at the inside part of your arm or your derriere! That's because areas with little to no sun damage don't suffer from the range of problems that stem from the cumulative damage of daily UV light exposure.

Anything you do that damages your skin will either cause you to have dry skin or make dry skin worse. Following are fundamental ways to stop the cycle of dry, uncomfortable skin. The first step is to **stop damaging the outer layer of the skin** by avoiding:

» Bar soaps/cleansers (all kinds—anything in bar form, natural or not).
» Drying, water-soluble cleansers that leave skin feeling tight and dry.
» Products with irritating ingredients, such as denatured or SD alcohol, peppermint, menthol, mint, citrus, eucalyptus, and fragrance—including so-called "essential" oils.
» Excessive exposure to hot water and hot steam.
» Abrasive scrubs. Think of the microdermabrasion-at-home type, or those that contain fruit, shell, or nut fragments.
» Loofahs.
» Tanning, indoors or out, which destroys the substances skin needs to be healthy. [16,17,137]

All of these items or activities cause damage and irritation, which disrupt the skin's surface. This disruption in turn leads to water loss and destroys the vital substances in skin that allow it to hold on to just the right amount of moisture.

The next steps are to give your skin what it needs so it can act like it did before it was damaged by the sun. Skin can also be genetically dry, dry from varying health problems, or dry as a side effect of medications. Regardless of the root cause, dry skin needs barrier-repairing ingredients that help it maintain a healthy moisture balance as well as help it "hang on" to the types of substances that keep it hydrated, smooth, pliable, and soft.

Following are some fail-safe ways to help you have beautifully-smooth, younger-looking skin:

» **Wear sunscreen rated SPF 30+ daily, even in winter:** Sun damage slowly makes your skin less able to hold moisture or feel smooth and damages the outer layer of skin—sun damage is insidious for all skin types, but especially for dry skin. [16]
» **Use state-of-the-art moisturizers (serums, gels, lotions, creams, antiwrinkle, anti-aging, firming, and so on are all just "moisturizers"):** Regardless of texture, moisturizers should be filled to the brim with antioxidants, ingredients that help skin hold on to water, skin-repairing ingredients, and anti-inflammatory ingredients. To ensure the stability of the light- and air-sensitive ingredients, make sure whatever moisturizer you choose does not come in clear or jar packaging. [16,17,137]
» **Exfoliate:** Shedding skin cells (exfoliating) is a function of healthy skin, but, primarily due to sun damage, your skin needs help with this process. Built-

up dead skin cells prevent moisturizers from absorbing, leaves skin feeling rough, and makes it look dull and uneven. A well-formulated alpha hydroxy acid (AHA) or beta hydroxy acid (BHA) product can help skin cells exfoliate in a more natural, youthful manner by removing the buildup of old skin cells and replacing them with newer, healthier, and smoother cells. [16]

» **For very dry skin, use pure plant oils** such as almond, coconut, or jojoba seed oil, applied after or mixed into your moisturizer.

» **Don't forget your lips:** Lips are the least capable of staying smooth and soft, so don't leave them naked, day or night. During the day, apply and reapply an emollient lipstick or gloss—preferably one that provides sun protection. At night, don't go to sleep without protecting your lips with an emollient lip balm. None of these should contain irritating ingredients like fragrance or menthol because they'll only make dry lips worse.

» **Never use products that contain drying or irritating ingredients:** But you already knew that, right? Still, we just had to mention it again!

» Constant exposure to dry environments, cold weather, or air from heaters or air conditioners can also be problematic. These can impair and degrade skin's outer protective layer and deplete the skin's natural moisture content—adding a humidifier to your home (at least in your bedroom) can make a world of difference! [16]

DOES DRINKING MORE WATER HELP?

Can't you just drink more water to eliminate dry skin? This is one of those beauty myths that refuses to go away, but here are the facts: Although drinking eight glasses of water a day is great for your body, **it doesn't improve or reduce dry skin.** [135,136] If all it took to get rid of dry skin was to drink more water, wouldn't it be wonderful? How simple, right? And no one would need to endure this frustrating condition and struggle with searching for the perfect moisturizer or worrying about any of the skincare products they use. Alas, drinking more water will only result in more trips to the bathroom; the water you drink doesn't go to your skin to keep it hydrated and eliminate dryness.

WHAT ABOUT FACIAL OILS?

You've likely noticed more and more brands launching pure facial oils like argan, jojoba, and coconut, or blends of oils with claims to treat everything from acne to rosacea and wrinkles. Are these worth exploring, and, if so, how do you know which one is right for you?

Non-fragrant plant oils or synthetic oils can be used anywhere on the face or body to help improve and even eliminate dry skin. As is true for all skincare products, it's important to remember that fragrance, whether natural or synthetic, is a problem for skin because of the irritation it can cause. This is even more important with these types of products because many facial or body oils contain "essential oils," which are just fragrance disguised with a pleasant name. We're not saying that a facial oil should smell bad, but shopping for a facial oil shouldn't revolve around whether you prefer a citrus or floral aroma you'll smell for hours after the oil is applied to your skin.

Many facial and body oils are sold with claims that the special oils they contain have miraculous properties. Examples are argan oil (also called Moroccan oil), moringa oil, coconut oil, and noni oil. There's nothing miraculous about any of these oils. Each is just a good, non-fragrant plant oil, but no better for skin than the less glamorous, but exceptionally wonderful, options like grape seed, sunflower, canola, meadowfoam, rosehip, and avocado oils. And there's no research to the contrary.

You can consider using a single pure oil, but many products contain a blend of oils so you'll get the best properties of each. Plus, you may find that, aesthetically, certain oils or blends work better for you than others, so experiment to see which you prefer.

How do you use a facial oil (or body oil)? If you have dry to very dry skin or seasonal/environmental dryness and find that your moisturizer isn't quite doing the job (especially during the colder months of the year or if you live in a dry part of the world), try applying or mixing a facial oil with your usual moisturizer. It may be just what your skin needs, and you can use these types of non-fragrant facial oils around the eyes, too.

Those with oily skin likely won't find facial oils helpful because the amount of oil their skin produces naturally will eliminate the need to add more oil.

If you have combination skin, you can benefit from applying the oil to dry areas. The trick is to keep it away from the oil-prone areas, which isn't easy because oils have movement and will slide to other areas after they're applied. A tip: Blend away from your oil-prone areas, which is typically the center of the face. So, blend an oil on your cheeks and smoothe it toward your ears, not your nose!

Although plant or mineral oils are helpful for boosting skin's moisture, they are rather "one note" on their own; that is, they don't provide the complete array of beneficial antioxidants, skin-repairing ingredients, and cell-communicating ingredients necessary to keep your skin younger looking and healthy. That's why we don't recommend replacing your well-formulated moisturizer with a facial oil! Facial oils are really additive products, not products to be used on their own as your only moisturizer.

Many plant oils are indeed rich in antioxidants, and some, like safflower oil, contain some very good fatty acids that can help repair skin's barrier. [138] However, as we've said, your skin needs more than any single oil or blend of oils can provide. Think of face oils as supporting players rather than as the centerpiece of a skincare routine.

Concerns such as sun damage and wrinkles, rosacea, and acne are all complex issues that require a combination of products to treat them. [5,9,33] The skin can never have all of its needs satisfied by a single ingredient (even with anti-aging powerhouses like retinol or vitamin C) or a single product. Yes, we've said that before, but it's important enough to bear repeating. The myth about some miracle ingredient being the only thing your skin needs is so pervasive, it drives us crazy!

If you're considering adding a facial oil to your routine, avoid fragrant oils, such as lavender, eucalyptus, or any type of citrus or mint. These fragrant, so-called "essential" oils do not have the same benefits as the non-fragrant variety because each contains compounds that have significant potential to irritate skin. For example, many citrus oils are phototoxic to skin when it is exposed to UV light (potentially leaving the skin discolored). [139] A surprising number of facial oils contain non-fragrant and fragrant oils, so choose carefully and opt for fragrance-free or, at the very least, minimal fragrance.

If you're not sure which oils to avoid because of their potential to irritate skin, see Chapter 16, *Cosmetic Ingredient Dictionary*, which includes the most common fragrant oils you'll come across when checking skincare product ingredient lists.

DRY SKIN VS. DEHYDRATED SKIN

"Dehydrated skin" is something we're asked about frequently, and there's quite a bit of confusion about it because the term is often used interchangeably with "dry skin." We're happy to tell you it's not as confusing as it seems! Let's see if we can help resolve your questions.

Unlike truly dry skin, dehydrated skin produces a normal or even excessive amount of oil, yet feels tight or dry, and can even be flaky. If you can describe your skin as dry underneath, oily on top, it can be a sign of dehydrated skin. It also tends to come and go depending on the climate, season, and your activity, such as swimming or using a sauna frequently.

Dry skin, on the other hand, has almost no oil present, and this situation rarely fluctuates. Dry skin may get worse depending on the climate, season, or activity, but regardless of those things, having dry skin along with minimal to no oil production is consistent. [16,17,137]

While dehydrated skin can be caused by different factors, quite often it's the result of using harsh or irritating products. It can also occur when you're using too many active products at once or applying them too often. For example, your skin may not be able to tolerate the combination of an AHA or BHA exfoliant, prescription retinoid, and vitamin C treatment every day, resulting in a dehydrated look and feel with the excess oil your skin produces sitting on top of it.

All that can be true for dry skin, too, but it will be worse for dry skin because of the lack of production of protective oil. For those with oily skin, it may seem impossible to believe there can be healthy, normal oil production, but for those with dry skin, that's one of the major problems that causes the dry skin type.

Irritating ingredients like SD or denatured alcohol can dry out the surface of skin and leave it feeling "dehydrated," yet also stimulate excess oil production at the base of the pore, so skin still ends up being oilier. [3,4,53] This is especially common with people who struggle with acne because they often use products that strip skin, leaving it tight, red, and flaky. It's not your fault—there are a lot of harsh anti-acne products out there that leave skin the worse for the wear!

The key to treating dehydrated and dry skin is to first stop using harsh, irritating products. [16,17,138] That means using gentle, yet effective, cleansers that don't leave skin feeling tight, avoiding harsh scrubs and/or rough cleansing brushes, using replenishing toners instead of skin-stripping astringents, and the judicious use of treatment products such as retinol. Once you cut out the irritation, you can better assess what your true skin type is, and begin to benefit from the recommendations outlined in this book.

For dehydrated skin, this change may be all you need to eliminate the problem, assuming you follow our other skincare routine recommendations. If you have dry skin, this all helps as well, but you'll probably still need to adjust the kinds of moisturizers you use and perhaps consider adding other supplemental products to your routine, such as a great facial oil or a booster that includes a high concentration of hyaluronic acid plus other skin-repairing ingredients.

What about dry, dehydrated skin and acne? That's up next, and the two definitely have elements that overlap...

DEALING WITH DRY, OILY, AND ACNE-PRONE SKIN

Although having dry skin, oily skin, and acne at the same time isn't typical, there are definitely those who struggle with this hard-to-treat problem. It's frustrating enough to have acne and oily skin, but dealing with all three is even worse!

We're not going to say there are easy solutions to these dilemmas; however, with some facts and by fine-tuning your skincare routine you can get beautiful results.

When all three conditions—acne, dry skin, and oily skin—are present, then in all likelihood your skincare routine could be the major cause of the problem, or at least the reason why your skin is dry. Using drying soaps or harsh scrubs, overdoing cleansing brushes like the Clarisonic, applying toners with alcohol or other irritating ingredients (think witch hazel or menthol), not using lightweight moisturizers (think gels) that contain healing ingredients, and not using sunscreen daily all add up to a disaster for your skin. [3,4,53]

Your skin simply cannot survive the onslaught of such an assault or neglect. As we've explained, research shows that the results can be increased oil production, dryness, and breakouts! In short, **the wrong skincare routine or overdoing things can cause skin to be both oily and dry, often in the same areas**. [3,4,53] The products you use matter a lot—and even one poor formulation can throw off the results of a routine that otherwise contains great products!

Another possible cause of dry skin in combination with oily, acne-prone skin is that anti-acne treatments, both over-the-counter and prescription, can be drying if used too often or if you apply too much at once—perhaps because you think if a little bit is good, then more must be better (or will work faster). Numerous studies have shown—with valid scientific research-based certainty—that salicylic acid and benzoyl peroxide are essential anti-acne ingredients, but you need to be the judge of how often you use these products or if you should use both for your particular skincare needs (some people do great just using one or the other). [33]

There's also the serious concern that many of the salicylic acid– and benzoyl peroxide–based products being sold also contain detrimental, skin-damaging ingredients like alcohol, menthol, witch hazel, peppermint, eucalyptus, or sulfur. These are always terrible for your skin because of the irritation they cause. Your skin will suffer if you apply these ingredients on a regular basis, even if the salicylic acid and benzoyl peroxide ingredients seem to be helping your skin. They will help even more if you cut out the problematic irritants!

Benzoyl peroxide is the gold-standard topical disinfectant for acne, but it can be drying for some people, especially if they start off using a 5% to 10% concentration rather than a lower 2.5% concentration to see how their skin responds to it. Those are some of the major issues for those with all three skin problems, but there are still a couple more to think about....

ARE YOU OVERDOING IT?

Even the best anti-acne skincare routines can go awry if you get overzealous, using too many anti-acne treatments or using them too often. Not everyone's skin can handle more than one anti-acne product at a time, some not even one product every day. So, think about it: Are you applying too many anti-acne products at the same time? If you're using a prescription retinoid, such as Retin-A or Differin®, and an antibacterial product containing benzoyl peroxide, and a BHA exfoliant containing salicylic acid—one right after the other—your skin most likely will not be happy, and will react negatively. Then, if you add "active" anti-aging products to the mix, such as a vitamin C or retinol serum, your skin may end up rebelling against too much of everything all at once. All of this is confusing—almost enough to make you want to stop using any products at all—but that won't help either, at least not in the long run.

You must experiment to see how your skin responds to different combinations of treatments. For example, for some people, it's best to apply retinoid products only once every other day. Others might get the best results by alternating the use of benzoyl peroxide and a retinoid, using one on one day and the other the next, applying either in the morning or at night after cleansing and toning. A BHA exfoliant then can be used during the day, perhaps every other day, applied morning and/or evening after cleansing and toning and before applying any prescription products.

WHAT KIND OF MOISTURIZER DO YOU NEED?

The truth is not everyone needs a moisturizer—at least not a traditional cream or thick lotion moisturizer, especially if struggling with acne. The ingredients that give a product a cream or thick lotion texture can worsen clogged pores or make skin oilier. Clearly, that's not the best for acne-prone, oily skin, even if dryness is also a concern.

What to do about the dryness? Use lightweight, liquid or fluid products! Lightweight gel moisturizers, toners and essences, serums, or thin lotions, all filled with antioxidants, skin-repairing ingredients, and anti-redness ingredients are perfect! Such products are just what the doctor *should* be ordering for your troubled acne-prone skin that's also dry. You can also consider layering some of these products to get the best results, without suffering from the problems that heavy, emollient moisturizers can cause.

WHAT TO DO WHEN YOU ONLY HAVE ACNE AND DRY—NOT OILY—SKIN

Despite the fact that excess oil is a chief contributing factor for acne breakouts, a small percentage of people find themselves with truly dry skin and acne. In fact, they have almost no surface oil, blackheads, or visible pores at all. They struggle to find a moisturizer that addresses the needs of their dry skin without aggravating breakouts, and continually worry that anything they try to get the breakouts under control will make their dry skin even drier. This scenario can be a paralyzing dilemma when shopping for skincare products!

Here's what you need to know: All the recommendations we make above still apply, but you may need a moisturizer that is more appropriate for dry skin and not oily or combination skin. This means you'll have to experiment to find an appropriately emollient moisturizer that doesn't trigger more breakouts. Another option is to layer a lightweight cream that you know won't make your breakouts worse (yet it doesn't supply quite enough moisture) with a lotion-textured moisturizer that kicks in the missing hydration without adding heavy, potentially pore-clogging ingredients.

RECOMMENDED PRODUCTS FOR CLASSIC DRY SKIN:

The following products are highly recommended for dry to very dry skin, but aren't necessarily ideal for dry skin that's also struggling with acne. If you have dry skin and acne, consider the lighter-weight moisturizers (both daytime and nighttime) we recommend in the chapters on oily skin and combination skin, and know that you may need to layer lighter-weight products for extra hydration rather than apply one richer, more emollient moisturizer to dry areas.

Cleansers
 » First Aid Beauty Milk Oil Conditioning Cleanser ($26)
 » Paula's Choice Skin Recovery Softening Cream Cleanser ($17)
 » Yes to Cucumbers Gentle Milk Cleanser ($8.99)

Toners
 » M.A.C. Lightful C Marine-Bright Formula Softening Lotion ($35)
 » Merle Norman Brilliant-C Toner ($22)
 » Paula's Choice Skin Recovery Enriched Calming Toner ($20)

AHA Exfoliants
» Olay ProX Anti-Aging Nightly Purifying Micro-Peel ($39.99)
» Paula's Choice Resist Daily Smoothing Treatment 5% AHA ($32)
» Peter Thomas Roth Glycolic Acid 10% Moisturizer ($45)

Daytime Moisturizers with SPF
» Olay Regenerist Superstructure Broad Spectrum Cream SPF 30 ($29.99)
» Paula's Choice Skin Recovery Daily Moisturizing Lotion with SPF 30 ($28)
» Rodan + Fields SOOTHE Mineral Sunscreen SPF 30 ($41)

Nighttime Moisturizers
» Clinique Even Better Brightening Moisture Mask ($36)
» Paula's Choice Resist Intensive Repair Cream ($32)
» Replenix Power of Three Cream ($70)

CHAPTER 11

Balancing Combination Skin

WHAT IS COMBINATION SKIN?

Traditionally, and throughout the cosmetics industry, combination skin is thought of as simply having oily skin in some areas of your face and dry skin in other areas. Although that's indeed the way most people (and the cosmetics industry at large) think of combination skin, we also define it as when someone is dealing with more than one concern or skin type. For example, it could be oily skin and sun damage with brown spots or dry skin with patches of rosacea and wrinkles.

Having combination skin that's a mix of oily and dry areas can be hard to identify and even trickier to treat if you don't exactly know what you're experiencing or seeing in the mirror. And perhaps you don't have combination skin in the classic sense (oily T-zone, dry cheeks), but your skin is more normal—what then? The answers are what this chapter aims to reveal!

IS THE GOAL TO HAVE "NORMAL" SKIN?

When you hear "normal" described as a skin type, you might envision someone with perfect skin. From that perspective, having normal skin would mean your skin is neither too oily nor too dry, has minimal to no signs of dryness or oily shine, has a smooth surface with no breakouts, blackheads, or visible pores, and has an even skin tone with no wrinkles or visible sun damage.

The problem with this description of normal skin is that such perfect skin doesn't really exist. It's the unicorn of skin types! It's not that some people aren't blessed with what appears to be flawless skin, but in the long run they too will struggle, at the very least with the unwanted side effects of sun damage or with problems that show up later in life. This is especially true as skin ages, from both the passage of time and cumulative sun damage. [5,7,9]

Everyone will get older and their skin will age to some degree even if they have been diligent about sun protection. Even the most neurotic use of sunscreen and being sun smart can't eliminate all of the sun's impact on skin. And think back to the times in our youth when getting tan or accidentally sunburned was something that happened to almost everyone. **Remember:** Sun damage is cumulative; it begins from the very moments your skin is exposed to the sun without protection and seeking shade—the visual result of this won't show up until later in life, but there's no question it will appear. [7,43,44]

Having normal skin ends up being a matter of degree and expectations rather than an actual skin type. It can also get confused with combination skin. For example, just because you see some shine on your nose doesn't mean you have oily or combination skin, and a little dry skin on your cheeks doesn't mean you have dry skin, especially if you have normal skin on the rest of your face. Plus, there's the issue of treating the skin you have now and working to prevent, or at least delay, what you may see on your skin in the future.

Here are some ways to determine if you currently have normal skin:

» You wouldn't describe your skin as being oily or dry; it just looks and feels equal (normal) in all areas.
» The little bit of oiliness or dryness you experience is rare and easily resolved.
» Products designed for oily skin feel too drying for you, but products designed for dry skin feel too rich or greasy.
» Your pores aren't invisible, but they're not enlarged or obvious, either.
» You rarely, if ever, feel you need to blot your skin to absorb oil or touch up your powder during the day.
» Your skin doesn't feel tight or dry at the end of the day, nor is it obviously shiny.
» You have minimal to no lines or wrinkles.
» Your skin tone is fairly even, with no brown or red spots.

If you can identify with most of the statements above regarding your skin, chances are good that you're dealing with normal skin. However, even if you can relate to all those points, you still have skincare needs because, as time goes on, as we mentioned (we do tend to repeat ourselves on important points so please forgive us), everyone accumulates sun damage that causes some amount of wrinkles, brown spots, dryness (especially around the eyes), and so on. [5,7,9] There's also the likelihood that even those with near-perfect skin will experience occasional breakouts.

Because truly normal skin (meaning perfect skin) is the rare exception rather than the rule, in reality, most of these people are really dealing with what we call "normal skin plus"; that is, normal skin mixed with other issues that are unrelated to skin "type" but rather skin concerns that occur over time. Essentially, your skin may feel normal, but it isn't perfect, and it is changing as the years march on. These distinctions are why so many people are confused about their skin type and why so many people truly have combination skin.

WHAT CAUSES CLASSIC COMBINATION SKIN?

A variety of factors contribute to the different forms of combination skin, and sometimes it just comes down to the luck of the draw—genetics. Generally, the areas around the nose, chin, and forehead have more active oil glands than other parts of the face. [140] So, from a physiological standpoint, most of us have combination skin!

Combination skin can also be a result of the skincare products you're using. For example, if you're using products that contain irritating ingredients, they can stimulate oil production in the T-zone area and at the same time create more dry skin and redness on the rest of the face. [3,4,53] Voilà: You have taken your relatively normal skin and made it combination!

You may also be using moisturizers that are too emollient, making your skin feel oilier and clogging up pores. All the products you use must be appropriate for the different skin types you're experiencing—even if that means using different products on different parts of your face, particularly if you have what we refer to as "extreme combination skin."

EXTREME COMBINATION SKIN

How is "extreme combination skin" different from regular combination skin? Those struggling with extreme combination skin experience an exceptionally oily T-zone, while the sides of the face remain *very* dry and may also be flaky or feel tight.

Treating this frustrating skin type means approaching your skincare routine strategically. While certain products can be used all over your face (gentle cleanser, well-formulated toner), you may need to spot treat your dry and oily areas with different products, or consider layering lighter products to moisturize the dry areas without making the oily areas feel extra-slick.

Keep in mind that avoiding fragrance and other potentially irritating ingredients is best for any skin type, but it's essential for getting extreme combination skin in balance—even the slightest irritation will exacerbate the oily areas and, at the same time, make dry areas worse.

What about extreme combination skin with breakouts? In this scenario, breakouts are very frustrating to treat because they can occur in the dry areas, too. Although it seems daunting, you *can* treat breakouts without making dry areas worse, and without shortchanging your dry areas of the extra moisture they need! See the section on dealing with dry skin and acne in Chapter 10, *Healing Dry Skin*.

HOW TO TREAT CLASSIC COMBINATION SKIN

The key thing to keep in mind with combination skin is that it isn't one size fits all and it isn't dependent on age. Oil-absorbing or matte-finish ingredients will be a disaster on drier areas of skin, while emollient, thick moisturizers will be a problem over oily areas of combination skin. Depending on the severity of your combination skin, you may have to use different products for different parts of your face, but the following guidelines will help get you on the right path with options that gently balance skin. The goal is unification to the extent possible, so that your combination skin looks and acts more like normal skin (though you may still have concerns like brown spots or wrinkles that can be treated with products added to the core routine below).

Cleanse

Gel-based or mild foaming cleansers are ideal for oily/dry combination skin. Regardless of the texture, it should be gentle; no irritants or fragrance.

Tone

Use an alcohol-free toner filled with a healthy dose of skin-repairing ingredients, antioxidants, and cell-communicating ingredients that normalize skin. A well-formulated toner really can help improve dryness and reduce oiliness at the same time—and won't make the dry areas drier or the oily areas oilier! Don't skip this step!

Exfoliate

Beta hydroxy acid (BHA/salicylic acid) is an optimal choice for gently exfoliating combination skin and both the dry skin and oily skin can benefit, albeit for somewhat different reasons. Both skin types need exfoliation, but oily skin needs deeper exfoliation in the pore and dry skin needs more surface exfoliation. When properly formulated, a BHA exfoliant does both, without being drying or irritating. Some people find that using an AHA on the drier areas and BHA on the oilier areas works best for them, so this is something you need to experiment with to see what's true for you. Opt for exfoliants in gel or liquid form if your combination skin leans more toward oily than dry. If your combination skin leans more toward dry than oily, a lotion form of these products is a better option.

A.M. Sun Protection

A lightweight sunscreen with a soft matte finish or matte feel can work all over the face for combination skin. If your skin leans more toward oily than dry, apply a super-light serum underneath. Over the dry areas, this type of sunscreen can also be layered over a moisturizer and serum. You would use the moisturizer only over the dry areas and the lightweight serum all over. You can use a moisturizing eye cream with sunscreen around the eyes because you don't want to forget sunscreen there. It shouldn't be necessary to wear two different facial sunscreens, regardless of how extreme your combination skin is, given that you can layer other products underneath.

P.M. Hydration

Your moisturizer and/or serum shouldn't feel heavy or greasy and you may need to layer two lightweight moisturizers over the dry areas; doing so ensures that the oil-prone areas won't become too slick. If you have very dry areas and you find that layering two lightweight formulas isn't enough, you may need to apply a richer, more emollient moisturizer just to those areas, being sure to blend away from the oil-prone areas, which may be fine with a lightweight moisturizer (gel or lotion) and/or a serum.

RECOMMENDED PRODUCTS FOR COMBINATION SKIN:

The products below are recommended for classic or extreme combination skin, meaning a mix of oily and dry areas, whether the dry areas are slightly or moderately dry. These products, especially the daytime and nighttime moisturizers, are also worth considering if you have dry skin that's prone to breakouts, but you may need to use richer cleansers and toners and/or layer lightweight moisturizers (or add a hydrating booster) to keep your skin comfortably balanced.

Cleansers
» Biore Combination Skin Balancing Cleanser ($7.49)
» Laura Mercier Flawless Skin One-Step Cleanser ($35)
» Paula's Choice Resist Perfectly Balanced Cleanser ($18)

Toners
» Clinique Even Better Essence Lotion Combination to Oily ($42.50)
» MD Formulations Moisture Defense Antioxidant Spray ($28)
» Paula's Choice Resist Weightless Advanced Repairing Toner ($23)

BHA Exfoliants
- » DHC Salicylic Face Milk (liquid lotion texture; $21)
- » Paula's Choice Skin Perfecting 2% BHA Gel (gel texture; $28)
- » Paula's Choice Resist Daily Pore-Refining Treatment 2% BHA (liquid texture; $28)

AHA Exfoliants
- » Alpha Hydrox Oil-Free Treatment 10% Glycolic AHA Anti-Wrinkle ($9.49)
- » Paula's Choice Skin Perfecting 8% AHA Gel ($28)

Daytime Moisturizers with SPF
- » Nia24 Sun Damage Prevention UVA/UVB Sunscreen SPF 30 PA+++ ($49)
- » Paula's Choice Resist Youth-Extending Daily Fluid SPF 50 ($32)
- » SkinCeuticals Physical Fusion UV Defense SPF 50 ($34)

Nighttime Moisturizers and Serums
> **Note:** *The products below may be applied on their own or layered; for example, one of these serums may provide enough hydration for oily areas, but you may need to layer a serum and a moisturizer for the dry areas of combination skin.*
- » Bobbi Brown Intensive Skin Supplement ($72)
- » CeraVe Facial Moisturizing Lotion PM ($12.99)
- » Clinique Super Rescue Antioxidant Night Moisturizer, for Dry Combination Skin ($47)
- » Estee Lauder Perfectionist [CP+R] Wrinkle Lifting/Firming Serum ($68)
- » First Aid Beauty Ultra Repair Liquid Recovery ($38)
- » MD Formulations Moisture Defense Antioxidant Hydrating Gel ($45)
- » Olay Regenerist Instant Fix Wrinkle Revolution Complex ($22.99-$28.99)
- » Paula's Choice Resist Anti-Aging Clear Skin Hydrator ($32)
- » Paula's Choice Resist Hyaluronic Acid Booster ($45)
- » Paula's Choice Resist Ultra-Light Super Antioxidant Concentrate Serum ($36)
- » Paula's Choice Skin Balancing Invisible Finish Moisture Gel ($28)

CHAPTER 12

How to Treat Special Skin Problems

Where skincare really gets complicated is when you're dealing with more than one skincare issue. We mentioned in the previous chapter that combination skin, as we define it, is more than just having dry skin in some areas and oily skin in others. As we see it, combination skin can encompass far more. Anytime you're dealing with more than one skincare concern, we think that's exactly what combination skin is all about, and why people are so confused about whether this is their skin type or not. In reality, most people have some kind of combination skin because most can have a variety of issues at the same time.

The skin conditions mentioned in this chapter can be present with any number of other skincare problems/concerns. It's important to realize that the medications or skincare recommendations below will need to be combined with other skincare recommendations in this book as part of a comprehensive daily skincare routine that contains core products suitable for your skin type AND the corresponding products needed to address your skin concerns.

These corresponding products should have **textures that work with your skin type**; for example, if you have oily skin and brown spots, use a lotion or gel-based skin lightener rather than a skin-lightening cream that's better suited for dry skin. Treatment products labeled "for all skin types" generally have lighter textures because they are more versatile and easier to combine with other products in your routine.

ROSACEA

Rosacea is a chronic, inflammatory skin condition of the face characterized by areas of pink to red color (called flushing) often spread out in a butterfly pattern over the nose and cheeks. In time, rosacea often progresses to the chin and central part of the forehead, too. In the beginning, this flushing can come and go, but over time it becomes increasingly persistent and will eventually stay. For some people, the flushing can be accompanied by bumpy skin, as well as acne breakouts or blackheads and oily or dry skin. Now that's a dilemma!

Quite typically, rosacea-affected skin starts off being sensitive, but sometimes not. In almost all rosacea cases, skin sensitivity shows up at some point down the road, and tends to progressively worsen without treatment. Often those with rosacea react strongly to internal or external changes in temperature as well as to eating spicy food. Rosacea is a very temperamental, frustrating skin disorder, and it happens to a lot of people! [141]

Rosacea affects primarily adults, usually between the ages of 30 and 60. It affects all segments of the population, but is most common in people with fair skin tones, especially those who tend to blush easily. In fact, depending on whose statistics you want to believe, it can afflict somewhere between 30 and 50 percent of the Caucasian population! Women are diagnosed with rosacea more frequently than men, but men tend to experience more severe symptoms, such as a swollen, distended nose area and more broken capillaries. The diagnosis differential between men and women can be at least partially accounted for because women are more concerned about their skincare problems and are more willing to see dermatologists for treatment than men. Guys, if you think you have rosacea, it's not something you have to "tough out." An increasingly red, ruddy complexion can be made better—and it's not the least bit unmanly to take steps to improve what you don't like about your skin!

Left untreated, the sensitivity of rosacea-affected skin can go off the charts, reacting to a random mix of stimuli, from the most gentle skincare products to sipping an iced tea.

We mentioned that those with rosacea can also have skin that's oily or dry (or both), with persistent flaking. The acne-like bumps that tend to accompany rosacea typically don't respond to over-the-counter or prescription acne treatments; in fact, such products may cause rosacea to become more inflamed and red, either immediately or later on. Adding to these frustrating symptoms is that some people who have rosacea also get acne, and while traditional treatments work to control the acne, they make the redness and sensitivity from rosacea worse, leaving the person feeling torn between not treating the acne so as not to worsen their rosacea, or treating the acne at the expense of making their rosacea worse.

No question—treating rosacea isn't easy and there's no known cure, but following the steps we present will get you closer to the beautiful, calm skin you want. First, let's discuss what causes rosacea, and then, most important, we'll tell you how to treat it.

WHAT CAUSES ROSACEA?

One of the main reasons there have been such problems finding a cure for rosacea is that no one knows, or at least not everyone agrees on, exactly what causes it. Many researchers think there's a genetic component to the development of rosacea. Others believe that elevated levels of an inflammatory peptide called cathelicidin or high levels of an enzyme known as KLK5 in the skin's uppermost layers play a role. [142,143]

Another theory is that a mite commonly found on human skin, *Demodex folliculorum*, triggers the inflammation that leads to rosacea. Research has shown that those with rosacea tend to have a finer layer of superficial blood vessels in their facial skin, and that these vessels are hypersensitive to internal and external factors. [144,145]

Last, some researchers believe that those with rosacea have a thinner, more delicate surface barrier than normal. Think of the skin's layers like the layers of an onion: On rosacea skin, the barrier is akin to the onion's paper-thin skin; on skin without rosacea, there are more layers (literally, thicker skin) offering enhanced barrier protection and, in turn, less reactive, more resilient skin. [146]

Though it's interesting to know the probable causes of rosacea, it really isn't helpful because no matter what you believe about the origins of the problem, it will take experimentation to see what skincare routine and what prescription options will reduce and possibly even eliminate your symptoms. It won't be a cure, so consistency of treatment is vital. The rest of this chapter deals with what you can consider doing and not doing to improve your skin's condition.

Let's start with the lifestyle issues that can make rosacea worse. Basically, anything that causes a rush of blood to the face can be an issue. All of the following are triggers.

» Sun exposure.
» Wind.
» Hot climates.
» Heavy or strenuous exercise.
» Emotional stress (or just emotions in general).
» Specific cosmetic ingredients, such as fragrant plant extracts or oils; various forms of mint and citrus; denatured alcohol, and witch hazel.
» Topical steroid creams and other topical medications that can thin the skin.
» Spicy foods, alcohol, coffee, or caffeinated teas, and hot beverages in general.
» Reactions to certain fabrics that might brush against your face, like wool or textured, scratchy-feeling fabrics. [146]

That's quite the lineup—and it's not even the entire list. Although some triggers are more obvious than others, it's hard to know what will spark a rosacea flare-up for you, as it can differ from case to case. What's on the list above may or may not apply to you and there may be other things that do serve as triggers but that aren't on our list. The variations of problems someone with rosacea may encounter is one of the stranger aspects of this disorder.

TYPES OF ROSACEA

Making rosacea even trickier to address is that it doesn't manifest itself in just one way; just like there's more than one type of acne, there's more than one type of rosacea! In its earliest stages, rosacea can be so subtle and fleeting that many people don't even know they have it. They tend to think they just have an uneven skin tone or sensitive skin instead of an actual skin disorder. That's a drawback because the sooner you catch and treat rosacea, the easier it will be to control the symptoms and, more important, to stop its progression!

From subtle beginnings to more advanced cases, here are the four different types of rosacea.

Erythematotelangiectatic: This long and hard-to-pronounce name is the most basic type of rosacea. It's characterized by flushing and persistent redness, often in a butterfly pattern on a person's nose, cheeks, forehead, and chin. Blood vessels under the skin may also be visible, and often are referred to as broken capillaries or spider veins. The affected skin may feel warmer to the touch than the surrounding skin, and often reacts strongly to stimuli such as steam from a hot stove or a few sips of red wine. [146,147]

Papulopustular: This form includes bumps and pimple-like eruptions in addition to redness, with some of the bumps becoming infected with acne-causing bacteria. This is what people mean when they say they have acne rosacea. As we stated above, oftentimes, conventional acne treatments only serve to make the redness and extreme sensitivity worse. [146,147]

Phymatous: Most common in men, this type of rosacea involves a thickening of the skin and hyper-growth of facial blood vessels, which can result in a bulbous nose from the excess growth of tissue in this area. Legendary comedian W. C. Fields, famous for his large nose, had this disfiguring type of rosacea. [146,147]

Ocular: This type of rosacea affects the eyes. Symptoms include dry eyes, tearing and burning, a sensation of the eyes feeling gritty, swollen eyelids, recurring sties (an inflammation of the eyelash hair follicle)—and even potential vision loss. Ocular rosacea often exists with another type of rosacea, so you're battling skin symptoms plus itchy, irritated eyes. If you suspect you have this type of rosacea, consult your dermatologist or ophthalmologist for prescription solutions. There isn't much that can be done via skincare to control ocular rosacea, though of course avoiding fragrance and irritating ingredients will help. [146,147]

SKINCARE FOR ROSACEA

Because rosacea is an unpredictable skin disorder, with just about anything capable of setting it off or creating extreme sensitivity, it's critical to assemble the most gentle skincare routine possible so as not to aggravate matters. All skincare products should be fragrance- and dye-free. "Fragrance-free" means avoiding fragrant plant oils, too, which surprisingly, and disturbingly, often show up in products labeled as being safe for sensitive skin. For example, lavender oil and citrus oils are definite no-nos due to the volatile fragrance components they contain! [148]

A skincare routine for anyone with rosacea must do the following:
» Eliminate irritating or sensitizing ingredients, which may include otherwise benign ingredients not known to be irritating (but they are for your skin).
» Include calming products that reduce redness and soothe skin.
» Improve cell turnover to remove the buildup of dead skin cells.
» Protect from sun damage without causing irritation.
» Fight wrinkles with products containing antioxidants and skin-repairing ingredients.
» Absorb oil if skin is oily, but not to the point where skin becomes dried out.
» Provide a steady stream of barrier-repair ingredients to help skin become more resilient, less reactive, and have a smoother surface. [149,150]

As is true for everyone on the planet, using sunscreen is one of the most important steps in your skincare routine! Unprotected UV exposure makes rosacea worse, so be sure to apply a sunscreen every day that's rated SPF 30 or higher to keep those damaging rays from harming your delicate skin. [151]

Generally speaking, those with rosacea or sensitive skin should check the ingredient label when selecting a sunscreen. Ideally, you should use only sun-protection products whose active ingredients are titanium dioxide and/or zinc oxide. These mineral sunscreens are gentle and are the least likely to cause a stinging or burning sensation, both of which can worsen the redness and irritation you're trying to minimize.

When it comes to enjoying time outdoors, don't forget that sunscreen can't do it all on its own. Consider sunglasses and wide-brimmed hats to further shield your face from UV radiation.

Here's a step-by-step routine you can follow to try to get rosacea under control:

» Use an extremely gentle, non-drying, water-soluble cleanser that is appropriate for your skin type. Choose an emollient lotion or cream cleanser if you have dry skin and a thin-textured, gel, foaming, or soft lather cleanser if you have oily or combination skin. No soaps or bar cleansers!

» Soothe and reduce redness with a gentle, fragrance- and alcohol-free toner that's loaded with anti-irritants and barrier-repair ingredients. This step may seem like extra work, but it can make a HUGE difference in the appearance and comfort of reddened, sensitized skin.

» During the day, apply a sunscreen with SPF 30 or greater whose only active sunscreen ingredients are titanium dioxide and/or zinc oxide, along with healing ingredients such as antioxidants and skin-repairing ingredients. If you have dry skin, choose a more emollient, creamy sunscreen; if you have oily or combination skin a more fluid, lotion texture is optimal. If your combination skin has markedly dry areas, layer a regular cream moisturizer or richer serum underneath your sunscreen only on the dry areas.

» For extra sun protection (and we love extra protection), if you normally wear foundation and pressed powder, select those that have sunscreen. Stick with makeup with sunscreen whose only active ingredients are titanium dioxide and/or zinc oxide as they present little to no risk of irritation. Look for foundation and pressed powder with sunscreen rated SPF 15 or greater, and be sure your daytime moisturizer is rated SPF 30 or greater.

» If you have rosacea with oily or combination skin and breakouts, makeup with sun protection can be the only sunscreen you need (though in that case try to find makeup rated SPF 30). If you have dry skin and rosacea, you can wear a moisturizer with sunscreen under makeup to add a layer of protection or a moisturizer without sunscreen and then the foundation with pressed powder and SPF. There are many foundations and powders with mineral sunscreen actives, so you'll have plenty of options!

» If you have oily or combination skin, in the evening apply a gel moisturizer or a light serum formulated with antioxidants and skin-repairing ingredients. A serum with retinol is fine because retinol has research showing it helps reduce the inflammatory factors that contribute to rosacea. [152,153] You'll probably need a separate, more emollient moisturizer for around the eyes because a gel or light serum is usually not enough for that area. If you have normal to dry skin, in the evening use a lotion or cream moisturizer formulated with soothing antioxidants and skin-repairing ingredients. It's OK if it contains retinol. You can also use a serum over or under your moisturizer for extra hydration, redness reduction, and protection.

» Regardless of your skin type, you'll want to consider using a BHA (salicylic acid) exfoliant once or twice a day. It takes experimenting to see what strength and frequency of application works best for you. BHA not only exfoliates skin, but also has anti-inflammatory properties that reduce redness and eliminate dry, flaky skin. BHA also works amazingly well if you have rosacea and acne or blackheads!

» Check with your physician to see which prescription medication is best to treat your rosacea. Topical options include MetroGel®, MetroLotion®, Tazorac®, Renova, azelaic acid (brand names Azelex® or Finacea®), brimonidine, doxycycline, isotretinoin, and low-dose minocycline. Oral options include tetracycline and metronidazole. These are considered the most reliably researched medical options. [152,153,154]

All of the topical medications should be applied as directed by your physician. Our strong recommendation is to apply any topical medication in the evening as the last step of your skincare routine, following your cleanser, toner, exfoliant, moisturizer, and/or serum. During the day, apply the topical medication before the sunscreen. Sunscreen is always the last skincare product you apply so as not to dilute its effectiveness.

PRODUCTS TO ELIMINATE IF YOU HAVE ROSACEA

Aside from what you should use if you have rosacea, it's critical that you eliminate the parts of your normal skincare routine that increase inflammation and worsen or trigger redness, such as the following.

» Harsh cleansers such as bar soap, bar cleansers, and cleansing scrubs.
» Drying liquid or lotion cleansers. (If your face feels squeaky clean after use, the product is too drying for your skin!)
» Toners with alcohol, witch hazel, rosewater, and fragrance.
» Abrasive scrubs.
» Rough washcloths or facial brushes such as the Clarisonic; the "sensitive" brush head of the Clarisonic is an option, but be aware that even that might cause a reaction.
» At-home facial peels, especially high-strength peels.
» Using too many products at the same time, particularly anti-aging products that contain higher amounts of active ingredients like vitamin C.
» Retinol products, especially high-strength formulas, may be problematic, but retinol products with lower concentrations are usually well tolerat-

ed. As mentioned above, some research has shown retinol to be helpful for those with rosacea; however, you'll want to be cautious with products whose retinol concentration exceeds 0.5%. [150,155]

PRESCRIPTION TREATMENTS FOR ROSACEA

Because rosacea is a chronic condition with no known cure, you'll most likely need to see a doctor to get it under control. The reality in most cases is that **skincare alone won't be enough.** A good dermatologist should know about the latest prescriptions and in-office treatments and techniques for dealing with rosacea, and can properly diagnose what type you have. Following are a few more details about the variety of medical treatments available for rosacea.

» **Oral antibiotics** like tetracycline or low-dose doxycycline (brand name: Oracea®) can relieve acne-like pustules and inflammation without aggravating rosacea symptoms. [152,153,154]

» **Topical antibiotics**, including metronidazole, have been shown to be effective in killing *Demodex folliculorum* and other microbes that may play a role in rosacea. MetroCream®, MetroGel®, and MetroLotion® contain this active ingredient. Your dermatologist or physician will prescribe based on the texture you prefer, which will be partly based on your skin type (dry, oily, and so on). [153,154,155]

» **Prescription-strength azelaic acid** (brand names Finacea® or Azelex®) can help reduce lesions and bumps and is also believed to play a role in controlling the inflammatory process that triggers rosacea. [153,154,155]

» **Mirvaso® Gel** is a prescription product from the Galderma brand (of Cetaphil fame). It's FDA-approved for treating persistent redness from rosacea. Although how this drug works isn't exactly clear, researchers believe it constricts the blood vessels that fuel facial redness, with results lasting up to 12 hours. Its chemical name is brimonidine, and, like all topical medications, it has side effects you must discuss with your doctor, particularly if you have circulatory system issues. [153,154,155]

» **Beta blockers** (prescribed in pill form; typically used to treat heart conditions and high blood pressure) have been shown in some studies to reduce rosacea's redness. [152]

» **The vitamin A drug isotretinoin, both oral and topical, can be effective. Oral isotretinoin** was first marketed as the anti-acne drug Accutane, but has been shown to help combat the pustules seen in papulopustular rosacea, although this oral medication typically is a last resort due to its many serious side effects. [156] Topical isotretinoin also has been shown to be effective, with far less severe side effects than the oral version. [154]

» **Salicylic acid**, also known as beta hydroxy acid (BHA), is not a medical solution, but we feel so strongly about its potential benefit that we include it in this list. Topical salicylic acid in 1% and 2% strengths has anti-inflammatory properties that can potentially reduce redness. It also gently exfoliates rosacea-affected, breakout-prone skin, which can mitigate the flakiness and/or breakouts that can occur with some forms of rosacea. BHA also has antimicrobial properties, and that can be helpful in reducing the microbes that may be associated with rosacea. [31]

LIGHT-BASED TREATMENTS FOR ROSACEA

Some of the best and most effective treatments for rosacea involve using light to target the blood vessels that cause the "red mask" and broken capillaries that are the hallmarks of rosacea. Special lasers or intense pulsed light (IPL) machines target capillaries and can diffuse redness in the upper layers of the skin. These light-based treatments cause the walls of blood vessels to heat up, which damages them, causing them to be absorbed by the body as part of its natural defense.

The catch? Repeated treatments (typically 4–6 spaced a few weeks apart) are required for the redness to disappear completely, and most people will need a maintenance treatment at least once per year. These light-based treatments aren't cheap—they can cost as much as $300 to $700 per treatment, and medical insurance often doesn't cover the expense (check with your health insurance provider).

Weighing the benefit versus the cost of light-based treatments is obviously a personal decision, but given the potential improvement, both to your skin and your self-esteem, it's something that should be given consideration. [157,158]

SUMMING IT UP

Although there's no simple, works-for-everyone solution for rosacea, you can take action and control its most telltale symptoms. Through trial and error, rosacea can be brought under control—no more hiding, no more embarrassment. Male or female, if you have rosacea, see your dermatologist for medical treatments (they will be needed), and keep your skincare routine gentle, gentle, gentle!

RECOMMENDED PRODUCTS FOR ROSACEA:

The products below include various cleansers, toners, moisturizers, and mineral-based sunscreens that we feel strongly are worth trying if you have rosacea. Because rosacea-affected skin can be incredibly finicky and capable of reacting to the most benign formulas, coming up with a definitive list is tricky and, unfortunately, not a sure thing. Therefore, please consider these recommendations knowing that, based on the frustrating nature of rosacea, your skin may respond unfavorably.

Cleansers
» Eucerin Redness Relief Soothing Cleanser ($8.79)
» First Aid Beauty Milk Oil Conditioning Cleanser ($26)
» Neutrogena Ultra Gentle Hydrating Cleanser, Creamy Formula ($8.99)
» Olay Foaming Face Wash, Sensitive Skin ($4.99)

Toners
» Bioelements Calmitude Hydrating Solution ($30)
» Paula's Choice Resist Advanced Replenishing Toner ($23)

BHA Exfoliants
» Paula's Choice Skin Perfecting 1% BHA Lotion ($26)
» Paula's Choice Skin Perfecting 2% BHA Liquid ($28)
» philosophy clear days ahead oil-free salicylic acid acne treatment & moisturizer ($39)

Daytime Moisturizers with SPF
» Exuviance Sheer Daily Protector Sunscreen Broad Spectrum SPF 50 ($42)
» MDSolarSciences Mineral Creme Broad Spectrum SPF 30 UVA/UVB Sunscreen ($30)
» Paula's Choice Resist Super-Light Daily Wrinkle Defense SPF 30 ($32)
» Paula's Choice Skin Recovery Daily Moisturizing Lotion SPF 30 ($28)
» Rodan + Fields Soothe Mineral Sunscreen SPF 30 ($41)

Moisturizers and Serums
» Arbonne Calm Gentle Daily Moisturizer ($36)
» Dr. Dennis Gross Skincare Hydration Super Serum Clinical Concentrate Booster ($68)
» Elizabeth Arden Ceramide Capsules Daily Youth Restoring Serum ($74)
» Olay Regenerist Micro-Sculpting Serum, Fragrance-Free ($23.99)

» Paula's Choice Calm Redness Relief Serum ($32)
» Paula's Choice Resist Intensive Repair Cream ($32)
» Paula's Choice Resist Intensive Wrinkle-Repair Retinol Serum ($40)
» Replenix Power of Three Cream ($70)

BROWN SPOTS

Regardless of your ethnic background or skin color, eventually most of us will struggle with some kind of brown or ashen pigmentation problem. The primary, if not exclusive, cause of these spots is sun damage. Skin will either appear lighter or darker than normal in concentrated areas, or you may notice blotchy, uneven patches of brown to gray discoloration or freckling.

No matter when or where these spots show up, chances are good that you want to get rid of them! Brown spots pop up on areas of skin that are always exposed to sun, and even if we try to be diligent about sun protection, years of prior unprotected and prolonged exposure to the sun will add up. But before we discuss treating brown spots, it's critical to understand more about how they got there in the first place!

WHAT CAUSES BROWN SPOTS?

Skin pigmentation problems occur because the body produces either too much or not enough melanin. Melanin is the pigment in skin; it's produced by specific cells known as melanocytes. An enzyme called tyrosinase, which is the catalyst that creates the melanin responsible for the color of our skin, eyes, and hair, triggers it. Excess melanin production is **caused primarily by chronic unprotected sun exposure** or by hormones (particularly during pregnancy or from taking birth control pills). [159,160]

As far as skin is concerned, depending on how much melanin is present, it provides some amount of sun protection by absorbing the sun's UV light and functioning as a built-in antioxidant. This explains why darker skin colors are less susceptible to sunburn and to the overall inflammatory, aging effects of sun damage. But, "less susceptible" does not mean "immune from problems." Also, for those who think getting a tan means you're getting protection from the melanin changing your skin's color, you're not! Tanning is the skin's response to damage, not a sign you're getting better protection!

TREATING BROWN SPOTS BEGINS WITH SUNSCREEN!

Without question, the first line of defense is sun-smart behavior, which means avoidance or, at the very least, careful exposure to UV light, and daily use (365 days a year) and liberal application (and, when needed, reapplication) of a well-formulated sunscreen. [161,162] Diligent use of a sunscreen alone allows for some repair as well as protection from further sun damage, which is what created the problem in the first place. [163] This is true for everyone!

No other aspect of controlling or reducing skin discolorations is as important as being careful about exposing your skin to the sun and using sunscreen, SPF 30 or greater, that includes the UVA-protecting ingredients of titanium dioxide, zinc oxide, avobenzone, Mexoryl SX™ (ecamsule), or Tinosorb listed as active. Using effective skin-lightening products, exfoliants, peels, or laser treatments without also using a sunscreen will prove a waste of time and money. Sun exposure is one of the primary causes of the skin discoloration disorder melasma, and treatments cannot keep up with the sun's daily assault on the skin. [164] Before you look at any other option for brown or ashen skin discolorations, start by applying sunscreen and reducing sun exposure. By "reducing exposure," we don't mean just spending less time in direct sunlight or tanning only in the early morning hours; it's about never getting a tan (indoors or out) and taking other precautions such as wearing a hat, sun-protective clothing, and sunglasses—each time, every time, from now on!

Scary but important fact: One bout of unprotected sun exposure can undo months of progress with a skin-lightening product. [165] There's simply no room for compromise here: Sun protection and skin lighteners are a package deal. When it comes to treating brown spots, one cannot work well without the other—both play critical roles in lightening the brown spots you see now AND preventing those you don't want to see later! It almost goes without saying, but we'll say it anyway: No skin-lightening routine will give you the results you want if you continue to get a tan; even "a little sun" can stall or reverse months of progress toward getting you the even skin tone you want. Stated bluntly: Failure to comply here can't be blamed on the skin-lightening product not working. You have to be willing to commit to avoiding further sun damage.

SKIN-LIGHTENING OPTIONS

The most successful brown spot treatments use a combination of topical lotions or gels containing melanin-inhibiting ingredients along with a well-formulated sunscreen, and a prescription retinoid (such as Renova or generic versions containing tretinoin, a type of retinoid). [160] Depending on how skin responds to these treatments, exfoliants, either in the form of topical skincare products or chemical peels performed by a physician, can also be included. Then there are lasers or intense pulsed light treatments to enhance the results from topical treatments and, in many cases, pick up where the topical treatments leave off. [166]

Topical **hydroquinone** is considered the gold standard for reducing or eliminating skin discolorations. [167] Despite the controversy surrounding the hydroquinone* ingredient, topical application has extensive research indicating it is a safe and effective treatment for brown skin discolorations for those with lighter skin tones, and many dermatologists agree. Topical hydroquinone in 2% concentrations from cosmetics companies is available over-the-counter, and 4% concentrations are available by prescription, and are definitely to be considered.

Plant extracts, such as *Uva ursi* (bearberry) extract, *Morus bombycis* (mulberry), *Morus alba* (white mulberry), and *Broussonetia papyrifera* (paper mulberry), as well as the plant extract arbutin are touted as being natural skin-lightening agents that don't have the problems (or at least the bad reputation) associated with hydroquinone. Ironically, these plant extracts actually break down into hydroquinone when absorbed into skin, which explains why they have a positive effect on brown discolorations. [168]

*See Chapter 16, *Cosmetic Ingredient Dictionary*, for information on the controversy surrounding hydroquinone.

Some research has shown that topical **azelaic acid** in 15% to 20% concentrations is as efficacious as hydroquinone and has a decreased risk of irritation. [169,170] Tretinoin by itself has also been shown to be especially useful in treating hyperpigmentation of sun-damaged skin. **Kojic acid**, alone or in combination with glycolic acid or hydroquinone, has shown good results due to its inhibitory action on tyrosinase; however, kojic acid has had problems in terms of stability and potential negative effects on skin and is rarely used nowadays. [171]

Several other plant extracts and many types of vitamin C (especially ascorbic acid) also have research showing them to be effective for inhibiting melanin production. [172] All of the above are valid considerations for those who want to avoid hydroquinone, or they can be used with hydroquinone, a combination that could provide even better results!

WHAT TO EXPECT WHEN YOU BEGIN USING A SKIN LIGHTENER

Of course, the obvious expected (and desired) result from using a skin lightener is for the dark or brown spots to get lighter, right? And, if they fade completely, hey, that's even better! With once- or twice-daily usage, you can reasonably expect a well-formulated skin-lightening product that contains proven ingredients to progressively lighten your dark spots. But, pack your patience (we know, easier said than done)!

Sadly, the lightening won't happen overnight, and it's important to keep that in mind. While we completely understand the desire to see those spots fade NOW, the truth is that it took several years of ongoing daylight exposure for the spots to form deeper in skin and then to show up on the surface. So, it stands to reason these slow-to-form brown spots will require patience and persistence as you wait for them to fade.

Most of us will need to use a lightening product every day, morning and evening, along with daily application of a great sunscreen rated SPF 30 or greater for at least 3 months before we see significant results. Some people do see results sooner, but maximum improvement and continued maintenance is a commitment to using these products regularly. None of these products are a cure.

As stated earlier in this section, but it bears repeating: What you shouldn't expect from a skin lightener is for it to work if you continue to expose your skin to UV light without sun protection or if you continue to tan, whether from sunlight or, even worse, in a tanning bed. No skin-lightening product will be effective if you're not willing to protect your skin daily from further UV damage. And, if you want to keep tanning, sorry, a skin lightener won't work at all—and it's not because the product is faulty. Sun protection (some dermatologists also stress sun avoidance) is a key part of lightening brown spots and preventing new ones from developing.

To repeat: The bottom line concerning getting rid of brown spots—if you're not willing to commit to daily sun protection and to not tanning no matter what, there's no sense in using any skin-lightening product. You'll be steadily undoing what they're trying to fix! Two steps forward, one step back isn't the way to get the best skin of your life—and that's what we want you to have!

WHY YOU MAY NEED MORE THAN ONE SKIN-LIGHTENING PRODUCT

Even if you're using one of the best skin-lightening products out there and being diligent about daily sun protection, you may not see much, if any, improvement in your dark spots. Why? Simply put, some discolorations are rooted deeper in the skin and, as a result, are much more stubborn and slower to respond to topical treatments.

What to do? Consider seeing a dermatologist for a series of light-emitting or laser treatments; using a prescription product with a higher amount of hydroquinone and/or a retinoid; or having a series of chemical peels—or all of these, spaced out over time. But, before you make an appointment, consider adding a second—or, potentially, a third—lightening product to your routine and see how your brown spots respond after several more weeks (sigh ... see what we mean by needing patience?).

Research has shown that for some people, a combination of active skin-lightening ingredients is needed for optimal results. [173,174] Hydroquinone or vitamin C alone might not be enough, but those two ingredients layered with products that contain other brown spot–fighters (and sunscreen, of course) may be the perfect combination to *finally* fade those brown spots.

ADDING A SKIN-LIGHTENER TO YOUR ROUTINE

OK, so you're ready to add a skin-lightening product to your skincare routine. Here's how to work it in to the skincare routines discussed earlier in this book:

Morning
» Cleanse your face.
» Apply toner (if used; if not, skip to Step 3).
» Apply your AHA or BHA exfoliant.
» Apply the skin-lightening product to the affected areas or all over your face. A lightweight lotion or gel can work for all skin types and layers well with Steps 5 and 6.
» Apply serum. (If you have oily or combination skin you may want to reserve this step for evening only.)
» Apply daytime moisturizer with sunscreen. Eye cream, if used, should be applied before sunscreen unless the eye cream provides sun protection.

Evening
» Cleanse your face.
» Apply toner (if used; if not, skip to Step 3).
» Apply your AHA or BHA exfoliant. If you prefer to apply your exfoliant only in the morning, skip to Step 4.
» Apply the skin-lightening product to the affected areas or all over your face.
» Apply serum and/or a nighttime prescription treatment, such as a retinoid.
» Apply nighttime moisturizer and/or eye cream.

You do not need to wait for the exfoliant to set or dry before you apply the skin lightener, but it's fine to do so if that's what you prefer. The same goes for applying serum over the skin lightener and the moisturizer (with or without sunscreen) over the serum.

What if you're also using a topical anti-acne product? Apply it before the skin lightener, either all over or just to the breakout-prone areas, morning and/or evening—whichever frequency of application you find works best to control your breakouts.

What if you're using more than one skin-lightening product? Simple: You can apply them in succession. Which one you apply first doesn't matter, but it helps to go from the lighter texture to the heavier texture; for example, liquid before lotion. It's also fine to apply one skin lightener in the morning and another one at night. Experiment to find what works best for you. There's no reason not to go after those brown spots with every potential ingredient proven likely to make a visible difference!

LASER TREATMENTS FOR BROWN SPOTS

Both ablative and nonablative lasers and light treatments administered by a dermatologist can have a profound positive effect on melasma and brown spots. However, the results are not always consistent, and problems can occur (such as hypo- or hyperpigmentation).

Laser treatments of this kind often are a problem for those with darker skin tones. Nonetheless, when laser treatments work, they can make a remarkable difference in the skin's appearance, especially when used in combination with the topical treatments previously mentioned. The results from lasers can be amazing and, although expensive, are absolutely worth a try for stubborn discolorations. There are many types of lasers that can be used for this purpose. Which one is optimal for you is best determined by a skilled dermatologist who has a practice that incorporates a variety of different lasers and/or light-emitting devices. Don't get caught up in a search for the perfect laser for your brown spots; in almost all cases, it's wasted energy because there usually are several options that might be equally effective. [166]

As effective as laser treatments can be, they're not cures. If you don't continue to follow the absolute rules—daily sun protection, use of melanin-inhibiting skincare products or topical medications, and not getting a tan—the brown spots will come back, no question.

Following a great skincare routine as detailed above will be helpful in improving brown skin discolorations, along with keeping it healthy and protected from further UV damage. In terms of inhibiting brown discolorations, the following are the best products we've found that contain well-researched ingredients that really can make a difference.

RECOMMENDED PRODUCTS FOR TREATING BROWN SPOTS:

» Alpha Hydrox Spot Light Targeted Skin Lightener ($9.99; hydroquinone)
» Black Opal Even True Tonecorrect Fade Creme ($10.95; hydroquinone)
» Black Opal Tri-Complex Tonecorrect Fade Gel ($12.95; hydroquinone)
» Dr. Dennis Gross Skincare Ferulic Acid & Retinol Brightening Solution ($88; arbutin)
» Olay ProX Even Skin Tone Spot Fading Treatment ($39.99-$44.99; niacinamide)
» Osmotics Lighten FX 3x Dark Spot Remover ($64; arbutin + niacinamide)
» Paula's Choice Resist Pure Radiance Skin Brightening Treatment ($32; niacinamide + vitamin C)
» Paula's Choice Resist 25% Vitamin C Spot Treatment ($55; vitamin C)
» Peter Thomas Roth De-Spot Plus ($78; hydroquinone)

MILIA/WHITEHEADS

Milia is the technical term for small, hard, white bumps that are rarely swollen or inflamed, and that don't change much once they show up—mostly on the face—in just about anyone, including infants, teens, and adults. These frustrating yet benign bumps are incredibly stubborn, and can last for weeks, months, and sometimes longer!

Though milia aren't harmful in any way, getting rid of them can be tough. There's a right way and a wrong way to remove them—and the wrong way can damage your skin. Following our recommendations should help you safely get rid of the bumps you have and possibly keep them from ever coming back!

Milia Are NOT Pimples!

If you've had milia, you likely wondered if they were some kind of pimple. While many people mistake the tiny, pearl-like bumps for acne, they're not the same thing. One of the easiest ways to identify milia bumps is by how they feel and look.

Unlike acne, milia are rather firm, and squeezing has little or no impact on them. Also unlike acne, these bumps can show up around the eyes and on parts of the face where there aren't active oil glands. Milia also don't have the pain and redness associated with acne nor are they due to inflammatory factors within skin. When a pimple forms, it quickly becomes inflamed, red, and sore; that doesn't happen with milia. In fact, milia just tend to sit there, minding their own business! [175]

YELLOW BUMPS UNDER THE EYES?

If you have yellowish, slight to obvious bumps without a depressed center around your eyes and/or on your eyelids, they aren't milia (which typically are a translucent flesh to white color). Instead, you may be dealing with a skin growth known as xanthoma. These bumps are common in people who have high cholesterol or high triglyceride levels. See your health care provider for a lipid panel, a test that involves drawing blood to analyze it for the amount of cholesterol and triglycerides that may be causing the bumps. Reducing the health problems associated with xanthoma can reduce the number and size of the bumps. [175]

WHAT CAUSES MILIA?

Milia occur when dead skin cells clump together and get trapped under the skin's surface, forming small, hard cysts. It's estimated that nearly 50% of infants in the United States get milia, in part because their young skin is still "learning" to exfoliate. As their skin matures, the milia will disappear on their own, no treatment necessary. Doctors don't consider infant milia a problem, and rarely prescribe treatment for it. Parents may find the bumps unsightly, but the baby isn't bothered by them, and they have no impact on the baby's health. [175]

Adults can get two forms of milia, most often seen on the cheeks and forehead: primary and secondary. Primary is the same type seen in babies, caused by skin cells that build up in the pore lining because they just didn't shed properly. Secondary milia occur when a skin condition or infection (such as herpes) that leads to blistering actually damages the pore lining. Burns or severe rashes can increase the number of skin cells trapped under the skin's surface, resulting in milia that form even after the trigger has faded. [175]

Sun damage is a contributing factor to milia because it makes skin rough and leathery, so it's more difficult for dead cells to rise to the skin's surface and shed normally. Clogs will ensure milia show up, and as mentioned they tend to stick around. [175]

Many people believe heavy moisturizers, foundations, or makeup in general are responsible for the problem, but that's highly unlikely. Given that 50% of all babies get milia, and men do as well, it clearly isn't related to skincare or makeup products. [175] Of course, if you're still concerned, you can experiment with changing your product selection or application method to see what works for you.

TREATING AND PREVENTING MILIA

Because milia often go away on their own without treatment, being patient and waiting it out is an option—but waiting is definitely not for everyone!

Because milia form when the skin's natural exfoliation process malfunctions, using a targeted exfoliating treatment with salicylic acid on a regular basis will immediately improve exfoliation. It may also allow the bump to dissolve on its own (relatively quickly, too) and prevent new ones from forming. [175]

If using a leave-on BHA exfoliant doesn't help, then you might consider seeing a dermatologist who can tell you which type of milia you have and perhaps even remove them right there in the office. Using a needle or a tiny lancing utensil, a dermatologist can easily remove the milia, leaving very little damage to skin and ensuring a fast healing time. [175]

SKINCARE FOR TREATING MILIA

Although there's not much you can do to prevent milia, maintaining a suitable skincare routine certainly helps minimize the chance of them appearing. Because deeper or larger milia can be caused by sun damage, always use a daytime moisturizer with SPF 30 or greater to protect your skin every day. This will give those annoying white bumps less of a reason to set up shop on your face!

Milia are a real pain to put up with, but there are things you can do to treat these white bumps. Remember: Patience, daily exfoliation, sun protection, and resisting the temptation to (literally) take matters into your own hands (unless you follow our suggestions) can go a long way toward having clearer, bump-free skin sooner!

REMOVING MILIA AT HOME

Removing milia at home is not for the faint of heart, or for those who tend to be overly aggressive with their skin. It also isn't something we encourage, but knowing that some of you will try it anyway, we figured we might as well explain how to do it the right way. Removing milia yourself is not like "popping" a pimple. In Chapter 7, *Stop Acne and Breakouts (No Matter Your Age)*, we explain how popping a pimple the right way (emphasis on the *right way*) not only gets rid of the unsightly red swelling and white sac, but also reduces the inflammation by releasing the pressure inside, and speeds up healing.

Milia are not pimples; in fact, in many ways they are completely unrelated. Unlike pimples, which for the most part can release somewhat easily on their own, milia actually need to be excised and that is more risky to your skin than popping a pimple, which is why doing it the right way is even more important.

There is only minimal benefit to be gained from removing milia, other than the aesthetics, of course. If aesthetics is important to you, we understand why you want to remove milia, and, just as with pimples, it's not always realistic to see a physician every time you get one. So, for those of you who aren't going to spend the money to see a physician to remove milia and are determined to do it yourself, here are the steps you need to take to do it the right way and minimize the risk to skin.

One important caveat: Our strong warning is that if you have many milia all at the same time, as opposed to just one or two that occur intermittently, don't even begin to do it yourself; it is best to see a physician. The risk of trying to remove lots of them all at once by yourself is just too great. Again, you really could make a mess of things.

Excise means you need to make a tiny tear in skin, directly on top of or near the milia, and then literally lift it out of skin with tweezers or use a comedone extractor with only slight pressure. Here are the steps to follow:

» Make sure you have on hand a sharp needle, very pointed tweezers (flat-ended tweezers will not work!), and/or a comedone extractor. You can buy a comedone extractor from Paula's Choice or at Sephora. Here's what it looks like:

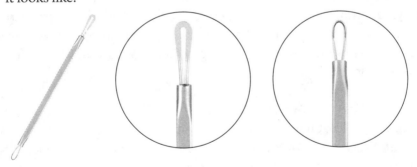

» Cleanse your face with a gentle water-soluble cleanser. Use tepid to warm water (not hot or cold, both of which are damaging to skin).
» Before rinsing, lightly massage skin with a soft, wet washcloth or a Clarisonic to remove dead skin cells from the surface to make excision and removing the milia easier. Do NOT over-scrub because that can damage your skin even before you've started.
» Dry skin gently. Do not do anything before you've dried your skin because skin is more vulnerable to tearing and creating a scab when it is wet.

» Rub the pointed needle, tweezers, and/or comedone extractor with alcohol to prevent infection.
» Then, gently, with either the needle or tweezers, make the teeniest tear in skin, either on top of the milia or right next to it. That should give you enough access to remove the milia.
» If you've made the teeny tear next to the milia, then, with very little pressure, use the comedone extractor to gently (and we mean really gently) coax the milia out through the small opening. If you've made the teeny tear on top of the milia, use the tweezers to lift it out. That should release the contents.
» Do NOT repeat this process over the same bump more than once or you will damage your skin, so be very, very careful, and go slowly.
» Remember to be gentle and make the teeniest possible tear in skin; the goal is to remove the whitehead without creating a scab or damaging the surrounding skin (scabs are not any better to look at than milia).
» When you're done, use a cotton swab with hydrogen peroxide or alcohol to disinfect the area. This is the only time we will ever recommend using either of those two skin-damaging products on your face (hydrogen peroxide generates free-radical damage and alcohol causes inflammation).
» You can then follow up with your usual skincare routine.

RECOMMENDED PRODUCTS FOR MILIA:

Other than a skincare routine that's best for your skin type and other concerns, as we explain in previous chapters, treating milia is really about adding a more potent salicylic acid exfoliant to your routine and using it as a spot treatment. Unfortunately, the list of products that stand a good chance of reducing and potentially eliminating milia is very short, largely because milia are unresponsive to most skincare products.

In our experience, and the experience of others who've tried these products, we believe they are among the best options. Once you get your milia under control, you can use other types of exfoliants mentioned throughout this book. Of course, daily sun protection and treating skin gently remain vitally important, but that's true for everyone!

» Paula's Choice Resist BHA 9 ($42)
» Paula's Choice Resist Weekly Retexturizing Treatment 4% BHA ($35)

SEBACEOUS HYPERPLASIA

If you have struggled with oily or combination skin for most of your life and are now over the age of 40, you may have noticed a series of small, stubborn, crater-like bumps with a whitish rim popping up randomly on various parts of your face. While these bumps may appear to be a type of blackhead, milia, or breakout, they aren't. The difference is that these strange spots just don't go away, no matter what you do. If you're seeing these spots, chances are you have sebaceous hyperplasia.

WHAT IS SEBACEOUS HYPERPLASIA?

Sebaceous hyperplasia is the technical name for a benign bump on the skin that forms over time as a result of damage to a pore caused by unknown factors. Randomly, a damaged oil gland (and often more than one) can become enlarged and clogged in a very specific manner, displaying a soft or firm white or yellowish outer rim typically with a tiny to wide depressed center. The depressed center of these bumps is one of the primary ways you can tell you're dealing with sebaceous hyperplasia, and not with something else such as a whitehead (milia, discussed above) or pimple.

It's not uncommon to have several of these bumps at once, sometimes spaced apart, but they can be clustered, too. Sebaceous hyperplasia is most often seen on the forehead and central part of the face, but can appear anywhere on the body, especially in areas where the skin has more oil glands. [176]

Cumulative sun damage is considered a co-factor of this condition because sunlight further damages skin and oil glands. [177] That's one more reason to make sure you're protecting your skin every day with a well-formulated sunscreen! It's also typically seen in people who have struggled with oily skin and large pores most of their lives, so getting this problem under control sooner rather than later is also important.

HOW TO GET RID OF SEBACEOUS HYPERPLASIA

Treating sebaceous hyperplasia usually requires a visit to the dermatologist, but now there are products available you can use at home to try and get these unsightly bumps under control—at the very least, you'll achieve noticeable improvement in skin tone and texture!

A dermatologist has several options for treating sebaceous hyperplasia. Before you consider any of them, however, know that, like many other skin disorders, sebaceous hyperplasia cannot be cured, only controlled. The bump can be reduced or eliminated, but the affected oil gland likely will produce a new bump if treatment isn't maintained, and even then it can recur. Therefore, even if you decide to see a dermatologist for treatment, you'll want to ensure your at-home skincare routine includes products to keep these bumps at bay, at least to the extent possible from skincare products.

When you visit a dermatologist for sebaceous hyperplasia, he or she may offer the following treatments, alone or in combination:

» **Facial peels**—This involves using salicylic acid or trichloroacetic acid (TCA).
» **Electric needle**—This causes the bump to break down and ooze, forming a scab that falls off in a week or so.
» **Photodynamic therapy (PDT)**—This is a light-emitting treatment where the skin is pre-treated with a special gel that reacts with the light. This option often requires several office visits.
» **Liquid nitrogen**—This potent option can be effective, but it's also risky because if it penetrates too deeply, you may be left with a scar or loss of skin pigment.
» **Prescription retinoid or azelaic acid**—These treatments are intended to reduce the appearance of the lesions, but they won't eliminate the problem.
» **Surgical excision of the bump**—This may lead to scarring, but the bump won't recur in the excised area. This is considered a last-resort option.
» **Antiandrogen medication**—This reduces testosterone, which may be stimulating enlargement of the oil glands. Examples of these medications are spironolactone or flutamide. This, like surgical excision, is a last resort. [178]

Note: Some sebaceous hyperplasia bumps can resemble a type of skin cancer known as basal cell carcinoma. [179] Your dermatologist will need to examine the area to make an accurate diagnosis. If you're unsure, don't assume it's not skin cancer.

SKINCARE FOR SEBACEOUS HYPERPLASIA

What about options outside the dermatologist's office? Although treating sebaceous hyperplasia yourself can be frustrating, and in almost all cases a dermatologist's care is required, there are a few key products to consider. Chief among them is a product we're very proud of, one that Paula uses for her sebaceous hyperplasia, and that's our Resist BHA 9 ($42). This clear, liquid-like solution contains a 9% concentration of salicylic acid. Despite its strength, it's still extremely gentle due to its time-release formula. Salicylic acid penetrates the oil buildup in the pore lining, increases cell turnover by exfoliating the surface of the skin as well as inside the pore to unclog these bumps, and reduces inflammation, all of which can diminish these bumps. There's no research directly linking salicylic acid in skincare products to treating sebaceous hyperplasia, but in theory and, as we've seen, in practice, it can and often does help a great deal!

You also can consider products that contain lower amounts of salicylic acid, but most cases of sebaceous hyperplasia won't respond as well to lower strengths; however, they can be extremely beneficial for daily maintenance all over the face. Most people struggling with sebaceous hyperplasia have other bumps and breakouts that can be successfully treated with lower concentrations of salicylic acid.

Other products to consider are those that contain retinol. Research has shown that retinol, which is another name for vitamin A, either in over-the-counter skincare products or in various prescription forms such as Tazorac or Retin-A, can reshape the pore lining and restore more normal pore function and size. Retinol works to control the growth of skin cells that can clog the pore lining, and encourages normal oil production. [95,180]

These factors, plus retinol's anti-inflammatory action, theoretically make it a powerful option to combine with salicylic acid for treating sebaceous hyperplasia.

Another skincare ingredient that may help improve sebaceous hyperplasia is the B vitamin niacinamide. This cell-communicating ingredient offers multiple benefits to skin, such as reducing inflammation and oil proliferation that accompany sebaceous hyperplasia. [181,182] Products containing salicylic acid, retinol, and niacinamide can be used once or twice daily after cleansing, and may help reduce sebaceous hyperplasia!

What about scrubs? No scrub in the world, regardless of claim or price, can remove these bumps. Sebaceous hyperplasia forms deep within the skin right at the base of the oil gland itself; scrubs simply cannot reach the source of the problem. Warning: Zealously trying to scrub away these bumps can lead to other skin issues, such as dryness, redness, and irritation.

RECOMMENDED PRODUCTS FOR SEBACEOUS HYPERPLASIA:

The list of products that can successfully treat sebaceous hyperplasia is fairly short, largely because most people dealing with sebaceous hyperplasia will require treatment from a dermatologist. These bumps rarely resolve on their own no matter what you use topically. However, skincare *can* play a role in terms of maintenance and in improving the appearance of sebaceous hyperplasia. The products below are those that can exfoliate inside the pore lining, unclog pores, and influence the pore lining, in the hope that they not only will reduce sebaceous hyperplasia but also prevent, to the extent possible, new bumps from forming.

» Olay Regenerist Regenerating Serum Fragrance-Free ($22.99; contains a high amount of niacinamide)

» Nia24 Skin Strengthening Complex ($93; contains a high amount of niacinamide)
» Paula's Choice Clinical 1% Retinol Treatment ($55)
» Paula's Choice Resist BHA 9 ($42; contains 9% salicylic acid)
» Serious Skincare A Force XR Retinol Serum Concentrate ($39.50)
» SkinCeuticals Retinol 1.0 Maximum Strength Refining Night Cream ($70)
» SkinMedica Retinol Complex 0.25 ($60)
» SkinMedica Retinol Complex 0.5 ($75)

KERATOSIS PILARIS (AKA CHICKEN SKIN)

Now let's leave the face and go on to the body to discuss a very common problem. If you're seeing large patches of little red or white inflamed bumps on the outside of your upper arms, thighs, or backside, you probably have a skin condition called keratosis pilaris. Also known as KP or as "chicken skin," this disorder affects 50%–80% of all adolescents and almost half of all adults, though no one knows exactly why this happens or why it's so prevalent. [183]

KP isn't a serious or harmful medical condition in the least, but it's a frustrating and undesirable one nonetheless. For many, these bumps are an embarrassment, and covering them up feels like the only solution. Thankfully, covering up isn't the only solution. But, as with so many other skin issues, before you understand how to fix the problem, it helps to understand what's causing it!

WHAT CAUSES KERATOSIS PILARIS (KP)?

Research has shown that there's a genetic component to KP; 50% of those who struggle with it have a family history of it. [184] There are a few different forms of keratosis pilaris. It can range from pink to red bumps on the cheeks (often mistaken for acne) to small, hard red bumps that aren't irritated to pimple-like bumps that feel rough and coarse but are inflamed and red. Most often, KP shows up on the upper arms and legs.

Regardless of the type, all forms are the result of the buildup of keratin, a hard protein (skin's surface is made up of cells known as keratinocytes) that protects skin from infection and harmful external substances. The keratin forms a plug that blocks the opening of the hair follicle, resulting in patches of bumpy, often inflamed skin.

Regrettably, there's no universally accepted treatment for chicken skin, though it's generally well accepted that unclogging hair follicles and reducing inflammation can make a big difference. [185]

GETTING RID OF KP

One of the best ways to get to the root of the problem is to use a beta hydroxy acid (BHA) leave-on exfoliant (active ingredient salicylic acid) that has a pH low enough for exfoliation to occur. [36] BHA is a wonderful multitasker because it penetrates beyond skin's surface to exfoliate inside the pore lining. It also has antimicrobial properties to kill bacteria that might be making matters worse. Plus, because salicylic acid is related to aspirin (aspirin is acetylsalicylic acid), it acts as an anti-inflammatory agent to reduce the redness that's often seen with KP.

What about alpha hydroxy acids (AHAs)? AHAs can help exfoliate skin cells, but only at the surface. However, they're an option for those whose keratosis pilaris does not respond well to BHA treatment. AHAs can be effective when the KP plugs are not very deep, and so the penetrating ability of BHA isn't quite as necessary. For best results, look for an AHA with glycolic or lactic acid (these may be combined in the same product) at a concentration of 5% or greater.

Because keratosis pilaris is an inflammatory disorder, reducing inflammation is vitally important. (Actually, reducing inflammation is important for skin, period!) You can do this by avoiding bar cleansers and bar soaps, as the ingredients that keep them in their bar form can clog pores and make matters worse. Also, avoid highly fragranced body creams and lotions, whose fragrance can cause irritation and worsen the itching that can accompany KP.

It's also important not to scrub skin. These bumps can't be scrubbed away because the problem is deeper than scrubs can reach. Plus, scrubbing only serves to further irritate and inflame skin, making matters worse. Ditch the body scrub and loofah and use gentle cleansers and moisturizers to keep skin smooth. If desired, use a damp cotton washcloth as a mild "scrub," but be aware that KP itself cannot be scrubbed away, and it's not the result of skin being dirty.

When it comes to treating KP, ongoing application of such products is required to keep the condition under control. If you stop using them, the condition will eventually return. Some people may find that applying a KP treatment a few times per week will keep the bumps at bay; for others, daily application (once or twice, morning and/or evening) may be needed. As with so many things for your skin, you'll need to experiment to see which product and what frequency of application works best for you.

TREATING KP WITH LASERS

If topical treatments prove ineffective after a few weeks of daily use, talk to a dermatologist about laser treatments. Several options are available, including photopneumatic therapy (PPx), intense pulsed light (IPL), pulsed dye laser, long-pulsed alexandrite laser, and the Nd:YAG laser. [186,187,188,189]

Laser or light-emitting treatments have an impressive-to-decent track record for improving KP, most notably for reducing its redness and, for those with darker skin tones, the dotted brown spots left behind by the bumps. They also improve skin's overall surface texture. If topical treatments don't work (and some cases of KP can be *very* stubborn), a lot of people find these alternatives are well worth the time and money! In most cases, once your KP is cleared up via laser treatments, you can keep it under control with topical treatments. That's great, as the ongoing expense of laser treatments adds up!

In terms of skincare, there are only a handful of products we've found that contain the types of ingredients that can adequately address the cause and symptoms of KP.

RECOMMENDED PRODUCTS FOR KERATOSIS PILARIS:

Note: All of the products below contain AHA (glycolic or lactic acid) or BHA (salicylic acid) ingredients in a lotion, cream, or wipe form. All are viable options for controlling keratosis pilaris; there isn't a single "best" option. We encourage you to try more than one to see how your KP responds. Whichever products you choose from the list below, apply at least once daily.

» Alpha Hydrox 12% AHA Silk Wrap Body Lotion ($11.99)
» CeraVe Renewing SA Cream ($21.99; BHA)
» DERMAdoctor KP Duty ($38; AHA)
» Paula's Choice Clinical KP Treatment Cloths ($32; AHA + BHA)
» Paula's Choice Resist Skin Revealing Body Lotion 10% AHA ($27)
» Paula's Choice Resist Weightless Body Treatment with 2% BHA ($25)

ECZEMA

Eczema (also known as atopic dermatitis) is a general term used to describe a strange variety of skin rashes ranging from small sections of skin that are slightly itchy, dry, and irritated to chronically inflamed, oozing, crusted areas covering the entire body and accompanied by incessant itching. [190] Pardon us for being blunt, but eczema just sucks!

Eczema can have multiple appearances, looking and feeling completely different from person to person. The most common areas for eczema to occur are in the folds of the arms and legs, the back of the neck, back of the hands, tops of the feet, and the wrists. It's estimated to affect up to 20% of children, and the research on how eczema improves and worsens throughout life is inconclusive—though symptoms do seem to become less intense when a child with eczema reaches adulthood. [191]

WHAT CAUSES ECZEMA?

One of the predominant theories is that someone with eczema has a short-circuited immune response, [192] where the skin reacts abnormally when a substance comes in contact with it. In severe cases of eczema, the substance can be as benign as water; for others, the trigger can be anything from clothing, detergents, soaps, grass, food products, allergens (including dust mites), a lack of humidity, or a combination of things. Even more frustrating is that the reaction can be intermittent, with no real rhyme or reason for why or when.

There also appears to be a strong hereditary component to eczema. [193] For example, children whose parents suffer from eczema run an 80% chance of developing it themselves. Further, in both children and adults, stressful situations tend to trigger, prolong, or worsen eczema flare-ups.

Regardless of the source, eczematous skin reacts to a substance or substances or to environmental conditions by spinning out of control and generating mild to severe inflammation, which leads to itching and subsequent scratching that damages skin's critical barrier function.

TYPES OF ECZEMA

There are several types and varying degrees of eczema, which, as you can imagine, makes diagnosis and treatment a bit tricky! The following are the most common types of eczema:

Atopic eczema (also referred to as atopic dermatitis): Perhaps the most pernicious and painful type of eczema, it's characterized by its severity and the intolerable sensation of itching and irritation, leaving skin raw, fissured, and vulnerable to infection. This is the type of eczema that many infants experience between the ages of two and six months. In infants, symptoms appear on the face, scalp, feet, and hands; in older children and into adulthood, symptoms appear in the fold of the arm and behind the knees, though particularly bad outbreaks can appear anywhere on the body.

Allergic contact dermatitis: This specific form of eczema often stems from a subset known as irritant contact dermatitis. It occurs when a specific substance comes in contact with the skin and causes the immune system to overreact. The result is inflamed and sensitized skin. [194] Most typically, allergic contact dermatitis is caused by fragrance, nickel, detergents, wool, grass, citrus, household cleaning products, and vinegar. Once you've identified the specific substance, avoiding it often solves the problem.

A subset of allergic contact dermatitis is **eyelid dermatitis**. Typically mild to moderate redness is present, as well as scaling, flaking, and swollen skin. This is extremely common and almost exclusively affects women in relation to their use of hairstyling products, makeup, and nail polish (even once it dries) when your manicured nails come in contact with the eye area. The best way to solve the problem is to stop using the offending product(s) and find options that don't trigger a reaction.

Infantile seborrheic eczema: Better known as cradle cap, this form of eczema generally affects only babies and children. [195] The crusty, thick, sometimes reddened lesions may look problematic, but this disorder is rarely itchy or even felt by the child. If you want to treat this, and success is limited, consider a 1% hydrocortisone or a 2% topical ketoconazole cream, which are available from your infant's pediatrician. [196]

Adult seborrhoeic eczema: This shows up for most people between the ages of 20 and 40, and is estimated to affect 5% of adults. It's usually seen on the scalp as mild dandruff, but can spread to the face, ears, and chest. The skin becomes red and inflamed and starts to flake. It's believed to be caused by yeast, but its precise cause remains unclear; stress may be a factor. If the area becomes infected, treatment with an antifungal cream, topical steroid creams, or immunomodulators may be necessary. [197]

Nummular eczema: Typically localized on the legs, nummular eczema is characterized by coin-shaped patches of pink to red skin that may take on an orange cast if crusting or scaling is present. Left untreated, the dry, scaly spots typically darken and thicken. This type of eczema is most common in adolescent girls and in women between the ages of 30 and 60, and the condition tends to occur in winter. [198]

TREATING ECZEMA

There's no cure for eczema on the horizon, but the good news is that there are a number of treatments that can reduce the symptoms and decrease the level of discomfort. Keep in mind that many people diagnosed with eczema when they are young eventually, for the most part, outgrow it. The primary treatment options for eczema are as follows:

Gentle, effective skincare: The first line of defense is a gentle, fragrance-free skincare routine that prevents or reduces inflammation and keeps skin moist and its barrier intact. [199] Improving the skin's outer structure by providing it with antioxidants, ingredients that improve the skin's barrier, anti-irritants, and emollients can have amazing results for most forms of eczema. In fact, it's been theorized that eczema makes skin more susceptible to oxidative damage, which in turn makes topical application of antioxidants even more important! [200]

Avoid irritants: In addition to using a gentle skincare routine and a well-formulated moisturizer, avoiding things that can trigger skin reactions is also of vital importance. Steering clear of known irritants and prolonged contact with water can be incredibly beneficial. It also helps a great deal to reapply moisturizer within seconds of washing any part of the body, but especially your hands, because soaps and cleansers are notorious for triggering a reaction in those struggling with eczema. [201] Try switching to a creamy, moisturizing body wash (Olay and Dove make good ones) and using that throughout your home as your hand soap. It works beautifully!

Topical steroids: The most typical and successful medications for eczema are prescription-strength topical steroids (cortisone creams such as Eumovate, active ingredient clobetasone butyrate, or various strengths of hydrocortisone). Over-the-counter cortisone creams can be effective for very mild or transient forms of eczema, but if those fail, prescription cortisone creams can save your skin. Although there are no short-term detrimental side effects of using most strengths of cortisone cream, it's still important to apply it only to the affected areas, and only as needed, because repeated, prolonged application of cortisone creams can cause thinning of the skin, prematurely aging it. [202,203,204]

Oral steroids: In severe cases of eczema, when topical steroids have failed to produce any relief, oral steroids may be prescribed, but only under a doctor's scrutiny due to the serious side effects associated with this type of medication. [205]

Topical immunomodulators: In 2000 and 2001, Protopic (active ingredient tacrolimus) and Elidel (pimecrolimus) were approved by the FDA as new topical drugs for the treatment of eczema. Not cortisones or steroids, these immunomodulators can regulate the skin's immune response, which plays a pivotal role in eczema. [206] Regrettably, in March 2005, the FDA announced a public health advisory for Elidel (pimecrolimus) Cream and Protopic (tacrolimus) Ointment "to inform healthcare providers and patients about a potential cancer risk from use of Elidel (pimecrolimus) and Protopic (tacrolimus)..." This risk is uncertain, and more recent studies have refuted it, but the FDA's precautions still advise that Elidel and Protopic should be used only as labeled, for patients who have failed treatment with other therapies. [207] The topical immunomodulators (pimecrolimus and tacrolimus) don't present the risk of skin thinning that's associated with topical corticosteroids.

Phototherapy: Research has shown that exposing skin to controlled wavelengths of UVA or UVB light can help reduce the symptoms of chronic eczema. [208] Under medical supervision, the use of specially designed bulbs can allow affected parts of the body to be exposed to the specific light source. More severe or chronic eczema can be treated with UVA light in combination with a prescription medication called psoralen. Psoralen can be administered either orally or topically, increasing the skin's sensitivity to light. [209] This treatment is known as PUVA (Psoralen + UVA light) and is administered more often to adults than to infants or children with eczema.

Phototherapy treatments are complicated and expensive. They are administered several times per week over a span of one week to several months at a doctor's office. As you might have guessed, the risk of accelerated aging of the skin and increased risk of skin cancer from UV radiation therapy can be the same as for sunbathing, so this isn't an optimal way to treat eczema, as it just replaces one problem (eczema) with another (UV damage). [210]

Non-fragrant oils and dietary changes: Evening primrose oil and borage oil contain gamma linolenic acid, a fatty acid that may play a part in general skin health and that has gained a reputation for reducing the occurrence of eczema when applied topically. Several studies, however, have shown that not to be the case. [211] Nonetheless, if you're interested in alternative treatments for eczema, this is one you can try with very little risk of adverse effects. Other non-fragrant plant oils, like safflower or jojoba, may also be worth experimenting with, and you can add a few drops of these to your regular body moisturizer, hand cream, or facial moisturizer.

There's also some research pointing to dietary considerations as a source of reactions. [212] It's worth experimenting to see if eliminating certain food groups, such as dairy, gluten, processed foods, or nuts, can decrease the severity and/or frequency of eczema outbreaks.

Skincare if you have eczema: From the neck down, treating eczema means being as gentle as you absolutely can, which almost always means avoiding bar soaps and scrubs. Below we list fragrance-free gentle cleansers and body lotions we strongly recommend. If you have eczema on your face, follow our recommendations in the sections that are appropriate for your skin type, also adding products to treat other concerns like rosacea, brown spots, and wrinkles.

DON'T BE AFRAID OF CORTISONE CREAM

Whether you have short-term or long-term bouts of eczema, rashes, or any kind of dermatitis, cortisone creams can be your best friend. Topical cortisone creams, which can be either over-the-counter (OTC) or prescription, are known by many names, including corticosteroids, glucocorticosteroids, and steroids. Without question, cortisone creams are truly the "gold standard" for treating eczema. When applied correctly, as directed, they're completely safe to use, even on children. [213]

We know that our "completely safe" comment may fly in the face of what you've heard about topical cortisones—that they're really terrible for skin—that's another myth that just isn't true. [214] In fact, believing this flawed information, and not using cortisone cream when it's called for, may lead to far more problems for your skin than you can imagine.

We are not saying that there are no risks associated with using cortisone creams, because there are; however, their benefits, when used correctly, will help prevent long-term damage to your skin by interrupting and reducing the cascade of chronic inflammation and itching caused by eczema. Here's what's happening:

Depending on the severity of the eczema, your skin can, seemingly for no reason, become red, inflamed, itchy, and flaky, on various areas of the face and body; sometimes accompanied by small sacs filled with fluid. This outbreak causes a great deal of damage to skin, both to the upper and lower layers of skin. More often than not, these eczematous areas are unbearably itchy, so maddening that it triggers uncontrollable and habitual scratching. This scratching further damages skin, causing pain, wounds, and even a risk of infection.

All these symptoms, and your reaction to them (scratching), reduce skin's ability to heal, cause collagen and elastin to break down, and make the skin more vulnerable to environmental damage, all of which are pro-aging. None of this is desirable, and it's clearly detrimental to the health of skin, over both the short term and long term. Regrettably, most alternative treatments (that is, those other than cortisone) for moderate to severe eczema are rarely, if ever, successful. They are always worth a try, especially if you have only occasional minor bouts of eczema, but when they fail to do the job, the only real relief will come from applying a cortisone cream that's appropriate for the type of eczema with which you're struggling.

So, you're wondering, what are the risks associated with cortisone creams? The primary risk, and what most people seem to be concerned about, is thinning of the skin. While that is indeed a risk of using cortisone creams it is only a risk from long-term chronic use. Yet, despite this fact, many people fear the thinning of skin will happen immediately and that is not the case.

For many people, cortisone cream is nothing less than a miracle; Paula can personally attest to that, as she's struggled with eczema to one degree or another for most of her life. Anecdotally, except for the areas where she used it chronically day in and day out for years there have been no negative consequences and the skin in those areas looks completely normal and healthy.

The real story about cortisone is that if it's used only intermittently for a few days here and there to relieve the symptoms, discomfort, and skin damage eczema can cause then there's no cause for alarm. Using cortisone creams indefinitely is the problem, not intermittent use to stop the symptoms and reactions so skin can begin to heal.

One strategy is to start with OTC options at your drugstore, but if they don't work, you may need to see a doctor for prescription-strength versions. In those situations, it's not uncommon for the doctor to prescribe two or more preparations of different strengths to be used at the same time, but on different parts of the body; for example, a mild cortisone cream for eczema on your face and a moderately strong version for eczema on the thicker skin of your arms or legs. A very strong topical cream is often needed for eczema on the palms and soles of the feet of adults because these areas have thick skin, and eczema in these areas doesn't respond as well to low-strength cortisone creams.

Topical cortisone creams should be used until the flare-up is completely gone, and then you should stop the treatment and only use it again when another flare-up occurs. Also, it's best to use the smallest amount possible that reduces the inflammation and itching; applying more won't make it work any faster or any better. In some cases, it might require treatment for as little as one day; in other cases, it may take up to 14 days to clear a flare-up. If it takes longer, you'll want to consult your physician. In all cases, apply it only as needed, and keep in mind that the sooner you apply it when you notice a flare-up starting—before it gets bad—reduces the amount of time you'll need to continue the treatment, and thus limits the potential risk of any skin-thinning.

When you weigh the pros and cons of cortisone creams, the research and results are clear that the damage that results from letting inflamed raw skin linger can be far worse than the effects of intermittent use of a cortisone cream, whether OTC or prescription-only. Don't let unbalanced, one-sided information prevent you from taking the best possible care of your skin.

RECOMMENDED PRODUCTS FOR ECZEMA:

» Aveeno Daily Moisturizing Body Wash ($8.99)
» Cetaphil Restoraderm Eczema Calming Body Wash ($17.99)

» Cortizone-10 Hydratensive Anti-Itch Lotion for Hands and Body, Healing Natural Aloe Formula ($10.49; this is medicated with 1% hydrocortisone and best for mild eczema)
» Eucerin Eczema Relief Body Crème ($10.49)
» Eucerin Skin Calming Dry Skin Body Wash ($8.79)
» Gold Bond Ultimate Eczema Relief Skin Protectant Cream ($11.99)
» Kate Somerville Eczema Therapy Cream ($48)
» Paula's Choice Clinical Ultra-Rich Soothing Body Butter ($19)

SCARS

Whether from an injury, surgery, or a skin problem such as acne, scars are something almost everyone has to deal with at some point or another. Although unsightly, they're an amazing example of the miraculous way skin heals itself when injured. Scars may be flat or raised, practically invisible or obvious, but what you do to assist the skin as it heals—and how you treat the scarred area afterward—makes a big difference in how the scar looks. Before you learn how to treat scars, you need to understand how they form, how to care for injured skin to minimize scarring, and what type of scar you're dealing with.

HOW DOES A SCAR FORM?

The scar that you see on the skin's surface is the result of a complex process the skin goes through as it recovers from damage. There are many factors that affect how a wound heals, and the way the wound heals affects how the scar ends up looking. How skin heals and scars varies from person to person, but it also depends on how you care for the wound *before* the scar is done forming.

The skin goes through three stages of repair before you see a scar. In the first stage, there's swelling, redness, and some tenderness or pain as a scab begins to form. A scab in and of itself is an amazing part of the healing process and must be protected, but more about that in the next section.

During the next stage, new skin tissue begins to form underneath the scab. The final stage involves rebuilding and reforming the outer and inner layers of skin.

What you do during the first days after getting a wound, what you do after the scab has formed, and what you do when the scab eventually falls off will greatly affect the appearance of the final scar.

WOUND CARE TO MINIMIZE SCARS

There's an easy-to-follow plan to minimize scarring. Although there's a lot of anecdotal information about specific ingredients (such as aloe and vitamin E) to reduce scars, most of it is not supported by research, and more often than not it's just a waste of time—time during which you could have used more effective remedies instead. Here's how to care for a wound to minimize scar formation:

» Allow the wound to "breathe" as much as possible. Do not gunk up the area with creams, oils, or vitamin E from capsules because these substances have occlusive textures that can impede the first stages of healing when skin is trying to repair itself. The fluid that is produced naturally around a wound (known as exudate) is fine by itself for the first few days.

» Don't soak the wounded area in water or get it wet for extended periods; doing so breaks down the scab and impairs the formation of the new skin below, risking scars that take longer to heal.

» Keep the damaged skin clean using a gentle cleanser, but don't over-clean or scrub it.

» After cleansing, cover the wound with a thin, light bandage that allows air to circulate.

» You may want to consider a specialty adhesive dressing, such as Nexcare Tegaderm Transparent Dressing or Convatec DuoDERM Extra Thin Dressing. These cost more than standard bandages, but are excellent at keeping wounds moist without letting them get wet.

» If you suspect there's a risk of infection, consider using an over-the-counter antibacterial liquid such as Bactine Original First Aid Liquid or Band-Aid Antiseptic Wash, Hurt-Free. If the redness increases or if the wound changes color, throbs, or swells, consult a doctor.

» After a day or two, apply a *thin* layer of a lightweight gel moisturizer or serum loaded with antioxidants (which are brilliant for helping skin heal) and other skin-repairing ingredients.

» If possible, rather than applying sunscreen to the injured area, keep it out of direct sunlight altogether, which means seeking shade or covering it up. Sun exposure makes scarring worse, so protecting the injured area from the sun (as you should be doing for your skin everyday even if you don't have a wound) is important.

» At night, change the bandage; if the wound is dry or itchy, apply a very thin layer of a lightweight moisturizer or serum, as mentioned above. Keeping wounds moist (but not wet) encourages healing. **Tip:** A lightweight moisturizer also makes the scab less itchy as it forms, and still allows the skin to breathe!

» Once a scab forms, **don't pick at it or even touch it**—ever! Any manipulation or removal is a serious impediment to the healing that is taking place underneath the scab, and **can cause scarring that otherwise would not have occurred**.

» **Do not irritate the skin!** Skin's primary, natural reaction to a wound is inflammation, so anything you do to irritate skin makes matters worse.

» Avoid soaps (they're too drying), highly fragrant products (whether natural or synthetic, fragrance is a skin irritant), and alcohol, menthol, citrus, eucalyptus, clove, camphor, or any type of mint, all of which increase irritation and make matters worse. [2,5,7]

TYPES OF SCARS

Depending on your genetic makeup and the depth and type of tear in your skin, scarring can range from a slightly reddish discoloration to a thick, raised red or dark scar. There are three main types of scars, generally described as flat, indented, or raised.

Flat scars are the most common, and usually occur from everyday injuries or minor burns. Depending on your skin color, flat scars may be pink to red (and eventually fade to very light pink or white) or tan to deep brown or black (eventually becoming lighter).

Note: The flat, pink-to-red or tan-to-brown marks left from a breakout are technically not scars. These marks are known as post-inflammatory hyperpigmentation.

Indented (atrophic) scars often result from cystic acne or a bout with the chickenpox virus. If you've ever had a deep, painful breakout or chickenpox, chances are you have at least one of these scars. Other names for indented scars are pockmarks, ice pick scars, and depressed scars. These scars result from the destruction of skin's underlying support structure, which is why they don't heal as well as flat or raised scars.

Raised (hypertrophic) scars result from overproduction of collagen in response to injured skin. This type of scarring can result from a slight tear in skin or from a deep wound, and everything in between. Sometimes referred to as keloid scars, they are more common in persons with dark skin. Raised scars flatten over time, but can take years to resolve. We explain how you can help this process along in the next section: Scar Treatments. Stubborn or large/long raised scars may require medical or surgical treatment.

SCAR TREATMENTS

Even when you take the proper steps to minimize scarring, once the wound has healed, you'll likely want to keep treating the scar to make it even less noticeable. You'll be happy to know there are products and medical procedures that can help—a lot!

Even if you choose to do nothing, a scar continues to heal and change, often for the better part of up to two years after the fact. With ongoing gentle skincare, sun protection, and patience (that's the hardest part), most scars do improve, becoming less apparent over time. If you don't want to wait it out, there are some things you can do to treat the scars you have now, as follows:

» Apply a silicone-based gel or scar treatment loaded with skin-healing ingredients and antioxidants such as quercertin. Eight weeks of once- or twice-daily application can make the scar less noticeable, especially if it's a fresh scar. This type of product shows the best results on flat scars, but also can be helpful on raised and indented scars. Always treat the skin gently and protect the scar with sunscreen rated SPF 30 or greater if it will be exposed to daylight.

» Watch out for scar gels that are little more than silicone, and there are a lot of them out there. Although pure silicone can help heal and reduce scars, silicone alone isn't all that the skin needs to improve scars. A range of anti-inflammatory, skin-healing, and skin-repairing ingredients will get you much better results because they work with the skin's natural repair process.

» **Raised scars can be flattened** to some extent with daily application of a silicone-based scar treatment gel and/or a silicone gel sheet, such as ScarAway Silicone Scar Sheets or Rejuveness Pure Silicone Sheeting (which is reusable). The sheet is worn for 12 to 24 hours at a time for at least three months.

» **Indented scars** respond best to a series of in-office laser treatments (including Fraxel), dermal fillers, fat grafting, or a combination of these. In extreme cases, surgery may be necessary; there are various methods that your dermatologist can discuss with you. How much an indented scar improves depends on its depth and on how well your skin responds to treatments. Although it's not realistic to expect 100% improvement, 50% improvement is possible.

What about Mederma for scars? Research on Mederma is conflicting; some research shows that it does work and some shows that it does not work, so the results are mixed. Yes, that's confusing, but it's what the science says. In short, Mederma is a product for which you must weigh the pros and cons yourself. [215]

RECOMMENDED SCAR GELS:
» Kate Somerville D-Scar Scar Diminishing Serum ($48)
» Kinerase Scar Healing Therapy ($48)
» Paula's Choice Clinical Scar-Reducing Serum ($24)

WHAT IS PSORIASIS?

Psoriasis is a complicated skin disease that is said to affect over 125 million people worldwide. It is a chronic condition resulting from what is thought to be an auto-immune disorder in which skin cells malfunction and reproduce much faster than normal, leaving thickened, raised patches or large areas of red or brown, wet-looking, scaly skin on the face and body.

There are several forms of psoriasis, ranging from mild to severe—and even disabling. Sadly, there is still no cure, but, thankfully, there is an immense amount of research taking place today that is seeking better medical treatments and potential cures. There are many different types of treatments available, ranging from over-the-counter (OTC) options to prescription-only treatments, both topical and oral. Depending on how your skin responds to the treatment, there is a very good chance you will experience improvement for extended periods of time and possibly even keep it that way.

There also are advanced medical options, such as immune-modulating drugs, but they can have long-term risks, which you should discuss with your physician. Experimenting with a variety of options will likely provide the best results, but regardless of what you decide to do, it will require regular and consistent behavior and usage.

TREATMENT OPTIONS FOR PSORIASIS

As mentioned, there are various therapies available to treat psoriasis, and our strong recommendation is to start with those that have the least-serious side effects, such as intermittent use of an OTC topical cortisone cream; vitamin D preparation, both topical and oral; retinoids; salicylic acid (BHA); and topical coal-tar creams, lotions, cleansers, and shampoos. [216,217,218,219,220]

It is important to point out that the vitamin D treatments for psoriasis, both oral and topical, are not the same as the vitamin D supplements you can buy in stores. Calcipotriene is the form of vitamin D used to treat psoriasis, and it has a very different action on skin and the body than the form of vitamin D in supplements (cholecalciferol).

Based on how your skin responds to the above treatment options, you then can decide if you want to consider higher risk treatments, such as UVB therapy. UVB therapy can involve merely exposing your skin to the sun's UVB rays (daylight) or to UVB emitting devices, or a combination therapy that involves UVB-emitting devices along with topical medications (immune-modulating medications). [221]

Keep in mind that successful treatment often requires a combination of methods. [224] Don't put off seeing a dermatologist to explore all your options. It is surprising how many people suffer with psoriasis without seeking medical options.

CHOOSING A SKINCARE ROUTINE WHEN YOU HAVE PSORIASIS

Several of the basic principles of skincare we discuss throughout this book apply when you have psoriasis. The exception is if your doctor has prescribed UVB treatment, with sunlight or with UVB therapies, in which case the UVB exposure must be carefully monitored by your physician due to its inherent risks to your health.

Overall, it is vitally important you don't do anything to irritate your skin, as this will only make matters worse. Avoiding all the things we repeatedly warn against, such as harsh cleansers, abrasive scrubs, hot water, and products with irritating ingredients, especially fragrance (both synthetic and natural), will not only improve how your skin looks and feels, but also help the other treatments you might be using work even better by aiding absorption.

Aside from a gentle, effective, and healing skincare routine, adding skincare products that contain salicylic acid or retinol (vitamin A) to your routine can be helpful in treating psoriasis.

The best skincare routines for those with psoriasis start with a gentle water-soluble cleanser followed by a skin-soothing toner. A leave-on topical salicylic acid (BHA) exfoliant comes next. [223] During the day, follow with a sunscreen, if approved by your dermatologist, and at night, your moisturizer (with or without retinol).

If you are using other topical medications, such as a vitamin D, cortisone, coal-tar, or prescription retinoid cream or lotion, apply them before your sunscreen during the day and before your moisturizer at night. If you are using prescription retinoids, use a moisturizer that does not include retinol.

HOW SALICYLIC ACID AND RETINOIDS HELP TREAT PSORIASIS

Salicylic acid is an extremely gentle exfoliant that can soften and remove the layers of scaly, thickened psoriatic lesions. Removing these layers not only improves the appearance of skin, but also allows other topical medications to better penetrate into skin.

In addition, because of salicylic acid's chemical relationship to aspirin (aspirin is acetylsalicylic acid), it has anti-inflammatory properties, which can reduce the redness associated with psoriasis. Given how salicylic acid functions, a leave-on salicylic acid–based exfoliant (2% to 6% concentration) is considered a viable skincare treatment for psoriasis.

Topical retinoids can significantly benefit psoriasis because of their ability to improve the way skin cells are formed. Prescription forms, like tretinoin Renova or tazarotene, can have impressive results for normalizing new skin cell production.

If you have psoriasis, you still must select skincare products based on your skin type—oily, combination, or dry. Especially important: You must be very careful to use only products that are free of potential irritants. (We are proud to say that Paula's Choice Skincare is one of the few truly fragrance-free, gentle skincare lines available that also has a wide range of retinol- and salicylic acid–based products.)

The battle against psoriasis is frustrating, and it will take experimentation to find the best options for your skin. Discovering what works best for you will be the result of trying one or more of the treatments we've mentioned, either alone or in combination. Experimentation takes patience, and a systematic, ongoing evaluation of how your skin is reacting and of your overall health. Successful treatment, as is true with all chronic skin disorders, requires diligent adherence to the regimen and a realistic understanding of what you can and can't expect. You also must be aware of the consequences and potential side effects of the various treatment levels.

For more information on the current status of the treatments available for psoriasis, visit the National Psoriasis Foundation (NPF) at www.psoriasis.org.

RECOMMENDED PRODUCTS FOR PSORIASIS:

Cleansers
» Neutrogena Ultra Gentle Hydrating Cleanser, Creamy Formula ($9.49)
» Paula's Choice Skin Recovery Softening Cream Cleanser ($17)
» The Body Shop Aloe Gentle Facial Wash, for Sensitive Skin ($17)

Toners
» derma e Soothing Toner with Anti-Aging Pycnogenol® ($15.50)
» MD Formulations Moisture Defense Antioxidant Spray ($28)
» Paula's Choice Resist Advanced Replenishing Toner ($23)

BHA Exfoliants
» Paula's Choice Resist Weekly Retexturizing Foaming Treatment with 4% BHA ($35)
» Paula's Choice Skin Perfecting 1% BHA Lotion ($26)
» philosophy clear days ahead oil-free salicylic acid acne treatment and moisturizer ($39)

Daytime Moisturizers with SPF
» MDSolarSciences Mineral Crème Broad Spectrum SPF 30 UVA/UVB Sunscreen ($30)
» Paula's Choice Skin Recovery Daily Moisturizing Lotion SPF 30 ($28)
» Rodan + Fields SOOTHE Mineral Sunscreen Broad Spectrum SPF 30 ($41)

Moisturizers and Serums
» Josie Maran Cosmetics Pure Argan Milk Intensive Hydrating Treatment ($56)
» Neutrogena Healthy Skin Anti-Wrinkle Cream, Night ($14.99)
» Olay Regenerist Micro-Sculpting Serum, Fragrance-Free ($23.99)
» Paula's Choice Calm Redness Relief Serum ($32)
» Paula's Choice Clinical 1% Retinol Treatment ($55)

CHAPTER 13

Botox, Fillers, Lasers, and Surgery

IS A PROCEDURE RIGHT FOR YOU?

This chapter is an overview and conversation about why cosmetic corrective procedures or surgery for the face might make sense; it is not, and not
meant to be, a comprehensive examination of all the various procedures available. We touch on what options are available, and in what combination you
may want to consider them, as you plan how to improve your appearance beyond what skincare is capable of providing (more on that in a moment). Before
we start sharing details, it's critical for you to understand that any one procedure never can do it all, just as any one skincare product cannot do it all. Even
a face-lift addresses only some of the things that make a face look older—the
procedure is not a cure-all for everything that causes skin to change because
of time and cumulative damage.

To be clear: Here at Paula's Choice, we are neither for nor against cosmetic
surgery or cosmetic corrective procedures. What we are always for is knowing
the facts—both the pros and the cons—rather than relying on the overhyped
promises made by some of those less-than-scrupulous cosmetic surgeons and
cosmetic dermatologists. (Unfortunately, some physicians and their assistants can hard sell their services and downplay the risks, just like salespersons
in other areas.) The only way to ensure you know what you are getting and
what you'll end up with is to have unbiased information and realistic expectations—and that information should be from multiple sources, not only from a
physician or a health care provider. You have homework to do, too!

DID SHE OR DIDN'T SHE?

In the world of beauty, nothing stirs up as much controversy as the topics
of cosmetic surgery and cosmetic corrective procedures. Everything, from Bo-

tox to dermal fillers and face-lifts, are claimed to plump up lines and thinning lips, eliminate forehead wrinkles, remove brown spots, tighten a sagging jaw line, and lift up sagging breasts; and others to cut away a flabby tummy or suck out fat with liposuction, and on and on.

Much of the debate about these procedures and surgeries revolves around celebrities, some of whom have distorted their faces and bodies by having so much "work" done. They have become little more than caricatures of themselves by cutting, pasting, filling, and Botox-ing their faces and bodies to the point of absurdity. Guessing and gossiping about who's had what done has become a popular pastime for lots of people.

A far more serious aspect of cosmetic corrective procedures and cosmetic surgery are the risks associated with these procedures. Taking such risks, some of which are significant, for the sake of beauty is understandably controversial. And being impulsive or uninformed about the risks of beauty enhancement is as shortsighted as dismissing them with disdainful judgment.

Beauty, and the desire to look young, is hardly novel. And nowadays, that desire to look young is starting at younger and younger ages, with many people in their 30s already undergoing a full menu of procedures. We all think about it to some extent, and probably act on it, at least to one degree or another. For example, even dyeing your hair to get rid of the gray or spending $200 on a wrinkle cream are attempts to look younger. The question that anyone who wants to look younger must answer for themselves is: What am I willing to do, and how much am I willing to spend, to look and feel more beautiful—what makes sense for me? Once you've determined how far you're willing to go, the next step is to be sure you have a thorough understanding of what works and what doesn't, then what procedures to consider and, finally, in what sequence do you want them—which can come down to your age and your expectations.

WHEN SKINCARE ISN'T ENOUGH

We here at Paula's Choice are the last people in the world to suggest that skincare can't do amazing things for skin, because it can. But it would be disingenuous of us to say that skincare can replace what cosmetic medical procedures or cosmetic surgery can do. Anyone who says otherwise is simply not telling the truth.

Skincare products that claim to work like cosmetic surgery, or Botox, or fillers, or lasers are making ridiculous, unsupportable claims. A comprehensive skincare routine with well-formulated skincare products (it always takes more than one product) can make a huge difference in the appearance of your skin, but it simply cannot come close to what cosmetic medical procedures or cosmetic surgery can do—it just isn't possible. The effects of aging, sun damage, gravity, genetics, and hormone loss due to menopause or health issues, among many other factors, cannot be erased by skincare products. Believe us, we wish we could say otherwise, but we don't want to mislead or delude you in any way.

It's also true that cosmetic corrective procedures and cosmetic surgery have limitations. Just because you've had dermal injections, Botox, and a face-lift doesn't in any way, shape, or form replace what great skincare products can provide going forward in life. You will still age, you will continue to sag and wrinkle, and brown discolorations will return. But, a brilliant skincare routine can slow that process, and help to maintain the results you get from medical procedures!

It's the combination of a great skincare routine complemented by the procedures that cosmetic dermatologists or cosmetic surgeons can provide that will give you the results many skincare ads allude to. It's important for everyone to realize the limitations of skincare as well as the limitations of corrective procedures and surgery—and to understand that one cannot replace the other.

Although it might seem as if cosmetic corrective procedures and cosmetic surgery are expensive, they don't have to be! In fact, if you take all the money you'd normally spend on overpriced skincare products (with rare exceptions, products over $80 are not providing value for the money), and put it in the bank, you may very well have enough money to invest in cosmetic procedures or surgery sooner than you think—and likely be more satisfied with the outcome!

WHAT ABOUT JUST AGING GRACEFULLY?

On the flipside of those who opt for cosmetic corrective procedures or cosmetic surgery are those who say we should just choose to "age gracefully." Rather than procedures or skincare products, focus instead on being healthy and don't bother trying to erase any signs of aging on our faces or bodies.

Without question, being healthy is fundamental to looking and staying beautiful regardless of your age, but whether you're pro- or anti-cosmetic surgery, the truth is that a combination of great skincare + cosmetic procedures can produce outstanding results. Procedures have their risks, yes, but there's no denying that they work. It's a personal choice, but if you decide to actually do something in the realm of medical cosmetic procedures or surgery, don't feel guilty or embarrassed—feel empowered!

In reality, lasers, Botox, fillers, and cosmetic surgery are the only ways to actually take years off your appearance between the ages of 40 and 70 (or before that, depending on the amount of sun damage you have). Skincare alone won't cut it (pun intended), and hoping that it would will just be a waste of your money—which could be better spent elsewhere.

As we've said, even the best skincare routines and products have limitations, but after a certain amount of time, it's the combination of a brilliant skincare routine coupled with surgical or corrective procedures that is the most realistic solution to looking younger, longer.

THE FEAR FACTOR

Not having some "fear" about cosmetic corrective procedures would be unwise, but being overly afraid is not necessarily wise either. If you're considering procedures or surgery, we think it's best to refer to this fear factor as "constructive concern," which can take some of the fear out of the process.

Having constructive concerns is helpful, and encourages you to be proactive in finding the right surgeon (not just automatically going with the first one you talk to), understanding before you make your appointment what sorts of procedures you're interested in, and to really know what your budget is or should be. (**Note:** Looking for a bargain in the realm of surgery or procedures is a *really* bad idea.)

When you finally do book your appointment, those constructive concerns mean you will be better prepared with questions about the risks of the procedures you're considering. Asking for the pros and cons and insisting the doctor not downplay the cons is all part of having constructive concerns. **The most important thing to remember is that getting answers for your concerns is part of being a great patient and getting the best results.**

One way to approach this objectively is to realize how many of these types of procedures are performed each year. Each year, millions of people in the United States alone have chosen to have cosmetic surgery or cosmetic corrective procedures. According to the American Society of Plastic Surgeons, the top five cosmetic surgery procedures in 2014 were: breast augmentation and breast lifts (386,000 procedures); nose reshaping (221,000 procedures); liposuction (200,000 procedures); and face-lifts (133,000 procedures). The top five cosmetic corrective procedures in 2014 were: Botox (6.3 million injections); dermal fillers (2.2 million procedures); and chemical peels (1.2 million procedures). If you're considering an elective procedure, you're not alone—many people have gone where you're thinking of going. The following information should help set you on the right path to getting the information you need to make an informed decision.

COSMETIC SURGEON OR PLASTIC SURGEON?

In the world of surgery, the terms *cosmetic* surgery and *plastic* or *reconstructive* surgery are often used interchangeably, but they are absolutely not the same. *Cosmetic* surgery is elective; it's performed to improve the physical cosmetic appearance of the face or body. *Plastic* or *reconstructive* surgery is a surgical procedure used to reconstruct facial or body defects due to genetic abnormalities, trauma, burns, or disease.

The training of a board-certified cosmetic surgeon and of a board-certified plastic surgeon differ significantly. A board-certified cosmetic surgeon's training is all about cosmetic surgery, while a board-certified plastic surgeon's training is only in part about cosmetic surgery. So, if a board-certified plastic surgeon is also a board-certified cosmetic surgeon, that individual is thoroughly trained in all aspects of the types of surgery that alter and improve the face and body, regardless of the cause or need. That combined training could mean that person has a superlative set of skills. Nonetheless, when considering surgery for your appearance, the most important thing to realize is that a board-certified cosmetic surgeon is the most important credential to look for because that encompasses the extensive specialized training needed for elective cosmetic procedures.

Both cosmetic and plastic surgeons can perform and are trained in an extensive array of procedures, ranging from invasive procedures (meaning surgery) to non-invasive procedures (meaning Botox and dermal fillers). Some would argue that surgeons should stick to invasive surgeries such as face-lifts and eye-lifts (blepharoplasty) and that cosmetic dermatologists should be sought for fillers, Botox, and laser procedures. There's no right answer to this one. However, what is 1000% true is that if you are having any kind of cosmetic surgery, the doctor you choose must be a board-certified cosmetic surgeon or board-certified plastic surgeon—and it's even better if he or she has both certifications.

BOARD-CERTIFIED SURGEONS—THE GOLD STANDARD

The difference between just any physician performing cosmetic or plastic surgery and a board-certified cosmetic or plastic surgeon performing the surgery is night and day! Training and credentials in surgery are the issues. Although a doctor may offer cosmetic, plastic, or aesthetic surgery, he or she may not be board-certified to perform that type of surgery. The person could be a gynecologist, pediatrician, or dermatologist with no training in cosmetic surgery whatsoever. Scary, huh?

Board-certified means the doctor has gone through very specific and extensive training in a specialized field and has passed a difficult examination administered by a board of experts in that field. A cosmetic or plastic surgeon who is not board certified may be self-taught, and may lack formal training in that field.

Why would anyone want cosmetic corrective surgery performed by someone who has never had any formal cosmetic surgery training? The answer is: You don't! At least not if you want the best possible outcome, which is why opting for a board-certified cosmetic or plastic surgeon is so important. We cannot stress that point enough.

One clear distinction that sets board-certified surgeons apart is that they have privileges to perform surgery at an accredited hospital. Although most cosmetic surgery procedures are performed in a doctor's office, you want to be assured that your surgeon has a level of skill that's accepted by an accredited hospital.

It's completely fair (and not the least bit rude) to ask any doctor you see for a cosmetic surgery consultation whether he or she is board certified, and, if so, which hospitals he or she is affiliated with. But that's not the end of it! With that information in hand, the onus is on you to check to be sure the hospital is accredited and that the doctor's certification is current and recognized by the appropriate board. For more information, visit the following websites.

» American Board of Cosmetic Surgery at
   www.americanboardcosmeticsurgery.org
» American Board of Plastic Surgery at www.abplsurg.org
» American Board of Medical Specialties at www.abms.org

Finding out first if the physician you are considering is board certified significantly reduces the odds of your getting someone who is inexperienced.

Although this section is about cosmetic surgery and board-certified cosmetic or plastic surgeons, it's important to realize that a board-certified dermatologist, even one trained to perform dermatologic surgery, does not have a certification that qualifies that doctor to perform cosmetic corrective surgery. Finding a board-certified dermatologist is vitally important for any cosmetic *corrective* procedures you are considering, but it is not enough for cosmetic *surgery* procedures.

COSMETIC DERMATOLOGIST OR MEDICAL DERMATOLOGIST

Similar to the confusion between a cosmetic surgeon and a plastic surgeon, there is equal confusion between the roles of a cosmetic dermatologist and the role of a medical dermatologist. The term medical dermatologist is the exact same thing as having the title dermatologist, but the term medical dermatologist is often used to make the distinction between the two relatively less confusing.

Unlike cosmetic surgery and plastic surgery, which are different, there is no such delineation between cosmetic dermatology and medical dermatology; they are indistinguishable. Ultimately, what that means is that medical dermatologists can call themselves cosmetic dermatologists, even if they have no special training or qualification, and they may choose their title based on the services they wish to offer. In other words, there is no specified certification that medical dermatologists must have to call themselves cosmetic dermatologists.

In many ways, the only real distinction between a cosmetic dermatologist and a medical dermatologist is financial (which we realize is a controversial statement that no doubt will raise the ire of many dermatologists, but it's a well-known and ongoing debate within the world of dermatology). Using the title cosmetic dermatologist is simply a way to indicate that a doctor's practice is mostly about elective procedures, such as Botox, dermal fillers, lasers, peels, light treatments, and the like. It also indicates that their services are primarily pay in advance, which means the doctor has far fewer insurance forms to fill out and there is no wrangling over how much to charge for a procedure.

Medical dermatologists, on the other hand, generally provide traditional therapies to treat skin disease, and then must wait for reimbursement from managed-care plans. This doesn't mean that medical dermatologists who don't refer to themselves as cosmetic dermatologists can't perform cosmetic corrective procedures, because they can and often do. The title medical dermatologist merely indicates the area in which the doctor chooses to focus: skin disease and disorders rather than cosmetic beautification.

So what does that all mean for you? It means it's a bit harder to determine what to look for when choosing a doctor to perform cosmetic corrective procedures because the only certification on the wall could be dermatology, and maybe some formal-looking "degrees" indicating training in specific procedures. In summary, there is no certification for cosmetic dermatology on the wall because such a certification does not exist.

Our personal recommendation: Find a board-certified dermatologist who describes his or her practice and/or themselves as cosmetic dermatology. That at least gives you some information about what you can expect when making an appointment; the doctor performs cosmetic corrective procedures more often than he or she treats skin disease. If your doctor frequently performs the procedures you want it means the doctor has at least some amount of experience in that area—and in the world of medicine, experience is everything, especially when it comes to beauty.

We also strongly suggest that you never have your dentist or gynecologist perform any cosmetic corrective procedure for you. [224] As shocking as it might seem, many physicians who are not board-certified dermatologists or cosmetic surgeons can also legally perform procedures. Although it might be hard to resist because it seems so convenient, cosmetic corrective procedures require extensive medical education, training, and experience in this very specialized field. Just because a dentist knows what to do when you open your mouth doesn't mean he or she has the extensive medical education and training needed to perform cosmetic corrective procedures. Do we even need to mention that getting cosmetic corrective procedures from your hairdresser is also a very bad idea?!

WHEN TO DO IT

In the not-too-distant past, most people waited until they were in their late 50s or 60s, and until their skin had noticeably aged, before they seriously considered cosmetic corrective procedures or surgery. All that has changed with the advent of relatively non-invasive, low-cost procedures such as laser resurfacing, Botox, and dermal fillers, as well as new and more advanced surgical techniques that leave barely noticeable scars.

Having procedures performed at a younger age, before you "need it," means having healthier, younger-looking skin continually for years, as opposed to having it done after you've begun to show signs of aging, which means there will be an abrupt change in your appearance. From our point of view, it doesn't make sense to wait until your skin is drooping and leathery before you do something about it. Think of it like waiting to quit smoking until your doctor breaks the bad news that you have lung cancer, instead of quitting years ago.

If your friends and family say you don't need surgery or a procedure yet, but there's something about how you're aging that bothers you (and is beyond the reach of a great skincare routine), then it's better to do something about it sooner rather than later. It's *your* face and neck, and *your* decision! And do you really want to wait until your friends and family begin saying you're looking old these days and you really should do something about it? Plus, having procedures or cosmetic surgery at a relatively younger age slows the way the skin will age, and when we're younger our skin is better able to heal. In short, the right time is when *you* are ready, based on your own feelings and finances.

Despite our strong recommendation that only you can determine when to start having cosmetic corrective procedures or surgery, it's also important to listen to your family and friends, especially if they start saying that you're distorting your appearance. You don't want to ever be a makeover nightmare, especially when it's a makeover you can't undo.

WHICH PROCEDURES ARE RIGHT FOR ME?

Probably the most fundamental question people ask when considering the vast assortment of cosmetic corrective and cosmetic surgery procedures is this: Which procedures are right for me? The number of ways the different procedures can be combined are truly mindboggling, so we understand the confusion. The simple answer: The choices depend on what you want to achieve and on your doctor's recommendation.

Perhaps the most difficult and discouraging part of all is to realize that no single cosmetic corrective procedure or surgery can do it all. Botox does not replace what dermal fillers can do, lasers do not replace what fillers or Botox can do, and surgery does not replace what fillers, Botox, or lasers can do. There can be some overlap of benefits depending on how much damage you've suffered or on how advanced the signs of aging are, but for the most part a little bit of each type of procedure, spaced out over a reasonable amount of time, will achieve the best results without looking overdone. For some people, especially if you are under the age of 40, one procedure may be all you need for a period of time to get the results you want—but nothing lasts forever. Overall, the less you are trying to correct, the fewer procedures you need to consider.

Another complication is that physicians often don't use the same machines, injections, peels, and surgical techniques available. There are literally hundreds for them to consider, receive training on, and then purchase. Given a doctor's investment in the equipment and in the training, each has his or her own favorites or the ones where they have the most skill. (**Remember:** There isn't time to receive training in or become an expert on everything.)

It's also important to realize that each physician has his or her own biases and sales pitch for the procedures they offer. That doesn't have to be bad; it's just that you need to know that a physician may recommend a specific type of laser or light machine or specific type of dermal filler over another because that's what he or she has available in the office. It's unlikely that a physician is going to tell you that there's a doctor next door or down the block who has a machine or injectable material that's better for you.

Before you even begin perusing our list of procedures and surgeries or begin your Google search, keep in mind that it isn't over until it's over. First, no procedure—surgical, invasive (deep ablative laser resurfacing), or non-invasive (Botox, dermal fillers, non-ablative lasers)—lasts forever. For example, Botox and some dermal fillers last no more than six months or a year. And, just having a procedure, or even several, doesn't mean you're going to stop aging. To maintain your results, you must have an ongoing plan of carefully selected procedures over your lifetime. You don't *have* to do any of it, but it's important to know that that is what it will take to keep up appearances and deal with further signs of aging with the passage of time.

Of course, if you don't use brilliant skincare products, including sunscreen unfailingly to fight off aging from UV light exposure and environmental damage, you will continue to age faster than you need to. Cosmetic corrective procedures of any kind do not in any way replace an exceptional skincare routine and daily, broad-spectrum sun protection.

OVERVIEW OF PROCEDURES

Following is an overview of what to consider when trying to understand your options for cosmetic corrective procedures and surgery for the face. Hold on to your hats—this is where it gets really complicated! Your doctor will have much to say about what to select to meet your specific needs and desires, but because doctors have only so much time to spend with you and because they often will oversell what they have to offer, you must be prepared with your questions and must do some preliminary research (this book will help).

Please note: In the list of procedures and surgeries below, we do not list specific lasers, intense-pulsed-light (IPL), radiofrequency, or ultrasound machines because there are just too many out there. Adding to the complexity, different types of lasers often are combined into one machine and new machines are being launched all the time. There also are numerous variations of modality, wavelengths, intensity, and brand names, making it impossible for consumers, even if they do extensive research, to follow. Even doctors find it difficult, if not impossible, to keep up, as we've been told by many a cosmetic dermatologist!

We start our list with Botox because it's the most popular cosmetic corrective procedure in the world.

Botox and Dysport are both drugs derived from the botulinum toxin Type A. Both are injected into various points on the face to temporarily paralyze specific facial muscles, which in turn erases lines almost immediately.

Although this sounds like a radical procedure, Botox has been in use since 1973 and has a long history of safety and effectiveness. [225,226]

Botox and Dysport, made by different companies, have been found to be equally effective, with very little difference. Both are used to eliminate horizontal lines on the forehead, to reduce or possibly eliminate the "11" lines between the brows (known as glabellar lines), and to reduce crow's feet by the eyes. [227] Some doctors also use Botox to lift the marionette lines (oral commissures) at the corners of the mouth, on the chin to reduce the "orange peel" look, to reduce puffiness under the eye area, to create an eye-lift appearance by injecting in areas above the brow, to reduce some deeper vertical lines around the mouth, and to soften the banding that can occur on the neck. The effects of Botox and Dysport can last for up to six months or a bit longer, and then begin to wear off.

Many people get both Botox and dermal fillers because the combination can produce a remarkably younger-looking face, but they do so in very different manners. Although both procedures involve injections, Botox is most often injected around the forehead and in wrinkles around the eyes to stop the muscle movements that lead to wrinkles (sometimes referred to as expression lines). Botox and Dysport injections have nothing to do with the plumping, smoothing effect of dermal fillers.

Dermal fillers are various kinds of injectable materials, either naturally derived or synthetic (including brand name fillers like Bellafill, Belotero Balance, Juvéderm, Perlane, Radiesse, Restylane, Sculptra Aesthetic, and Zyderm), that are suitable for and approved to be injected into the skin; some are better for specific needs or for specific areas of the face. [228] Dermal fillers have a very specific function that is unrelated to other medical corrective procedures. Dermal fillers are used to plump up deep creases that run from the nose to the mouth (called nasolabial folds or laugh lines), to plump thin lips and smooth out vertical lines around the edges of the lips, to augment the cheeks to improve their shape, to fill out depressions under the eye area, to fill in depressed scars such as from acne or chicken pox, and to add volume to a gaunt look in the lower cheek or temple area, which most often occurs due to fat pads shifting beneath the surface of skin. Depending on the filler, the effects can last from six months to two years; for semi-permanent or permanent fillers, the effects can last up to five years, and there are reports of even longer-lasting results.

Laser is an acronym for Light Amplification by Stimulated Emission of Radiation. There are many forms of lasers and there is no single best one (wouldn't it be nice if there were?). Depending on your needs and concerns, you might need more than one laser to achieve the best overall results. The following overview of lasers will highlight the different categories of lasers and what they can do.

Ablative lasers (also called ablative non-fractionated lasers), including the CO2 laser and Er:Yag laser, work in a very precise manner to destroy the entire top layers of skin with intense heat. This results in a deep wound over the treated areas that lead to the formation of relatively thick scabs, which eventually heal, revealing new skin. Ablative lasers are used to deeply resurface skin on the face, neck, or chest, removing sun damage, greatly smoothing skin's texture, improving skin tone, tightening skin, building collagen, and, to some degree, improving the appearance of wrinkles, scars, and brown discolorations. Of all the laser and light modalities available, ablative lasers produce the most dramatic and immediate results; however, they also have more serious risks. [229]

Ablative fractional lasers have results similar to those of ablative non-fractionated lasers, but work in a different, and relatively less invasive, manner. Where ablative lasers target the entire surface of the area being treated with deep, intense heat, ablative fractional lasers deliver deep, intense heat into the skin via thousands of tiny pixilated dots. The area around the dots remains unwounded, so healing time is considerably less than for ablative lasers, where the entire area of skin being treated is "wounded." Ablative fractional lasers work well to reduce the appearance of wrinkles and brown skin discolorations, and to produce a smoother skin texture. [230]

Non-ablative lasers (also called non-ablative nonfractionated lasers) can treat many aspects of skin rejuvenation without requiring much, if any, downtime because they do not put out as much heat as ablative lasers and thus rarely wound skin. Overall, depending on the machine and its settings, non-ablative lasers can reduce brown spots, surfaced capillaries, and redness from rosacea or post-acne marks, build collagen, tighten skin, improve skin texture, and, to varying degrees, improve scarring.

Non-ablative fractional lasers are said to combine the best of the relatively more gentle and safer aspects of both ablative and non-ablative laser technologies. [231] Non-ablative fractional lasers deliver a high degree of heat, similar to, but not as strong as, ablative lasers, to the skin in tiny pixelated areas (think of a grid). While hundreds of tiny areas of skin are vaporized, as they are with traditional ablative lasers, there is a difference in that the entire surface of skin is not wounded, which makes recovery much faster. [232] The trade-off is that this type of laser procedure often requires multiple treatments to achieve the desired results. They can work very well for mild skin tightening (think first signs of sagging), some collagen rebuilding, mild to moderate wrinkles, improving sun-damaged skin, some types of scarring, and various skin discolorations. [233]

Intense pulsed light (IPL, also referred to as a photofacial or photorejuvenation) is a type of non-ablative laser that emits multiple wavelengths and intensities of light that can be targeted to "zap" red blood cells in surfaced capillaries or the brown color (melanin) in sun-damaged spots. The results can be relatively immediate, but depending on the number of brown spots or surfaced capillaries and on the degree of redness, three to five treatments may be necessary, and the treated areas may worsen before they improve. When IPLs are used for overall "photorejuvenation" to reduce wrinkles and tighten skin, it definitely requires three to five treatments, usually once every three to six weeks. [234,235] The amount of improvement obtained from IPLs in regard to rejuvenation is considered impressive, although not as dramatic as the improvement from ablative fractional or non-fractionated lasers. [236,237,238]

Radio-frequency (RF) machines work on the same principle as lasers, except that the heat is delivered via RF waves rather than light waves. The two most well-known RF devices are Thermage and Pellevé. RF machines improve some amount of sagging skin, smooth out stretch marks, and tighten other areas of loose skin. Like non-ablative lasers, RF machines can require multiple treatments to achieve optimal results. [239,240,241]

Microfocused ultrasound is performed using a machine called Ultherapy, which works differently from all other forms of lasers and RF devices in that it uses ultrasound energy to generate heat in the skin. The heat from lasers and RF devices targets the surface layers of skin, but Ultherapy bypasses the surface layers and delivers heat to the deepest layers of skin, directly targeting and stimulating collagen production. The primary use of Ultherapy is for skin tightening and for mild to moderate sagging, and the results are considered impressive. Ultherapy is considered one of the more painful non-invasive treatments. You should discuss your pain tolerance levels and medications with your physician before having the procedure. [242,243,244]

Chemical peels are a way to resurface the top to the deeper layers of skin to improve the appearance of wrinkles, make skin smoother, tighten skin, and reduce skin discolorations. Lighter chemical peels have a temporary smoothing effect that can last from a few days to two weeks. Results from deeper peels can last from several months to one or two years. There are various types of peel solutions used in these treatments, including glycolic or lactic acid (AHAs), salicylic acid (BHA), or trichloroacetic acid (TCA).

Superficial peels, often referred to as lunchtime peels, use low concentrations of glycolic, lactic, or salicylic acid and act relatively gently to quickly improve skin texture, minor skin discolorations, and wrinkles. They can minimally tighten skin and improve the appearance of acne scars.

Medium-depth peels use the same acids as superficial peels to exfoliate past the superficial layers of skin into the middle layers of skin for more pronounced results. Medium-depth peels have the same overall impact as superficial peels, but with far more noticeable and longer-lasting results.

Deeper peels almost always involve trichloroacetic acid (TCA), which penetrates into the deeper layers of skin. This enhanced penetration provides far more and longer-lasting improvement than superficial or medium-depth peels. Not surprisingly, the recovery time and risks for deeper peels increases as the penetrating depth of the peel increases.

Face-lift, technically called an upper rhytidectomy, and **neck-lift**, technically called lower rhytidectomy, are fairly straightforward and are almost always done at the same time. They're perfect if you have extreme sagging skin at the jaw, neck, under the chin, or middle area of the face, or if you need to improve facial contours. A skilled, board-certified cosmetic or plastic surgeon should perform face-lifts and neck-lifts. The surgeon deftly cuts away just enough excess skin to make the face look younger without over-pulling and removing too much skin, which can create a distorted appearance.

During the surgery, the doctor also tightens the muscles under the skin, repositions or adds to the fat layer of skin, and then stitches everything back together again. Incisions are hidden along the inside of the ear, back of the ear, and along the back of the neck at the hairline. Depending on the amount of sagging, surgery might be the only option that makes sense.

Lasers and other types of machine-oriented or injectable procedures can tighten and restore volume to skin, some rather dramatically, but if you've waited too long and have pronounced fallen skin, corrective procedures might be a waste of your money, when a face-lift could produce the desired results in one fell swoop—albeit one with a much longer and more involved recovery time.

Eye-lift or eye tuck, technically blepharoplasty, is a surgical procedure performed either on the upper eyelid or the area under the eye. It's a perfect procedure for removing excess fatty deposits that appear as puffiness around the eyes, bags under the eyes, drooping lower eyelids, and wrinkles around the eye. It's the same basic process as a face-lift, but performed as an eye-lift: Excess skin is cut away, muscles are tightened, fat pads are either reduced or repositioned, and then everything is stitched back together.

A skilled surgeon will hide the incision for the lower eye-lift on the inside portion of the lower eyelid or directly along the lash line in such a way that it's almost imperceptible after healing. For the upper eyelid, the incision is carefully placed in the crease of the eye, and also barely perceptible after healing.

Whether you want to improve the appearance around your eyes or you're experiencing functional problems (such as reduced vision) with your eyelids, an eye-lift can be a stunning success. If the problems are with the functional aspects of the eye that may require surgery, they are often covered by your health insurance.

Forehead lift or brow lift is surgery performed to minimize or eliminate horizontal forehead lines and wrinkles, raise drooping brows, and open the eye area by lifting sagging skin on the upper eyelids. There are various forehead lift procedures, the different ones involve the surgeon making different length incisions in different locations along the scalp or hairline. A variation of this procedure, known as an **endoscopic forehead lift**, is intriguing because it's minimally invasive. This procedure uses an endoscope (a threadlike tube with a tiny camera on the end) along with specialized surgical instruments placed through very small incisions directly at the hairline. By looking at a screen, the endoscopic camera shows the surgeon where to adjust fat pads, reposition skin, and tighten muscles. Now that's a great surgical assistant!

Another type of forehead lift is a **coronal incision forehead lift**. This procedure is performed by creating an incision ear to ear across the top of the head about one to two inches behind the hairline. The forehead skin is then lifted and cut away at the incision line, making it possible to adjust muscles or fat pads with everything revealed (unlike the endoscopic technique, which, despite its cool factor, limits the doctor's overall view of the area).

The resulting scar from a coronal brow lift is well concealed within the hair, and when the hair grows back the scar is not visible, assuming you have enough hair growth to hide the scar. Either type of brow lift is perfect to improve a sagging or furrowed forehead, sagging brows, or upper eyelid, as well as to improve the shape of the forehead.

Chin augmentation, technically genioplasty or mentoplasty, is a surgery that involves inserting an implant into the chin area to improve the structure and appearance of the jaw and chin area. The implant material can be harvested from bone from the patient's body or from donor bone.

Ear surgery, technically otoplasty, is typically performed to "pin back" naturally protruding ears or to lift sagging ear lobes, which are often caused by years of wearing heavy earrings, although it might be a genetic feature for that individual. While ear surgery is not a popular procedure, it can be performed at the same time as a face-lift to improve the overall appearance and symmetry of the face.

Rhinoplasty, often referred to as a nose job, involves surgery to reshape and restructure the nose. The procedure typically is performed through incisions on the inside of the nose, so the scars won't be visible after healing. A skilled surgeon then remakes or reshapes the bone and cartilage of the nose by removing the cartilage that is not needed and then adding or rearranging the bone and cartilage to create a newly shaped proboscis (nose).

WHAT CAN GO WRONG

In short—everything can go wrong, or nothing can go wrong. Each procedure comes with its own risks and rewards. It turns out that there are far more positive results with any cosmetic corrective procedure or surgery than there are negative outcomes. In fact, negative outcomes are relatively rare, ranging from 1% to 5% depending on what you have done.

The rewards are obvious once recovery is complete; when you look in the mirror, you will look younger and likely see yourself as more beautiful. However, it's not a good idea to ignore the potential negatives; in the world of cosmetic corrective procedures, ignorance is not bliss!

The risks we describe in the following section sound pretty dire, but keep it in perspective and remember that, statistically, the positives far outpace the negatives, and sometimes there are no negatives. We also don't want you to base your decision about cosmetic corrective or surgical procedures on headline horror stories, which are all over the Internet and in the media. There are, indeed, rare horrendous outcomes, often due to an unqualified doctor performing the procedure and botching the work. There also are people, fortunately only a small minority, who become addicted to procedures, having things done repeatedly to their face. Unfortunately, their skin and the underlying structures can take only so much, and eventually they start looking plastic, distorted, and peculiar.

Following is a basic list of things to keep in mind when considering the types of medical treatments we discuss throughout this chapter. We do not mean to scare you, but these are the facts and the risks you must consider before booking your appointment.

The overarching risk for all procedures is being disappointed with the results. It might be that it wasn't worth the cost, that no real improvement was seen, that the pain was overwhelming, that the face seems now to have an uneven or distorted appearance, that skin discoloration or an unwanted texture to the skin appeared, or that the scarring takes too long to heal or heals in a ropey or raised manner— those are all possibilities.

As a general rule, the more invasive the procedure, such as a deep laser treatment or surgery, the higher the risk of complications and pain during recovery. The less invasive the procedure, the lower the risk of problems. However, pain is always a risk, and it varies from person to person and procedure to procedure.

Cosmetic or plastic surgeries—face-lifts, neck-lifts, eye-lifts, forehead lifts, and nose jobs—have a scary list of complications, so brace yourself! This is surgery, and there's a lot involved when you cut into skin and stitch it back together, no matter how superficial or deep the surgeon goes. Typical problems are scars that don't heal well, becoming ropey or thick; a numbing sensation that can last for a long period, or that doesn't ever go away; a feeling of tightness that lingers or doesn't go away; and pain in the area of the incision or surrounding area, which also can linger or never go away. Scars can be improved with different treatments or procedures, but the numbing and tightness that persists is not easily, if ever, resolved.

For cosmetic or plastic surgeries that require anesthesia or sedation, there are potentially serious risks, involving allergic reactions or breathing problems, and you should thoroughly discuss these with the anesthesiologist well in advance of the procedure—not wait until the day of the operation!

Bruising and blood loss during and after cosmetic surgery is considered normal, but excessive and continuing blood loss, especially once you're back home, is not normal and requires immediate medical attention. Don't wait—call the doctor!

There's also the possibility of infection, which is a risk after any type of surgery. Any sign of infection must be dealt with immediately because if left untreated, it can quickly spread and cause serious complications. If a severe infection does occur, additional procedures or surgery may be needed to remove the dead skin that can build up around or along the area of the incision.

A strange, and fortunately rare, negative outcome of eye-lifts is something called ptosis. This appears as unwanted sagging and drooping of the eyelid post-procedure, and can be corrected with additional surgery.

Depending on the extent of the surgery and the amount of correction needed, the list of potential disappointments can increase considerably. That's why you should discuss every potential side effect with your surgeon before you agree to have a cosmetic surgical procedure.

For **dermal fillers**, the most common issues are initial discomfort that lingers or temporary swelling or bruising that lingers. Fillers can also result in cysts, bumps, lumps (called nodules), skin irregularities, and/or inflamed tissue that persist, even with semi-permanent fillers. Allergic reactions can happen, but are rare. If you tend to get cold sores, dermal fillers can trigger a new breakout. Infection also can result, but it's extremely rare and easily treated. Not surprisingly, the most typical complaints about dermal fillers involve the results of the procedure.

Problems such as poor or inaccurate placement, unevenness, and overfilling the area are not unusual. Skilled doctors can correct some of these complications; for shorter term fillers, you just have to be patient and wait for the filler to dissipate as it is absorbed by your body. If hyaluronic acid–based fillers are used, errors sometimes can be corrected by injecting an enzyme into the affected area, which breaks down the material without causing any further problems.

Botox and Dysport have the most interesting potential downsides because of how they impact the muscles of the face. As mentioned in the previous section, most injections of Botox or Dysport are to treat lines and wrinkles on the forehead, including between the eyebrows. When done right, they definitely get rid of wrinkles, but can also result in what some people think looks like a stiff, immovable, and expressionless appearance. It's a trade-off that you must decide whether it's right for you.

The "Spock Effect" occurs when one or both eyebrows become overly arched and elevated, causing a surprised, unnatural appearance. If the doctor or practitioner doing the injections knows what he or she is doing, this is easily correctible with one or two expertly placed injections.

Eyelid or facial ptosis (drooping) occurs only rarely, but there are reported cases, and this is the most serious and obviously undesirable risk—and one more reason you want to ensure that the person doing the injection is well trained and experienced. There are prescription drops that will temporarily help counter the drooping until the effects of the Botox are gone; it takes about three to six months for most people.

In attempting to smooth the entire face, especially around the mouth, doctors and practitioners can get carried away and inject areas of the face that are probably best left alone. This is especially noticeable around the mouth and cheeks, where the procedures can lead to a flat smile as opposed to one that turns up. It can smooth out the wrinkles, but the overall appearance can be a negative for some people.

Developing "bunny lines" on the sides and the top area of the nose is a curious side effect of Botox and Dysport injections. Although these injections prevent muscle movement of the forehead and eyebrows, they don't stop the face's natural autonomic response to raise or furrow the forehead or eyebrows.

The face responds to these attempted movements by engaging and eventually overusing other muscles, resulting in bunny lines.

Minor discomfort and bruising often occur from the injections, but usually resolve quickly; pain during the procedure is typically minimal and easily avoided by applying a topical numbing cream pre-injection.

Depending on where you have the injections, some extremely rare, but possible, side effects include dizziness, difficulty swallowing, headaches (although Botox also has been used to reduce migraines), eye irritation, reduced blinking, and muscle weakness.

IPLs (intense pulsed light) and non-ablative lasers present the lowest risk of negative side effects, but they also have less dramatic results. The unwanted side effects can be pigment problems, ranging from reddened or purplish discoloration (known as purpura) to lighter patches of skin (hypopigmentation) in people with medium to darker skin tones or when the procedures are done on people who have tans.

Infections from IPL are rare. They occur primarily when the treatment is used around the mouth for hair removal, to reduce redness, or to improve collagen formation because the heat generated by the IPL can stimulate a dormant infection such as the herpes simplex virus.

A few minor transient problems can be a sunburn type of reaction, where the skin either feels hot or looks burnt. Swelling and bruising is possible, but again, almost always resolves quickly. As for pain, the sensation from each pulse (and there will be over a dozen pulses during each treatment) is most often described as similar to snapping a rubber band against your skin—more a discomfort than truly painful.

Ablative lasers have a far more scary list of side effects than IPLs because the depth of the treatment is greater and the manner in which skin is wounded is more serious. The deeper the resurfacing, the more severe the side effects. Immediately after ablative laser resurfacing, one can experience itching, swelling, redness, weeping skin, blisters, redness, acne, rashes, infection, changes in skin color (either lighter or darker than normal), and severe peeling, which can last for several days. Ablative laser resurfacing also poses a risk (although rare) of permanent scarring. If the resurfacing is around the eye area, a condition called ectropion can occur. Ectropion is where the lower eyelid and sometimes the upper eyelid turn outward, leaving the inner eyelid surface exposed, causing a strange look around the eye. Ectropion can be corrected with surgery, but it also can be prevented in the first place if the doctor takes precautions to stitch the back corner in such a way that it prevents it from occurring. (Paula's surgeon took this precaution when she had her ablative laser resurfacing.)

Finally, if you see any signs of infection, or if any of the other conditions persist, you must see your physician immediately.

Chemical peels have risks that vary with the type of peel. Superficial peels present minor risks, including redness, irritation, flaking, dryness, and, rarely, blistering for one day up to a week. Medium-depth peels have similar risks, but the intensity of the side effects increases and the length of time it takes to heal can be at least a week, possibly two. Because a deep peel literally causes a second-degree burn of the skin, all the side effects for the other types of peels will occur, plus a scabbing over and weeping of the skin. There also is a greater risk of infection and scarring with the deeper peels, and healing can take anywhere from two weeks to two months.

GENERAL TIPS BEFORE HAVING ANY PROCEDURE

Stop taking medications and supplements that increase bruising, swelling, or bleeding. Definitely talk with your doctor if it's absolutely necessary for you to continue to take any medications daily. Also ask your doctor if any other supplements or medications you're currently taking, or habits (such as smoking), could increase the risk of side effects post-procedure. Be 100% honest; tell the doctor about everything you use. The risks to your outcome depend on it, so this is not a time to be coy or embarrassed.

At least one to two weeks prior to your appointment, **stop taking aspirin, ibuprofen (Advil), naproxen (Aleve)**, *Ginkgo biloba*, St. John's wort, vitamin E, fish oil (omega-3) pills, ginger, and garlic. All of these are known to increase the risk of bruising and bleeding.

Do not drink alcohol for at least 24 hours prior to the procedure and, depending on what procedure you're having done, for up to several days (or weeks) afterwards, as alcohol inhibits the body's ability to heal.

Consider taking **arnica**. Because arnica has anti-inflammatory properties when taken orally, it may help if you begin taking this supplement up to two weeks before your procedure(s). Check with your physician to get his or her approval and a recommended dosage. Do not apply arnica to wounded skin, as it can be irritating.

It goes without saying, but just in case: **DON'T TAN** and **DON'T SMOKE!** This precaution is warranted because many people still tan and smoke, despite the fact that there are mounds of research showing that both of these lifestyle choices have a negative impact on skin. Tanning and smoking contribute significantly to skin discolorations, increase scarring, and delay healing, which is counterproductive to your skin's ability to heal. Plus, why engage in two such aging behaviors when you're paying good money for procedures to look younger, longer?

In regard to smoking, a doctor should ask a smoker to stop for at least three weeks before having surgery or an invasive corrective procedure. For many people, some of the more detrimental effects of smoking are greatly reduced after three weeks. Smoking has serious consequences because it introduces carbon monoxide into the body, which reduces the amount of oxygen available to the tissues, greatly inhibiting healing. Nicotine is also an issue because it restricts blood flow within the blood vessels. All this adds up to a greater risk of complications, none of which are pretty.

SKINCARE BEFORE HAVING A CORRECTIVE COSMETIC PROCEDURE

Generally, when it comes to cosmetic corrective procedures, there are no absolutes or special skincare steps or products you must add to or remove from your existing daily skincare routine. This, of course, assumes you are following our product recommendations and advice for taking brilliant care of your skin. The mantra here is (with very few exceptions) to **continue to take great care of your skin!** Doing so encourages faster healing and can also make recovery far easier.

Despite the fact that there are no pre-procedure musts for your skincare routine, some physicians do have opinions about your skincare routine and may ask you to change it. You should follow your doctor's advice on what he or she thinks is best, but, if in doubt, be sure to speak up and ask your physician why he or she is making the recommendation. Even if you don't agree, it's still wise to follow your doctor's advice.

Both before and after the procedure, discuss with your physician the **topical prescription medications** you use because they may interact with the surgery or procedure you're having done. For example, topical cortisone creams (over-the-counter or prescription-strength) can impede healing. Doctors also occasionally want their patients to stop using retinoids, such as Renova, Ret-in-A, or retinol-based products one to two weeks before a procedure because they may increase post-procedure inflammation. They also may tell you to wait a few weeks post-procedure before resuming topical medications.

Many doctors feel as we do and believe it's best to continue to use retinoids, whether prescription-only or in serum or moisturizers in the form of retinol, because retinoids strengthen the skin in significant ways that can reduce the risk of complications.

No matter what, be sure you're up front with your physician about any topical medications you use and share the details on any oral medications you take, including supplements bought over-the-counter from health food stores or drugstores. Many oral medications can interfere with recovery from a cosmetic procedure, so, as we mentioned above, it's critical for your physician to know exactly what you're taking.

It's also critically important to **protect your skin from the sun**, even more so than usual. It's best to be very afraid of the sun (really) before a cosmetic corrective procedure of any kind, whether invasive or non-invasive. Sun damage, whether you see it on the surface or not, hurts the skin's ability to heal, increases the risk of inflammation, and can make scarring worse. For some laser or light procedures, tanned skin can be more susceptible to complications than untanned skin.

Ask your doctor whether or not you should continue to use an **AHA or BHA** up until the procedure, and when you can add them back into your routine afterwards. Some doctors feel you should give up your daily topical exfoliants containing AHAs (glycolic or lactic acid) or BHA (salicylic acid). On the other hand, there are physicians who feel as we do; continuing to use your AHA or BHA exfoliant helps to gently remove the buildup of dead skin cells these procedures cause, and removing the buildup accelerates healing. However, if your physician urges you to skip this step for the time being, follow his or her advice.

SKINCARE AFTER HAVING A CORRECTIVE COSMETIC PROCEDURE

You've had a procedure (or multiple procedures) done. Now what? Here's what you need to do (or plan for) when you're recovering from minor or major procedures.

Apply cloth-wrapped ice packs as directed. One of the most important things you can do is to apply ice packs following Botox and dermal filler injections as well as other non-ablative laser- or light-based and intense pulsed light (IPL) treatments. Continue to use ice on and off throughout the day that you had the procedure.

For other procedures, such as chemical peels, ablative laser resurfacing, or cosmetic surgery such as a face-lift, **follow your doctor's instructions precisely** for at-home care. Generally speaking, the more involved or extensive the procedure, the more involved the post-care. There's a big difference between post-care following a Botox treatment and post-care following a face-lift!

Avoid activities that raise body heat. Depending on the procedure, your doctor may advise you to avoid raising your body temperature for the next few days. This means no strenuous exercise, no hot yoga, no soaking in the hot tub or sitting in the sauna, and no extended cooking over a hot stove.

Sleep with your head elevated. After any cosmetic corrective procedure, it can be exceptionally helpful to sleep with your head in an elevated position as much as possible. This reduces swelling and can significantly speed the healing process. If this proves too uncomfortable for you, try propping pillows against your sides so your arms can rest more easily with your head elevated.

Add a rich, emollient moisturizer. Many of these procedures can leave skin scaly and dry for several days, so if your skincare routine doesn't include a rich moisturizer, it should—even if your skin is usually oily. The moisturizer doesn't have to be heavy and occlusive like Vaseline, but it does need to be emollient and loaded with skin-healing antioxidants and skin-repairing ingredients. Once skin has healed you can go back to your usual moisturizer that is suitable for your skin type and concerns.

Along with moisturizer, consider using a silicone-based serum. Silicone ingredients, such as cyclopentasiloxane and dimethicone, have a proven ability to help protect and heal skin, and a silicone-based serum loaded with antioxidants and skin-repairing ingredients can be a wonderful addition to your post-procedure skincare. You'll want to keep using it after your skin has healed, too!

Stop using scrubs or the Clarisonic. Scrubbing your skin is a problem after most cosmetic corrective procedures because it can cause microscopic tears, which slow the healing process, especially after laser resurfacing and chemical peels. You can begin using these again only after your skin is completely healed.

After the initial healing process, you can return to your normal skincare routine, which we hope dovetails with the advice in this book. Once you begin using your AHA or BHA exfoliant again, pay attention to how your skin responds, and adjust the frequency of use accordingly. Discontinue use if you notice any signs of irritation. Many people find that these products enhance healing and lead to an even better outcome, but others do not. Our advice? Experiment to see what works best for you!

IT'S UP TO YOU!

There's no question that having the best skin of your life includes a combination of great skincare, a healthy lifestyle, and, potentially, cosmetic corrective procedures of some kind. We consider it a trifecta that can keep you looking beautiful and young for years and years. Cosmetic corrective procedures are not for everyone, but if you do choose to have something done, what you do to help your skin through the process will make it easier for you to see the results you want faster and more safely.

We're in a new era where cosmetic surgery and corrective procedures are widely available and getting better every year. Some people are pleased to know their face doesn't have to reflect their real age, and that they have a choice about what to do about it. As long as the results are impressive (and they often are), most people will want to maintain their youthful appearance via procedures that are relatively low risk and relatively permanent.

Wondering about that word "relatively" above? We use it because cosmetic surgery has duration limitations; that is, having a procedure will not keep your skin age-free forever. That's neither bad nor good, but many of these procedures, both invasive and non-invasive, are legitimate options for creating the look you want. Plus, it beats wasting money on creams and lotions that might do nothing for the wrinkles or sagging or pouching that bother you the most.

Skincare can do a lot to prevent and repair signs of aging, but any cosmetic surgeon worth getting to know would agree: When it comes to correcting signs of aging, the combination of a brilliant skincare routine (we can't say this enough) with the right cosmetic surgical (or non-surgical) procedures is what research has shown to be best for reducing and potentially eliminating many of the most bothersome signs of aging.

MICRO-NEEDLING

Micro-needling is a general term for a process that involves moving a special device over your skin that has a roller with many tiny needles embedded in it. There are different kinds of micro-needling devices with different product names. One is the manual version of micro-needling called a Dermaroller. There are also motorized devices such as the Dermapen or Dermastamp.

For the most part these micro-needling devices have reasonable science behind them indicating they may help in reducing the appearance of scars, but there is far less support for their ability to address wrinkles or for their ability to help anti-aging ingredients absorb better into skin.

It's tricky to weigh the pros and cons of such devices because when something sounds possible for one thing, many people often assume it must be good for everything. Another obstacle to obtaining the facts about micro-needling is the skewed information from the people who sell the device or use it in a spa versus having it done as a medical treatment by a physician. The exaggerated and misleading information we've seen is over the top!

A serious issue with these devices is you can buy them yourself and cause far more damage than any possible and even remote benefit. We'll do our best to make it easier for you to distinguish the real possibilities from the foolishness, but, for certain, micro-needling isn't for everyone, it can damage skin and make things worse not better, and for certain it doesn't perform miracles.

Dermarollers resemble small paint rollers you would use to get into tight spots, and they act as miniature aerators, like something you'd use on your lawn. They have a round, rotating cylinder with at least 200 tiny needles protruding from it, and a handle for moving it around your face. And that's exactly what you're supposed to do with it: You roll this quasi-aerator over your skin with some amount of pressure, puncturing hundreds of tiny holes wherever it goes.

Dermapens look exactly like a pen, with a circular head studded with tiny needles. The head and needles are motorized. The motor-driven needles move in and out of the skin in a stamping motion piercing it with thousands of tiny punctures.

Dermastamps resemble Dermapens but have a larger head with more needles protruding from the device and may be motorized or manual. They work exactly as the name implies: Rather than rolling needles over the skin or being moved over skin by a motor, you stamp the needles into skin. It's a bit like a tattooing machine, but with many needles puncturing skin all at once rather than a single needle (and obviously minus the ink deposit).

There are three primary uses for micro-needling devices. The first, which has some good research behind it, is to break down the thick collagen that causes some types of scarring. [245,246,247] The other two are more questionable, especially in terms of wrinkles and those are to stimulate collagen production by wounding skin and thereby improving the appearance of wrinkles, and the last is to deliver skincare ingredients into skin.

It seems clear from research that medical treatments using either the Dermastamp or the Dermapen to reduce scarring have the potential to produce good results. Whether or not the Dermaroller produces the same results is unclear because there is almost no published research available, but theoretically it should have the same results. Whether or not micro-needling of any kind can work on cellulite is at best dubious, but given that cellulite occurs on areas such as the thighs and not the face any downside would be far less evident.

In terms of building collagen, the Dermapen and Dermastamp have emerging research about their benefits for wrinkles as an easy procedure that is far less expensive than other devices or treatments. In contrast, the Dermaroller has no such research, though again, theoretically there is logic to the concept.

The Dermaroller is often touted as being better than chemical peels or resurfacing lasers for wrinkles because it doesn't remove the epidermis, but that it works in the same way to promote collagen production to repair the wounds it causes. However, removing the surface layer of skin is a primary benefit of chemical peels and resurfacing lasers. Resurfacing the skin creates a notably smoother outer layer of skin removing layers of sun damaged skin. Building collagen is only one way to improve wrinkles. Plus there many other types of lasers, light, radiofrequency, and ultrasound machines that don't resurface skin.

It's vitally important to keep in mind that if you constantly wound skin on a regular basis, eventually you will experience negative consequences. That's one of the major concerns about using any repeated treatment that constantly wounds skin, and why we're not enthusiasts of micro-needling devices for at-home use because of the risk of abuse. We describe the physiology of how this can happen below.

In wound healing and the formation of scar tissue, there's a change in the relative amounts of type I and type III collagen (for quick reference, there are at least 16 types of collagen in the body; types I and III are most prevalent in skin). [248] When skin is wounded, the amount of type I collagen increases and the amount of type III collagen decreases. When type I and type III are in balance, skin is healthier and looks younger; when they are out of balance, because of injury or aging, especially if the skin is repeatedly being reinjured, then type I is more prevalent. The result? Skin becomes stiffer and looks unhealthy. It's the balance between type I and type III collagen that comprises young skin. When skin is "wounded" during laser procedures or chemical peels, type I collagen increases as a response to skin's healing process, but then during the healing process skin starts producing lots of type III collagen to bring it back into a healthy state (skin loves being repaired if we don't get in its way).

Because it's the balance between type I and type III collagen that makes skin healthy, look younger, and radiant, continually wounding skin makes it almost impossible to regain or maintain a healthy balance between these two types of collagen. Peels and lasers are performed intermittently, while most needling devices come with instructions to use them daily and it's just too easy to think if a little is good a lot would be better.

Another claim about the benefit of micro-needling is to enhance the penetration into skin of prescription ingredients or cosmetic ingredients. While there is definitely research showing the potential benefit of micro-needling as a means for delivering prescription drugs into skin this is developing research and is not a standard practice by any means. [249,250,251,252]

In terms of skincare ingredients penetrating "deeper" by using the Derma-roller or similar tools, the benefit is at best dubious and minimally studied. Much of this research uses a small number of people and is often done by people (even doctors) representing the companies selling these machines.

The major issue, as we mentioned, is the risk of constantly re-wounding skin, which eventually damages it. The second issue is in regard to what skincare ingredients are going to be absorbed further into skin—and is that even a good thing?

The claims are usually around improved penetration of everything from hyaluronic acid to retinol, and vitamin C. There are even claims that human or plant stem cells and growth factors can be used at home with these devices to absorb better into the skin. [253] By the way, even if skincare products claiming to contain stem cells or growth factors could work they would have serious risks to the health of your skin, but they can't work so it's really more a waste of your time and money than it is a real risk.

Gaining the benefit of toners, moisturizers, or serums with anti-aging ingredients is not just about maximum penetration. Many ingredients, like antioxidants and skin-identical ingredients, must stay in the top layers of skin to have benefit, including defense against environmental free-radical damage (which encounter skin's surface first). Then there's the risk of getting unwanted ingredients (like preservatives or problematic plant extracts) deeper into skin, where their negative effects may be worse. Even beneficial ingredients like hyaluronic acid, vitamin C or retinol can be more sensitizing if they penetrate through a wound (i.e., when applied over broken or "punctured" skin), rather than being able to do their work in the uppermost layers of skin or penetrating deeper naturally through intact skin all on their own.

The fine point (sorry, we couldn't resist) on micro-needling is that in some situations it can have benefit especially for scarring and remotely but possibly cellulite, but there is absolutely not enough research to support a recommendation to use such tools as part of an anti-aging routine or to gain better results from deeper penetration of cosmetic ingredients (and we are all about the research). From what science has shown to be true about the types of collagen in the body and how the types of collagen in skin work in balance, there's a real risk to frequent use of micro-needling devices, powered or manual, in terms of throwing off the balance of healthy, youthful collagen production.

AT-HOME LIGHT DEVICES FOR WRINKLES OR ACNE

You may have heard about high-tech light devices for acne and wrinkles advertised for use at home. Alternatively, you can have a procedure in a spa or clinic setting called light-emitting diode (LED) therapy. Also known as photodynamic therapy (PDT), these light-emitting devices have a decent amount of research showing they can be effective for reducing acne and wrinkles. Even more impressive? There doesn't seem to be any risk associated with these treatments!

As positive as the research for these devices looks (and these aren't large studies by any means), they shouldn't be confused with, nor do they work or share strong similarities with, more sophisticated medical devices. **LED light devices do not in any way replace medical options, such as ablative lasers, non-ablative lasers, IPL, radiofrequency machines, or ultrasound machines, for treating wrinkles**. They also don't replace the need for a well-formulated skincare routine.

LED devices can be used at a doctor's office, but it's not necessary unless you are also being treated with a topical medication that then requires you to sit in front of an LED-emitting device for about 30 minutes to an hour. This treatment and medication, referred to as topical 5-aminolevulinic acid (ALA) with mediated PDT, can be effective for moderate to severe acne. [254] In contrast, at-home LED devices for acne tend to be best for mild or sporadic acne, and do not require concurrent use of a topical medication during treatment.

But, back to the at-home devices: There are mostly pros and only one con to consider, but if your expectations are realistic (these are not a cure for acne and the results for wrinkles are relatively subtle) the research is promising. That means there's almost no reason not to give these devices a try if you have the patience and the time!

Blue LED treatments for acne use specific wavelengths of blue light to target and kill the *Propionibacterium acnes* bacteria that play a pivotal role in causing acne for many people. It also can reduce inflammation. Although it sounds strong, this light doesn't damage healthy skin in any way; in fact, there's research showing it can reduce oil production. Other research shows that blue LED treatments can be helpful to reduce thickened scars. [255,256,257,258,259]

Not everyone will respond the same way to this kind of treatment; however, because the devices are reasonably priced (at least compared with repeated medical treatments), there's almost no reason not to see how this treatment works for you. Just keep in mind that blue LED treatments don't replace a great skincare routine for acne. [260] Plus, this treatment requires a time commitment: You must hold the device to your skin or sit in front of a panel of lights for several minutes once or twice daily, on a regular basis, to obtain results. Important tip: Be sure to protect your eyes from exposure to the light.

Two more points: Blue LED devices without ALA are not considered effective for cystic acne, and they have no impact on blackheads or whiteheads (milia)—one more reason to keep using effective skincare products along with LED treatments.

Red LED devices for wrinkles are identical in practice to the blue LED treatment devices, except that they emit red light. Like blue LED light, you expose your face to red LED light by moving a handheld device over your face or by sitting in front of a panel of lights. Red LED treatments have a relatively extensive amount of research showing they can help heal wounds and reduce wrinkles. Red LED devices are also believed to target the skin's oil glands to reduce cytokines, a class of pro-inflammatory substances believed to play a role in chronic acne and rosacea. [261,262,263,264,265,266]

The treatments can be performed at home or in a doctor's office, but there's no reason not to consider doing this at home given the relative affordability of at-home devices and the fact that when you follow the usage instructions there are no known side effects. If there's any downside, it's the fact this requires multiple treatments several minutes once or twice daily on a regular basis. Just like when using blue LED devices, you also must protect your eyes from the light.

What to buy? If you are considering an at-home LED device for anti-aging or clearing acne, we recommend shopping carefully and buying only from reputable manufacturers. Due to concerns over liability issues, many manufacturers of at-home devices limit their intensity, sometimes to a much lower strength than the LED-emitting machines your dermatologist uses. In a sense, that's good news because, although side effects are nil if used correctly, it's possible to overdo these treatments and end up damaging your skin, which is never the goal.

Some of the LED devices available to the public actually do have the strength of those used in dermatologists' offices. If that's the case, caution is warranted: To get the best results while minimizing, if not eliminating, risk, be sure to read all accompanying instructions and follow the usage directions to the letter!

At-home blue LED devices we recommend for treating acne: Quasar MD BLUE ($595); Quasar Baby Blue ($349); Quasar Clear Rayz for Acne ($249); Tria Acne Clearing Blue Light ($299).

At-home red LED devices we recommend for treating wrinkles: Quasar MD PLUS ($795); Baby Quasar PLUS ($399); Tanda Luxe Skin Rejuvenation Photofacial Device ($195).

Don't get caught up in making a decision based on the "FDA approved" label for what's known as a "Class II medical device." All that means is that the FDA approved the device for safety, **not** for effectiveness.

At-home diode lasers for wrinkles are very different from the blue or red LED devices discussed above. Products like Tria's Age-Defying Laser and Palo-Via's Skin Renewing Laser are both at-home diode lasers. They are not LED (light emitting diode) devices, which is what makes them completely different from the blue and red LED treatments we discussed above.

What makes these diode devices unique is their energy output and the wavelength of light they produce. PaloVia's device has a maximum energy output of 15 megajoules (mJ, a measure of energy) and a wavelength of 1410 nanometers; Tria's has a maximum energy output of 5–12 mJ/pulse and a wavelength of 1440 nanometers. Technically, this makes them similar to the type of non-ablative laser treatments you can receive in a doctor's office. These at-home devices have some advantages over the in-office versions: They can provide results similar to those you get from in-office treatments, without the repeated cost (most non-ablative laser treatments require multiple treatments over time). The downside is that similar does not mean the same. The energy output is the major difference and the versions in a doctor's office are far more powerful and effective, are used by someone who knows what they are doing, and can be calibrated to offer a customized treatment. [267]

The fact that the energy output of the Tria and PaloVia is less than that of the in-office devices doesn't mean that the diode devices don't have an impact on wrinkles. The technology behind these devices is sound, and if used following the instructions, if you can put up with the discomfort (it hurts), and if you make the time commitment, you can get reasonable results.

Both the Tria and PaloVia devices, not surprisingly, come with unrealistic claims. The question of whether or not these work better than retinoids, such as prescription tretinoin or over-the-counter retinol, is irrelevant because a laser or light treatment of any kind isn't skincare. How lasers or light treatments work is completely different from the benefits you get from great skincare products or topical retinoids. Lasers and light treatments remodel and stimulate increased collagen production, but there is much more to taking care of skin than that. Retinoids help skin cells make healthier cells and skincare products formulated with potent antioxidants and skin-repairing ingredients reduce further damage. AHAs and BHA exfoliants also keep the surface of skin smooth, something diodes or LED devices cannot do. And, of course, neither LED nor diode devices can protect skin from UV light, which is the leading cause of all signs of skin aging and a detriment to those struggling with breakouts.

We also wanted to compare stronger types of in-office procedures, such as much stronger lasers, IPL, ultrasound, and radiofrequency treatments to at-home LED and diode devices, but there's very little published research to be found. That means your guess is as good as ours! However, given that a doctor can customize and strengthen treatments and that users of at-home devices cannot, we suspect in-office procedures, even those that are similar to at-home devices, will retain their edge. Being able to "dial in" these treatments allows for more targeted results in much less time—which is good to know if you're dealing with more pronounced wrinkles, acne, or sun damage.

Which way to go? This is a decision you need to make based on how much time you have, how much money you're willing to spend, and the results you're hoping for. The Tria and PaloVia devices each cost about $500, and they require a minimum of several treatments over a period of weeks. And, most important, don't expect miracles—modest, incremental improvements after several weeks of use is a realistic expectation that will ensure you don't end up disappointed.

AT-HOME LASER HAIR REMOVAL

Perhaps no other form of light-emitting at-home device has shown more consistent promise and improvement in the research than laser hair removal devices. Among our favorite brand for this time- and money-saving procedure is Tria.

The Tria Laser 4X is a relatively new incarnation of the 810-nanometer diode laser device you can buy for use at home. As surprising as it sounds, it really is virtually identical to the laser hair removal machines used in doctors' offices or clinical/spa settings, which means it works to permanently remove hair! With a retail price of $449, the Tria Laser 4X isn't cheap, but it's definitely cheaper than repeated treatments for laser hair removal from a physician, especially if you have particularly stubborn hair growth that will require more than the usual number of treatments. Most will find this device worth the investment—at least if you can figure out how to use it! One drawback of the Tria device is that you must follow the instructions exactly or the device won't produce even minor results. This is not pain-free, but the treatment at the doctor's office isn't pain-free either. If you can keep up with the treatments and are patient, you could be pleasantly surprised and end up never having to use a razor again.

CHAPTER 14

Common Beauty Questions Answered and Myths Debunked!

The world of beauty can indeed be beautiful. All too often, however, the information you get is anything but beautiful; actually, it can be downright ugly! Sometimes the advertising and sales pitches you read and hear are minor distortions of facts or merely deceptive; in other cases, they are out-and-out lies (and those really get us worked up!). Whether the information comes from a cosmetics company, aesthetician, advertisement, physician, or from a well-intentioned website, we spend a lot of time untangling the senseless information to help you get to the truth.

In this chapter, we bust the most popular beauty myths (some are outright concocted stories) that many unsuspecting people believe. We give you the facts behind the industry hype so you can make the best decision for your skin.

IF I CAN'T SEE IRRITATION ON MY SKIN, THERE'S NOTHING TO WORRY ABOUT, RIGHT?

Any and all types of irritation, whether you see it on the surface of your skin or not, triggers inflammation and, as a result, is terrible for your skin, impairing healing, damaging collagen, and depleting the vital substances your skin needs to stay young and healthy.

Avoiding such things as hot water, harsh scrubs, sun exposure, and products with irritating ingredients (especially fragrance, whether synthetic or natural) will help save your skin. When it comes to skin, it's best to eliminate, as much as possible, the use of known skin irritants, especially when there are brilliant formulas available that do not include these problematic ingredients. Knowing this, it simply doesn't make sense to take the risk. [2,5]

DO I REALLY NEED A PRODUCT LABELED "EYE CREAM"?

All of the marketing hype you've heard about how eye creams are specially formulated for the sensitive, thin skin around the eyes, and that they can get rid of puffy eyes, dark circles, and sagging skin is, for the most part, simply not true. In fact, most of us don't need a product labeled eye cream (or eye gel or eye serum). The perfect "eye treatment" is likely already in your beauty routine; your facial moisturizer or serum can provide the same anti-aging and reparative benefits when applied around your eyes!

Most eye creams are not specially formulated, nor do they contain any unique ingredients that distinguish them from the ingredients in facial formulas. In fact, it takes only a quick look at the ingredient list of the majority of eye creams to see that their ingredients don't differ in any significant way from the ingredients of comparable facial moisturizers.

Also important to note: Most eye creams don't contain sunscreen, which means that during the daytime you're leaving the already wrinkle-prone eye area vulnerable to sun damage, which causes eye-area sagging, darkening, and yellowing, and can worsen puffiness. So, if you're using an eye cream, you should be applying a sunscreen rated SPF 30 or greater over it.

Very few studies identify any specific ingredients or combination of ingredients that the eye area needs (or should avoid) that are different from those that the skin on other areas of the face needs or doesn't need. When it comes to moisturizing skin, reducing wrinkles, building collagen, brightening, and improving skin tone, your skin needs the same ingredients, whether that skin is around your eyes or elsewhere on your face.

What about the claim that eye creams are better suited for the delicate skin in the eye area? Every part of the face needs stable, potent, and GENTLE state-of-the-art ingredients. It doesn't make any sense that the eye area should get the good, non-irritating ingredients, and that the face should get the bad or potentially troublesome ingredients—ironically, many eye creams contain irritating ingredients, such as fragrances, essential oils, and alcohol-based formulas.

If the face product you're using or considering is well formulated for fighting dry skin and wrinkles, repairing the skin's barrier, creating healthier skin cells, improving dark circles (to some extent) and preventing further sun damage, then use it in the eye area, too. You will be doing the most you can via skincare for the eye area! All of those benefits have nothing to do with what the product is called—it is all about finding brilliantly formulated products, whether labeled "eye cream" or something else.

You can indeed buy a well-formulated eye cream, but please stay away from ones that come in jars, contain irritating ingredients, or don't have sunscreen for daytime use.

CAN EYE CREAMS TREAT PUFFY EYES AND DARK CIRCLES?

Dark circles and puffy eyes are two common problems that most of us will have to face at some point in our lives, but can an eye cream, eye gel, or eye serum really eliminate puffy eyes or dark circles? Depending on what is causing your puffy eyes or dark circles and what your expectations are, the answer is: Maybe.

Dark circles have several causes; skincare products can address some of them, but, unfortunately, not all. There are things you can do to improve dark circles as well as to keep them from getting worse, but you won't find your solution in a specialty product that comes with miraculous claims or a "miracle" ingredient.

The most common causes of dark circles include sun damage, irritation, allergies, heredity (genetics), and veins/capillaries showing through the surface layer of skin. If heredity and surfaced blood flow are causing your dark circles, they aren't going to respond to topical treatments, but if caused by sun damage, they can be treated by **daily use of a mineral-based broad-spectrum sunscreen rated SPF 30** or greater during the day. For some, sunscreen ingredients other than zinc oxide and titanium dioxide can cause irritation around the eye, which would be counterproductive and make dark circles worse, so check the ingredients on the SPF product you are using.

Next, **use a brightening treatment during the day**. A well-formulated skin brightener loaded with antioxidants, skin-repairing ingredients, and cell-communicating ingredients can help improve skin texture, lighten sun damage–induced dark circles, reduce wrinkles, and brighten the under-eye area all at the same time. As mentioned in the previous section on eye creams, you can look for facial formulas (no need for a special eye-area product) that contain the same anti-aging ingredients we've discussed throughout this book, including vitamin C and retinol. [97,268]

If you find your dark circles truly bothersome, and you want to stop your seemingly endless search for a new eye cream that works, consider speaking to a cosmetic dermatologist about options, such as dermal fillers (like Radiesse), lasers, light treatments, radiofrequency treatments, and chemical peels for lightening dark circles and reducing wrinkles. [269,270,271] A dermatologist experienced with the various lasers used to treat skin will be able to tell you which option is best for your dark circles as well as for your skin color. The Q-switched ruby laser is the most common choice for treating dark circles, but even then, don't expect a dramatic improvement. [272] The best "treatment" product for stubborn dark circles is a good full-coverage concealer!

Puffy eyes are most often caused by fluid retention, allergic reactions, skin inflamed by irritation (including absentminded eye-rubbing), fat pads distending around the eye area, or a combination of these factors.

The cosmetics industry's frequent solution—eye serums or gels, dispensed through rollerball applicators that you massage on—only redistributes the fluid around the eye; it can't do anything for the other causes of puffy eyes, especially age-related redistribution of fat pads. The main causes of puffy eyes, along with what you can do to help treat them, are as follows:

» **Inflammation** can cause temporary puffiness around the eyes, usually the result of allergies or external irritants (think contact lenses, fragrances, essential oils, or alcohol-based products). Another culprit? Not removing every speck of your eye makeup at night!

» **Sun damage is a major culprit** because it causes wrinkles, loss of skin elasticity, and skin discolorations. If you suffer from puffy eyes, be aware ... your eye area is even more susceptible to the negative impact of unprotected sun exposure. The resulting sun damage causes the skin around your eyes to lose its elasticity, which in turn allows more fluid to accumulate in the area. [5,6,273] In addition, sagging skin just tends to look puffier. To protect your eye area, daily use of a broad-spectrum mineral-based sunscreen rated SPF 30 or greater is critical.

» For some people, puffy eyes may just be their natural appearance, the result of genetics. **Typically, this results from overly large fat pads** around the eyes or because the fat pads, over time, have pouched through the facial muscles and begun to distend (commonly referred to as under-eye bags). [5,6,273] If that is the case, the only way to send those bags packing is with cosmetic surgery, which usually is quite effective. [273] The procedure, known as blepharoplasty, is among the most common cosmetic surgical procedures, for both men and women.

» **Allergies can be a major cause of puffy eyes.** According to the American College of Allergy, Asthma, and Immunology, 30% of all adults have some type of allergy. Even low-level allergies can cause puffiness around the eyes. Talking to your doctor about daily use of antihistamines or using artificial tear drops or eye-lubricating drops can make all the difference in the world.

ARE "HYPOALLERGENIC" PRODUCTS BETTER FOR SENSITIVE SKIN?

"Hypoallergenic" is a term meant to imply that a product is unlikely or less likely to cause allergic reactions and, therefore, is better for allergy-prone or sensitive skin types—it isn't true. There are no accepted testing methods, ingredient restrictions, regulations, guidelines, rules, or procedures of any kind, anywhere in the world, for determining whether or not a product qualifies as being hypoallergenic. [274,275]

We have reviewed hundreds of products labeled "hypoallergenic" or "good for sensitive skin" that contain seriously problematic ingredients that actually trigger allergic breakouts or sensitive skin reactions. And many of us have used products labeled hypoallergenic that have caused a reaction of some sort.

If sensitive or allergy-prone skin is one of your concerns, then the **#1 thing to look for is products that are free of irritants**. The major irritants that show up in an astounding number of products, especially in products labeled organic or natural, are fragrance (both synthetic and natural fragrance are equally bad for all skin types), alcohol (isopropyl, SD, or denatured alcohol), and harsh cleansing agents. ALL of these ingredients may also appear in products labeled *hypoallergenic*.

IS ALCOHOL IN SKINCARE REALLY *THAT* BAD?

There is so much incomplete and/or misleading information online, it's easy to believe that a high amount of alcohol in skincare products, even in moisturizers, isn't *really* all that bad for your skin. But first, let us clarify what we mean by "alcohol."

When we complain about the presence of alcohol in skincare products or makeup, we're referring to ethanol, which you'll most often see listed as SD alcohol, isopropyl alcohol, or alcohol denat. (denatured alcohol) on the ingredient label. These types of volatile alcohols give products a pleasing, quick-drying finish that makes it feel weightless on skin, so it's easy to see their appeal, especially for those with oil-prone skin. When this type of alcohol is listed among the first five ingredients on an ingredient label, without question they will cause irritation, and that's bad for all skin types. It causes dryness and free-radical damage, and hurts the skin's ability to heal.

In contrast, there are other types of alcohols, known as fatty alcohols, that are NOT irritating in the least. Examples you'll see on ingredient labels include cetyl, stearyl, and cetearyl alcohol. All of these are good ingredients for dry skin, and in small amounts fine for any skin type. It's important that you not confuse these good forms of alcohol with the problematic types of alcohol.

Surely, you think, there must be a good reason so many skincare companies include alcohol in their products, especially given that some of these products are quite popular. There are indeed reasons, but it's not about good skincare; rather, alcohol is often used to keep a formula stable and/or to make an otherwise thick formulation feel almost weightless, creating a deceptively pleasant aesthetic. That's good for the product, but it's bad for your skin.

You may have seen information that alcohol is a good ingredient because it helps other ingredients like retinol and vitamin C penetrate skin more effectively. Although it's true that it does enhance absorption, the alcohol also destroys skin's barrier, the very substances that keep your skin healthy over the long term. [276] There are other, more gentle ways to get good ingredients to penetrate skin, without damaging and causing more problems than benefits.

Alcohol immediately harms skin and starts a chain reaction of damage that continues long after it has evaporated. A 2003 study, published in the *Journal of Hospital Infection*, found that with regular exposure to alcohol-based products, the skin is no longer able to keep water and cleansing agents from penetrating, thus further eroding the skin's barrier. [277]

If your skin is oily, it can be tempting to use alcohol-based products because they provide an immediate matte finish, essentially de-greasing the "oil slick." The irony of using alcohol-based treatments is that the damage they cause leads to an increase in breakouts, enlarges the pores, and makes inflammation worse, the consequence of which is that the red marks stay around for much longer than they would otherwise. [28,29]

And get this: Alcohol can stimulate oil production at the base of the pore, so the immediate de-greasing effect is eventually counteracted, prompting your oily skin to produce even more oil. [27,278] Talk about spinning your wheels!

In many ways, alcohol-based products are the handsome bad boys of skincare—flashy, attractive, even dangerous, but we all know it's a relationship that's going to do more harm than good. The research is clear: Alcohol harms your skin's protective barrier, triggers free-radical damage, makes oily skin and redness worse, and is best described as "pro-aging." Why bother, given the damaging effects of topical alcohol and the hundreds of skin-friendly alternatives that are available?

WHY IS JAR PACKAGING BAD FOR YOUR SKIN?

Innovations in skincare have led to formulations that can dramatically improve your skin, making it look less wrinkled, younger, healthier, and super-smooth and radiant. The primary ingredients responsible for these advancements are antioxidants, cell-communicating ingredients, anti-irritants, and skin-repairing ingredients.

Products loaded with these are the absolute best for all skin types at any age, but your skin won't reap the benefits from most of these brilliant ingredients if the product comes in a jar.

The ingredients that are most beneficial for your skin are not stable when exposed to light and air, which is exactly what happens when you take the lid off a jar. [279,280] No matter how great the formula, these amazing, but unstable, ingredients will begin to break down when you first open the jar! There is also the issue of hygiene; dipping your fingers into a jar transfers bacteria from your hands into the product, which causes the important ingredients to further deteriorate.

One of the critical factors in any anti-aging or skin-healing formula is the amount and variety of antioxidants, cell-communicating ingredients, and skin-repairing ingredients—the more the better. These ingredients function in a variety of ways to reduce the effects of the constant environmental stresses on your skin.

Antioxidants, cell-communicating ingredients, and skin-repairing ingredients not only can help prevent free-radical damage, but also, to a fairly impressive extent, help repair that damage. Surprisingly, all of these ingredients are just as vulnerable to sun exposure, pollution, and cigarette smoke as your skin. [279,280] So, once you open that jar, you immediately compromise the stability of the anti-aging superstars it contains. (Visualize their benefits disappearing like puffs of smoke each time you open the lid!)

With most skincare formulas, all that's necessary to protect these beneficial ingredients is a container that minimizes exposure to air and that keeps light, and your fingers, out of the product. A pump or an airless jar (meaning you can't take the lid off) design or an opaque tube with a very small opening is sufficient to keep these important ingredients protected and effective during the product's life span, and allow your skin to reap the rewards.

Remember, no matter how great a product's formula, jar packaging, and to a lesser extent clear packaging (which lets light in), is always a deal-breaker. Given the number and variety of products available today that come in air-reducing or airless packaging, why waste your money on products whose most beneficial ingredients will lose their effectiveness soon after first use? Yes, jars can be pretty, but so what if their contents aren't going to help your skin as much as they would if they were in air-resistant packaging?

What about the claims that some cosmetics brands make about using specially "encapsulated" antioxidants that are protected from air exposure when formulated in a jar-packaged moisturizer? The notion that encapsulating an antioxidant somehow keeps it from breaking down with exposure to air is actually counter to their primary function in skincare products. The ingredients that "encapsulate" an antioxidant are also supposed to break down to release the antioxidant, and they do so in the presence of air (oxygen). So, jar packaging also allows the encapsulating ingredients to deteriorate as well. [5,15,279,280]

We are asked all the time: Given the research that's out there about jars, why do so many companies continue to use them? We can guess, but, in truth, we don't know because this research about jar packaging is no secret. If those companies aren't aware of the research, that makes us even more worried because then we wonder what else they don't know.

No matter the rationale, jar packaging means a product is far less beneficial for your skin than one that is in air-resistant packaging.

What to do? Avoid buying products that come in jars, especially if they contain beneficial, but unstable, ingredients (which all the best anti-aging products do). Look for products packaged in tubes, pumps, airless jars, and airless containers. Because there are so many companies whose packaging keeps the beneficial ingredients stable, spend your beauty dollars on those products.

CAN I GET CANCER FROM SUNSCREEN?

Fears about sunscreen ingredients causing cancer are endlessly paraded in the media, fueled by lobbyist groups with dubious goals. The scientific-sounding allegations are frightening enough to leave you wondering which sunscreens are best for you and your family—or whether you should skip sunscreen altogether!

At first glance, these sunscreen concerns appear legitimate, but when we investigated the research, we found that the claims are either misleading or have nothing to do with how these ingredients are used in skincare formulas. Following is the information you need to make wise and safe decisions for your skin.

The benefits of daily sunscreen use are absolutely clear. Research shows—unquestionably—that when you wear a broad-spectrum sunscreen rated SPF 30+ properly (applied liberally, reapplying every two hours in direct daylight) every day, your risk of deadly or disfiguring skin cancer dramatically decreases. It also decreases premature signs of aging, such as wrinkles, brown spots, and sagging skin. [281]

An Australian study carried out in 2013 showed that a well-formulated sunscreen applied to exposed skin as directed **blocked the effects of DNA damage that can lead to skin cancer**. [282] What's more, regular use of sunscreen also protects an anti-cancer gene in the skin, known as p53, from becoming damaged, and destroying an anti-cancer gene can be deadly. Sunscreen does a lot more than just protect against sunburn and premature aging!

A randomized, 10-year study of 1,600 adults, published in the *Journal of the American Medical Association*, noted that even using a product with only an SPF of 16 reduces your risk of skin cancer. [283] Despite these long-established benefits of using a sunscreen daily, there is still ongoing controversy about their safety. If you've bought into this fear and stopped using sunscreen, we implore you to read on for the facts.

If these unsubstantiated claims about sunscreens causing cancer (meaning they are carcinogenic) were actually true, one would expect cancer rates to be higher among those who work in the cosmetics manufacturing industry because they are surrounded by high concentrations of these "suspect" ingredients. Yet, the medical data do not support this, as the **overall incidence of cancer has declined in the United States**, according to 2013 statistics from the American Cancer Society. [284]

Below we discuss the ingredients that are present in many sunscreens that are among the most disparaged for their alleged lack of a safety profile. We look beyond the distortions to see what the research *really* says.

First, we discuss not a sunscreen ingredient, but a vitamin A ingredient that appears in many sunscreens—retinyl palmitate. Ironically, **retinyl palmitate** is a healthy fatty acid form of vitamin A that is found naturally in skin. It provides multiple benefits, from neutralizing free radicals to reducing the risk of sunburn. [285] As a cosmetic ingredient, retinyl palmitate is **approved globally** for use in sunscreens. Yet, this essential vitamin has been said to increase skin cancer risk because of a **single, 16-year old study** that has not been reproduced or tested under real-life conditions that even remotely resemble how humans use sunscreen. [286]

Researchers in that study didn't test sunscreens containing retinyl palmitate (which contain very small amounts for their antioxidant benefit); rather, they applied high concentrations (much higher than the concentrations found in cosmetics products) of retinyl palmitate directly to rodents who were bred to get cancer. [286]

These conditions are not at all representative of how retinyl palmitate is used in skincare formulas—and, get this, researchers used a breed of rodent that is predisposed to skin cancer (80% of the mice who were exposed to UV light alone, without the retinyl palmitate, developed skin cancer anyway). [286,287] Following is what the published research on this controversy has concluded:

» The Skin Cancer Foundation's Photobiology Committee states: "There is no scientific evidence that retinyl palmitate causes cancer in humans...." and "no published data suggests that topical retinoids increase skin cancer risk." [288]

» The Memorial Sloan Kettering Cancer Center, in its 2011 peer-reviewed study, published in *Photodermatology, Photoimmunology and Photomedicine*, after reviewing the data stated: "In conclusion, the available evidence from *in vitro* and animal studies fails to demonstrate convincing evidence indicating that retinyl palmitate imparts an increased risk of skin cancer." [289]

» The Memorial Sloan Kettering Cancer Center also noted, "decades of clinical observations support the notion that retinyl palmitate is safe for use in topical applications such as sunscreens." [289]

Oxybenzone, a sunscreen active that's been in use for over 20 years, consistently comes under fire, despite the fact that the safety data on it are exhaustive. It's also globally recognized as a safe and effective sunscreen agent. Headlines hoping to get your attention just love to regurgitate the fact that minute levels of oxybenzone are absorbed by skin, and that trace amounts (parts per *million*), which is infinitesimally small, can be detected in urine (per a 2008 CDC report). [290]

While that may sound alarming, the presence of substances like oxybenzone in urine doesn't denote anything on its own. Research on volunteers has looked at the effect, rate of absorption, and potential of oxybenzone to accumulate. Otherwise, it is just your body metabolizing and excreting an unneeded substance, as it should.

A 2004 study in the *Journal of Investigative Dermatology* and a 2008 study in the *Journal of the European Academy of Dermatology and Venereology* demonstrated that applying a full-body application of a 10% concentration of oxybenzone over the course of 4 days had no negative health effects, and that it did not accumulate in the body. [291,292] Other points to confirm the safety of oxybenzone include the following:

» The American Academy of Dermatology states, "No data show that oxybenzone causes any significant health problems in humans." [293]

» The Skin Cancer Foundation Photobiology Committee agrees, noting, "There is no evidence that oxybenzone, which is FDA-approved and has been available 20 years, has any adverse health effect in humans." [294]

» The Memorial Sloan Kettering Cancer Center 2011 study in *Photodermatology, Photoimmunology and Photomedicine*, concludes, "the available evidence does not demonstrate biologically significant hormonal disruption with topical application of oxybenzone in humans." [289]

» The scientific and regulatory bodies of the European Union (EU) produced a 2008 report, *Opinion on Benzophenone-3* (another name for oxybenzone), which found that oxybenzone in sunscreens "does not pose a risk to the health of the consumer." [295]

Numerous investigative studies spanning the globe continue to confirm oxybenzone's place as a long-established and safe UV protectant. There is no reason to avoid it unless you know from experience that your skin is sensitive to it, which can occur for some people.

Octinoxate, also known as **octyl methoxycinnamate or ethylhexyl methoxycinnamate**, is also consistently under fire as a sunscreen active. As it turns out, octinoxate is the oldest and most common sunscreen active worldwide, with a solid record of safety, decades of research, and thousands of studies establishing its safety in sunscreens as indisputable. [296] Unfortunately, unfounded claims that this staple of SPF formulas "causes cancer" have made many afraid of their sunscreens.

Let us be clear: No studies demonstrate that octinoxate, when used in your SPF products, causes or increases the risk of developing any type of cancer. In the sole studies cited when the "octinoxate = cancer" claim is made, the studies' conditions are completely inapplicable to how sunscreen ingredients are used in skincare products.

For example, such studies use octinoxate in high concentrations (much higher than would ever be used in sunscreens) applied directly to skin cells, or fed in high concentrations to lab animals. The truth is: Octinoxate is safe as long as you aren't drinking it!

No studies exist that support the claim that octinoxate has any link to causing cancer or other illnesses when used in sunscreen formulas. In fact, the EU's usage level for octinoxate in sunscreens is higher than what is permitted in the United States (10% versus 7.5%), and sunscreen ingredient regulations typically are more stringent (though often for no valid reason) in the EU than in the States. [297]

The mineral actives titanium dioxide and zinc oxide have become controversial when **nanotechnology** is used to make these ingredients into what's known as **nanoparticles**, which allows these mineral-derived sunscreen actives to be more cosmetically elegant (less white cast) and better able to protect skin from UV damage. Sounds win-win, but not so fast....

Nanotechnology, which is about making things very small, is used in various industries, such as medicine and manufacturing, and sometimes in the cosmetics industry. One nanometer is one billionth of a meter, and nanotechnology generally refers to particles that range from one nanometer to 100 nanometers. For comparison, a piece of paper is about 100,000 nanometers thick.

Given the vast range of applications of nanotechnology and the substances that are made into nanoparticles, it is meaningless to categorically state that "all nanoparticles are dangerous," just as it is to say that "all red things are hot." The size and the substance make all the difference! So, when asking the question of whether or not nanoparticle-size sunscreen actives such as titanium dioxide and zinc oxide can penetrate skin and enter the bloodstream, it's important to ensure we're looking at the right information. Here are the facts:

» Titanium dioxide and zinc oxide are sized (at the high end of the scale, toward 100 nanometers) and then are coated with polymer or silicone to ensure they remain on the surface of skin—if they didn't remain on the surface, they wouldn't be very effective as sunscreen actives.

» In a 2007 study published in *Critical Reviews in Toxicology*, it was demonstrated that these particles do not penetrate through human skin, concluding, "nanoparticles currently used in cosmetic preparations or sunscreens pose no risk to human skin or human health." [298]

» Australian and Swiss research teams, using excised human skin in two separate 2011 studies, published in the *Journal of Biomedical Optics*, established that neither nano-size titanium dioxide nor nano-size zinc oxide penetrated beyond the superficial layer of skin (stratum corneum). **They did not and do not enter the body**. [299]

» The U.S. Environmental Protection Agency released a 2010 case study of nano-scale titanium dioxide in sunscreen formulas, stating there is no health problem or concern associated with its use. EPA's findings also confirmed that nano-size titanium dioxide does not penetrate beyond the superficial (dead) layer of human skin. [300]

» The Memorial Sloan Kettering Cancer Center published a review of nanoparticle titanium dioxide and zinc oxide in *Photodermatology, Photoimmunology and Photomedicine*, stating, "It has been established that the stratum corneum is an effective barrier preventing the entry of nano-ZnO (zinc oxide) and -TiO$_2$ (titanium dioxide) into deeper layers of the skin." [289]

In summary: There is no evidence that nano-size titanium dioxide or zinc oxide sunscreen actives pose any health risk (certainly not in comparison to skipping, or skimping on, your SPF).

It is worth mentioning that the discussion above also shows that research into the safety and applications of cosmetic and skincare ingredients is ongoing; it never stops. **Globally, extensive and continuous scientific and medical research has shown your sunscreen remains safe to use**, and that unprotected exposure to the sun itself is the "toxin" about which you should be concerned. **Disturbing fact:** As good as the sun can feel when you're basking in its warm glow; its UV light is the most pervasive carcinogen people worldwide face every day. [301]

Along with other practices, such as limiting sun exposure and wearing sun-protective clothing, hats, and sunglasses, reapplying sunscreen as often as needed is critical to reduce your risk of skin cancer, immune system damage, and numerous signs of aging.

DOES SUNSCREEN BLOCK VITAMIN D?

This really isn't a myth as much as it is a complicated issue, but because myths are often tied to complicated issues, we felt this topic belonged here. The answer to the question is, yes, there is growing research showing that wearing adequate amounts of sunscreen (meaning liberal application) can block the production of vitamin D, and, yes, it is critically important for the body to have sufficient levels of vitamin D. But, the subsequent question of what to do about it lies in balancing the facts, not just reacting to one side of the issue.

The dilemma facing all of us is that vitamin D is one of the few nutrients the body can't make on its own, and the "natural" way to get vitamin D is to expose skin to the sun's dangerous UVB rays, which cause sunburn, cell damage, skin cancers, and, possibly, other cancers. [302] Not maintaining sufficient vitamin D levels, however, is associated with risks of bone loss, cardiovascular disease, auto-immune conditions, and some cancers.

Adding to the conflicting research—and we are overwhelmed by the vast number of papers and studies on this—is that even though sunscreen can block vitamin D production, it is also well known that most people don't wear sunscreen as they should (or at all). Therefore, sunscreen application cannot explain the vitamin D deficiency issue. [303,304] Meaning, just because you wear sunscreen and live a smart-sun lifestyle doesn't mean you will have inadequate levels of vitamin D. Even in countries where almost no one wears sunscreen and where there is a great deal of sun all year long, there are people who have deficient levels of vitamin D. [303,304]

To many researchers and dermatologists the question is not whether or not to wear sunscreen, but rather to ask yourself how you can protect your skin from the serious problems that unprotected sun exposure causes and still get enough vitamin D.

We believe strongly that you can do both, and you should. It would be shortsighted to try and solve one problem (getting enough vitamin D) and cause an equally serious problem (skin damage and skin cancer). This would be especially wrong if the recommended solution to not wear sunscreen (rather to just suffer the damage of unprotected sun exposure) did not resolve the vitamin D deficiency problem anyway, so you'd be suffering from both!

You may have heard the recommendation that you need 15 to 30 minutes of unprotected sun exposure per day for your body to produce all the vitamin D it needs. There is no evidence showing that to be the case, especially considering that dramatically different amounts of sunlight are present in different parts of the world at different times of year. For example, 30 minutes of sun exposure at noon during nine months of the year in London, Paris, Moscow, Beijing, Seattle, Toronto, or New York won't do you much good because the amount of daylight present is minimal and the sun is never directly overhead, so the rays of the sun are diminished. So, it would be ill-advised to just count the minutes you are in the sun without protection to determine how much vitamin D you're getting. [305,306]

There is also the issue of how large an area of your skin must be exposed to the sun for your body to manufacture sufficient vitamin D. Is it enough if you only expose your face and hands, or should you expose your face, arms, and chest? Or should it be your face, arms, chest, and legs? No one knows (suggesting otherwise is not supported by any research) and just guessing would be dangerous, for your skin and for getting enough sun to create vitamin D.

Summer or vacation sun-tanning is certainly not an answer. Darker skin color, whether genetic or darkened by sun exposure, provides some amount of UVB protection, which in turn slows the production of vitamin D by the body. So, seriously damaging your skin by exposing it to the sun without achieving higher vitamin D levels is at best counterproductive and at worst dangerous.

Here's what you can do to take the best care of your skin and to make sure you have sufficient levels of vitamin D in your body.

At your next physical examination have your vitamin D levels checked. You may not be deficient or you may need far more.

If your vitamin D level is low, be diligent about taking vitamin D supplements. Ask your doctor to find out how many International Units (IU) of vitamin D you should be taking because overdosing with vitamin D supplements isn't healthy either. [307,308]

The amount and frequency of the supplements will depend on many factors, including your blood level of vitamin D, your geographic location, and your overall health.

Most important: Do not give up on sun protection and being sun smart! You can have the best of both worlds: adequate levels of vitamin D without having your skin suffer the aging and cancer-causing consequences of unprotected sun exposure.

One more important point: Fear of not getting enough vitamin D is causing a frightening increase in the use of tanning beds; many tanning salons are taking advantage of this fear by advertising that they provide the added benefit of increasing vitamin D levels in the body. Aside from the terrible risks associated with using tanning beds, they do not lead to the body producing vitamin D. As it turns out, UVB rays are responsible for stimulating vitamin D production in the body, and tanning beds emit almost entirely UVA rays! This terrible misinformation is killing your skin, and it's not getting you more vitamin D. [309]

SHOULD I AVOID PARABENS IN BEAUTY PRODUCTS?

If you've shopped for makeup or skincare products over the past few years, you've probably noticed more and more brands are advertising that their products are "paraben free" or "formulated without parabens."

You might be wondering what that means—and why companies think it's so important to put this on their product labels. The truth? This is the result of years of misinterpretation and misinformation that has given parabens, which are a group of cosmetic and food preservatives, an undeserved bad reputation.

Despite the media frenzy surrounding parabens, the published research and global cosmetics regulatory organizations are making the answer clear: **parabens, especially in the small amounts used in personal-care products, do not pose a health risk**.

Parabens come in various forms, such as butylparaben, isobutylparaben, ethylparaben, methylparaben, or propylparaben. Their bad reputation is a misunderstanding resulting from a 2004 research study, where these chemicals were mistakenly linked to breast cancer when their metabolites (not parabens themselves) were detected in breast cancer tissue samples. [310]

Soon after the panic over parabens began, the researcher who conducted the 2004 study (P. Darbre) responded in the *Journal of Applied Toxicology* to the media-drawn connection between parabens and cancer with a clear statement, "Carcinogenicity was not considered in this study and the presence of parabens was not claimed to cause breast tumours." [311] In fact, as considerable global research has subsequently, and exhaustively, demonstrated, parabens are broken down, metabolized, and excreted harmlessly by the body.

Another cause for concern for some people is the fact that parabens belong to a class of chemicals known as phytoestrogens—essentially, compounds that mimic the effect of the female hormone estrogen. And estrogen has been linked to some of the deadlier forms of breast cancer.

Sounds like a convincing connection, right? Not so fast: Many plants are also high in phytoestrogens, including apples, blueberries, carrots, oats, pomegranates, rice, soybeans, and yams. Researchers have actually found that the estrogenic effects of parabens on the body are 10,000 times weaker than the effects of some of the foods many people eat every day, and that when parabens are applied topically to skin they break down immediately, and are no longer "parabens." [312]

Following is what the U.S. and global science community has found on this issue:

» **The U.S. Food and Drug Administration** found, after reviewing the global research in 2006, 2007, and again in 2014, "that at the present time there is no reason for consumers to be concerned about the use of cosmetics containing parabens." [313]

» **The European Union**, in its 2013 official statement, *The Scientific Committee on Consumer Safety: Final Opinion on Parabens*, supported the unequivocal safety of parabens in skincare, cosmetics, and personal-care products. [314] This summary of decades of long-term and short-term safety data reinforced the EU's previous decision that parabens are safe in personal-care products.

» **Japan's Ministry of Health, Labour and Welfare**, in its Standards for Cosmetics, also considers parabens safe for use in personal-care products. [315]

» **Health Canada**, the Canadian equivalent of the U.S. FDA, also finds that, "Currently, there is no evidence to suggest a causal link between parabens and breast cancer." [316]

» **The American Cancer Society** has concluded, based on its research findings, that the scientific and medical research "studies have not shown any direct link between parabens and any health problems, including breast cancer." [317]

» **The Cosmetic Ingredient Review**, an organization that reviews and assesses the safety of ingredients used in cosmetics in an open, unbiased, and expert manner, consolidated more than 265 studies in *The Journal of Toxicology* that noted a woman's daily cosmetic regimen using products that contain parabens caused no adverse reproductive effects and confirmed the safety of parabens. [318]

Ironically, parabens are naturally occurring chemicals. It's ironic because many natural skincare brands claim that ingredients like parabens are dangerous, when, in fact, parabens have exhaustive safety data AND are naturally produced by vegetables and fruits. As mentioned above, many foods, including beans, blueberries, carrots, cherries, cucumbers, and soy, contain parabens and other chemicals that mimic estrogen—to a much greater degree than the minuscule amounts of parabens present in skincare, hair-care, and makeup products. [319,320,321,322,323]

Despite the presence of parabens in these common foods, when was the last time you read a media report or received a forwarded email about the breast cancer risk from beans, carrots, or berries? In contrast, you've likely seen media reports or emails regarding parabens and their link to estrogenic activity. Kind of puts it in perspective, doesn't it?

On a global scale, there is an exhaustive number of scientific and medical studies demonstrating the safety of parabens used in skincare and other types of cosmetics. **The bottom line:** Parabens in your personal-care products are not harmful.

CAN BEAUTY PRODUCTS OR SPA TREATMENTS DETOXIFY SKIN?

No! Despite the claims of many cosmetics companies and spa services, you cannot "detox" your skin. In fact, the brands, cosmetics salespeople, and aestheticians who make this claim never specify which substances their product or service supposedly banishes—which makes sense, as your skin isn't capable of storing any sort of toxin. An actual toxin is a poison, and we're talking REAL poisons, such as those produced by plants, animals, insects, reptiles (think snake venom or bee stings), or other organisms.

So-called toxins cannot leave your body through the pores or through your skin, whether via sweat or other means—they're filtered, broken down, and removed by the kidneys and liver. Heavy metal toxicity, for example, can't be "sweated" or otherwise drawn out of skin; it requires medical treatment to remove the toxins from your body.

Regardless of the skin concern you're battling, "toxins" aren't to blame. If you're serious about wanting results, stick to what the research says really works, and ignore the fantasy claims about "detoxifying" cosmetic products.

DOES BHA (SALICYLIC ACID) MAKE SKIN PURGE?

The answer is: Maybe, but only because it depends on your definition of purging. If the expectation is that the oil and dead skin cells clogging a pore will purge to the surface and be eliminated, the answer is yes, BHA will help purge the pore. Because BHA is oil-soluble, it exfoliates not only on the surface of skin, but also inside the pore lining. That kind of exfoliation can trigger a mass exodus of the inflammatory substances and the oil that, under certain conditions, can create more breakouts.

Essentially, because salicylic acid helps skin cells turn over at a faster rate, a concentrated BHA formula can bring pimples that were already brewing to the surface more quickly than they otherwise would have appeared. It sounds counterintuitive, but it can happen for some people.

The breakouts you see after you start using a BHA would have shown up eventually anyway, or simply would have remained deep in the pore, keeping it clogged and enlarged. In other words, it's actually good to see all this movement, even though a fresh crop of breakouts can be alarming!

Our recommendation? Give your BHA exfoliant a couple weeks of once- or twice-daily use before deciding whether or not it's working for you. If it seems to be too much for your skin, decrease the frequency of use (once a day instead of twice a day, or once every other day). It's highly likely that the "purging effect" is temporary, and that you'll begin seeing smoother, clearer skin within a short period of time.

HOW LONG DO I HAVE TO WAIT BETWEEN APPLYING SKINCARE PRODUCTS?

We have a simple answer you're sure to love: You don't have to wait at all! If you're using gentle, well-formulated skincare products (and you should be), then in most circumstances, waiting is about personal preference (what works best for you) than about necessity.

One question we're asked repeatedly is whether or not a person's skin can handle so many ingredients all at once. As it turns out, skin is capable of handling a lot—and 99 percent of the time, any one product in your routine doesn't get in the way of the others you are using. Think of it like your diet: Whether you eat all your vegetables at once or take small bites of them as you enjoy the other food on your plate, your body is going to get the same nutritional benefits from the veggies in your meal.

Ultimately, it is more about the product's feel and your preference than it is about how the products absorb or set. Some people just like the feel of waiting between skincare steps, while others prefer layering one product on right after the other; some mix products like moisturizer and exfoliant in the palm of their hand before applying. All of those methods are fine. Of course, there are a few exceptions, as follows:

» If you notice that the combination of products you're using, when applied one right after the other, tends to roll or ball up, then it's probably best to allow the first product to dry before applying the next product.
» Because sunscreen should always be the last skincare product you apply, it's a good idea to allow a few minutes for it to set before you apply your make-up. If your foundation or tinted moisturizer contains sunscreen, there's no need to wait.
» The final exception to the rule is to not apply an antioxidant-rich product at the same time you apply a product with benzoyl peroxide, unless you're willing to wait for the benzoyl peroxide product to absorb before applying the antioxidant product. Don't want to wait? Switch to applying the benzoyl peroxide product in the morning and the antioxidant product at night.

Last, it's worth mentioning that applying skincare products with **different pH levels** doesn't reduce the products' effectiveness. For example, there's no harm in applying a moisturizer or serum immediately after an AHA or BHA exfoliant, which, when well formulated, will have the low pH it needs to exfoliate.

How do we know this? Any water-based product (like most moisturizers) has its pH firmly established during the formulary and mixing phase, long before it reaches your home. Once that pH range is set, its narrow parameters are very difficult to alter, and impossible to alter with other skincare products applied on top; there simply isn't enough water present to cause the lower-pH (more acidic) product's pH to budge.

Cosmetic chemists know that few consumers use only one product, that we usually apply several, often one after the other. Therefore, a good chemist will take steps (known as a buffer solution) to stabilize their formula's pH to ensure that it remains compatible with other types of products, regardless of when they're applied. There you have it, one less thing to worry about when it comes to your skincare routine!

WHEN SHOULD I TOSS OUT BEAUTY PRODUCTS?

We've all been there. You *really* love that eyeshadow or lipstick you've been using for the past two years. You can't bear to toss that skincare product—you don't remember when you bought it, but you're certain you'll use it again at some point. Either way, these are products you really need to toss.

If you're hanging on to a skincare or makeup product past its prime, chances are that microbes and bacteria have taken their toll, and might even be contributing to the skin problems you're trying to solve. With either makeup or skincare, the consistency of the product will change (not for the better), and specific to skincare products, the beneficial ingredients, which often are unstable, will lose their effectiveness.

Expired beauty products can carry a range of bacterial baddies. A 2013 study published in the *International Journal of Cosmetic Science* evaluated the makeup routines and habits of 44 women (ages 18 to 28)—the results were more than a little cringe-worthy. Of the women in the study, 70% used some type of expired product—mostly eye makeup such as mascara, eyeliner, or eyeshadow. The researchers tested the eye makeup for contamination, and found that 67% contained potentially harmful levels of microorganisms, including *Staphylococcus* species, *corynebacterium* species, and *Moraxella* species, all of which are common in bacterial skin infections. [324]

Whether in moisturizers or mascaras, preservatives last only so long after a product is opened, and the other ingredients have a shelf life as well—for effectiveness, stability, or both. The tricky thing is that only products regulated as over-the-counter drugs, such as sunscreens and anti-acne treatments, have official expiration dates stamped or printed on the packaging. The average beauty product's expiration date depends on **when you first use it and on how the product is packaged and stored**. Using a product beyond its expiration date risks irritation, rashes, breakouts, and various skin or eye infections. [324] Yuck!

To make it easier for consumers to determine when a product is approaching its "use by" date, the Period After Opening (PAO) symbol was established in Europe and should be present on any skincare or makeup product sold there, including on U.S.-based brands that are sold in Europe. A PAO symbol is an open jar with an associated number and letter, such as "12M." The letter M stands for "mensis," the Latin word for month; the number 12 refers to how many months after opening you should throw it out. So, a product labeled "12M" means you should throw the product out 12 months after you've opened it.

The problem with the PAO system is that it's not a 100 percent sure bet. The symbol gives you a general idea of how long you should keep using a product after opening it, but should not be taken to mean the product isn't any good or that it becomes harmful after that date. The truth is cosmetics companies pick these dates not based on hard science, but rather based on estimates, usually for no other reason than to meet EU regulations.

The PAO indicators do provide some guidance, but there's also a lot that consumers can do during the time they own the product that can affect how long it lasts. For example, not recapping or closing the product after each use or storing it in an environment with wide swings in temperature can have a negative impact on a product's stability and lifespan, no matter the PAO date. Plus, if you never buy a skincare product packaged in a jar again, that alone will keep it stable far longer because when ingredients aren't exposed to air they last longer.

Although products vary greatly, as do the conditions of consumer usage and storage, following is a helpful guide for determining what you need to toss now and/or how long you can continue to use it:

Makeup:
» Mascara (regular or waterproof), liquid or gel eyeliners: 4–6 months (always toss out dry mascara—never add water to extend its life)
» Cream, liquid, or stick foundations, blush, and eyeshadows: 6 months–1 year
» Powder-based products (including mineral makeup): 2–3 years
» Lipsticks, lip gloss, and lip pencils: 2–3 years

Skincare (assuming you're avoiding jar packaging):
» Cleansers and scrubs: 1 year
» Toners: 6 months–1 year
» BHA or AHA exfoliants: 1 year
» Facial or body moisturizers and serums: 6 months–1 year
» Skin-lightening treatments: 1 year
» Lip balms, lip treatments: 1 year
» Sample packets: 1 day (Really, only 1 day!)

What about storing beauty products in the refrigerator? Don't do that! Skincare formulas are designed to withstand average fluctuations in temperature, but not long-term heat or cold storage. That means that keeping your products in the fridge will *reduce* their life span and stability. The work done to stabilize a formula (along with extensive testing) is done during the development process. Once this stage is complete and the product passes all testing, there are no special precautions for storing your products, save for keeping them out of long-term storage in very hot (a steamy bathroom doesn't get hot enough) or very cold environments. To get the most from your beauty products, keep them at room temperature and secure the caps tightly after each use.

WHAT ARE BB CREAMS, CC CREAMS, AND BLEMISH BALMS?

Curious about the BB creams and CC creams, or DD, EE, and even A to Z creams you've read about? We were too. You've probably heard these products can do everything, from creating a flawless complexion to reducing pore size, healing breakouts, controlling oil, correcting an uneven skin tone, and lightening dark spots. That's quite the to-do list!

Originally developed in Germany and called blemish balm, BB creams have since crossed borders and rapidly become extremely popular, must-have products in East Asian countries such as South Korea. As they became a hot commodity throughout Asia, it wasn't long before U.S.-based cosmetics companies picked up on the trend, with a slight change in the product name—blemish balms became beauty balms once they started being developed for Western markets.

Why "blemish balms?" In East Asian cultures, the term *blemish* refers to almost any skin flaw; in Western countries and throughout North America, the term generally means an acne-like breakout (pimple or blackhead), a condition that these creams cannot help. This name change gradually took hold in Asia as well, and eventually was shortened to what's seen in North American markets: BB cream.

Despite the hoopla fueled by the cosmetics industry and by many beauty bloggers, BB creams (and the host of initials used for this "alphabet cream" category of products) are not must-have products. Essentially, BB creams sold in Western countries are little more than tinted moisturizers, often with the addition of sunscreen.

In contrast, many of the BB creams sold in East Asia have much thicker textures and higher levels of titanium dioxide and zinc oxide to provide sun protection. They're also meant to leave a slight white cast on skin as this is a desirable trait for many Asian cultures. Most East Asian BB creams are very tricky to apply if the goal is a natural, "imperceptible" finish. Another distinguishing factor is that BB creams sold in East Asia are also (usually) formulated with antioxidants and skin-lightening ingredients because the marketing for these products in Asia is mostly about lightening skin.

In the United States, whether you use a BB cream or a tinted moisturizer, these products are all about convenience: sun protection, moisture, and sheer skin tone–correcting color from one product. The formulas differ widely from company to company, but sun protection and light-coverage color are the norms—they are nearly indistinguishable from tinted moisturizers with sunscreen, save for providing a touch more coverage.

Now turning to CC creams: CC typically stands for "color and correct" and, not surprisingly, these tend to look and act much like standard liquid foundations. Sometimes they offer sun protection (just as there are many liquid foundations that provide this benefit) and sometimes they contain a smattering, or even a beneficial amount, of helpful anti-aging ingredients for skin. Whether or not they're worth using instead of liquid foundation depends completely on the formula; some are great, some aren't.

There is no set standard for any of these products regardless of the letters on the product—some do go beyond the norm of providing sun protection, light coverage, and moisturizing ingredients, and some don't. Some BB and CC creams contain beneficial ingredients that can improve dark spots, brighten an uneven skin tone, or help further reduce signs of aging, and some don't.

The most important thing to keep in mind is that just because a product is labeled BB, CC, or any other letter does not guarantee you're getting a superior "does-everything" product destined to speed up your morning routine. A product's value for your skin is always about the formula, and skincare formulas are rarely created equal; variations abound, for both the good and the bad.

WHAT ABOUT GETTING RID OF CELLULITE?

Shockingly, cellulite shows up on the thighs of more than 85% of females past the age of 18 (only 5% of men have cellulite), and even though cellulite is more noticeable for Caucasian and Asian women, it affects every skin color and ethnicity. [325] Despite what you've heard to the contrary, cellulite is nothing more than normal fat stored beneath the skin distributed on the thighs in pockets and is dependent on estrogen, which is why women have more cellulite than men. [326,327] Ironically, weight is not part of the problem. Rather, any amount of fat (and we all need some of it in our bodies) can show up as cellulite on women's thighs; it's just that being overweight makes the cellulite more noticeable.

While there are cellulite treatments with some potential (and we say potential in a very limited sense), many rarely live up to the claims asserted, or the improvement is at best minor or temporary. The nonsense you see on many websites, even those with a seemingly quite medical appearance, have minimal substance or independent research.

For example, drinking lots of water doesn't help. If water could change skin structure and reduce fat, no one would have cellulite, and no one would be overweight for that matter. Some websites tout the need to drink more water to get rid of cellulite, others say that water retention is the cause of cellulite—neither is true. Fat cells actually contain only about 10% water, so eliminating excess water won't make a difference, and any measurable result would be transient at best.

A major myth about cellulite is the notion that you can eliminate it by detoxifying the body by wrapping the leg in plastic or that applying special masks can reduce the appearance of cellulite. Fat does not accumulate because of toxins—that's complete nonsense. If losing fat by these bogus detoxing treatments worked, who would be fat? More significantly, there are no studies showing that toxins or detoxing of any kind affect cellulite in any way. There are also a bevy of skincare lotions or creams, with varying ingredients (there is no consistency among products), making claims of reducing cellulite—which, unfortunately, do not work. [326,327]

What does work in the battle against cellulite? Most studies about cellulite treatments are sham-science, are poorly designed, and/or are paid for by the company that's selling the machine or product, which means that the results could only lean toward the positive; otherwise, they wouldn't have published the study. A medical journal article that reviewed 67 studies on cellulite concluded that there is no "scientific evidence of the efficacy of treatment for cellulite reduction. No clear evidence of good efficacy could be identified in any of the evaluated cellulite treatments." [326,327]

Other treatments, such as mesotherapy, a procedure that repeatedly injects skin with different substances, are at best questionable. There isn't any consistency, disclosure about what substance is being injected, safety data, or research showing this works. There also are claims about a rolling machine called Endermologie. Spas, salons, physicians, or just about anybody else with the money to buy one of these machines want you to believe in their exaggerated, over-the-top claims. There is limited science behind this, and the research that does exist was performed by the people who are promoting the device. The Endermologie device is often touted as being FDA-approved as a Class 1 medical device to make it sound as if that means it works. A classification as a Class 1 medical device simply means that there is "minimal potential for harm to the user." No other aspect of the machine is approved or sanctioned by the FDA. Examples of other Class 1 devices include elastic bandages and latex gloves.

In terms of liposuction, a medical procedure to suck fat out of the body, it turns out that the removal of large quantities of fat can sometimes worsen the appearance of cellulite by creating unsupported and slackened skin, which will allow any remaining fat (and some always remains) to show through. If there is any reality to the reduction of cellulite, it seems to lie with laser or radiofrequency procedures performed at doctors' offices. [328,329] There is a bit of research about retinoids being beneficial, but those studies were small in number and not particularly reliable. [330]

IS MINERAL OIL BAD FOR SKIN?

Find the answer to this and other ingredient-specific questions in our *Cosmetic Ingredient Dictionary* in Chapter 16.

CHAPTER 15

Professional Makeup Secrets

THE BEST MAKEUP OF YOUR LIFE STARTS HERE!

Part of having the best skin of your life, at least for many people, also includes enhancing it with beautifully applied makeup. Now that you've discovered (in reading the previous chapters) how to have clearer, smoother, and more radiant skin, applying makeup just became much easier and more enjoyable as part of your beauty routine.

Skincare is essential, while makeup is more of an accessory. Skincare has very specific rules when it comes to having healthy, young, perfected skin. Makeup is just the opposite, where everything is optional, and personal taste and experimentation are all part of the process—and the fun.

Makeup can be anything you want it to be, from alluring to classic, sensual to casual, or minimal to dramatic. In this chapter, we go beyond the normal step-by-step routine makeup information you typically see, and instead focus on the most helpful, unique makeup tips we've learned over the years. We've joined forces with some of the top makeup artists around the globe to give you the best makeup advice, tricks, and tips available.

Much of what you're about to read was inspired by the questions we receive from fans like you, asking us to help with the makeup problems you just can't seem to find solutions for. Most of these tips apply to everyone, to one degree or another, so we urge you to try at least a few of them—you might just be surprised at the results.

One crucial tip before we start: As wonderful as it can be to put makeup on, it is also vitally important to make sure you take it all off at night. Leaving makeup behind can cause irritation and make eyes puffy, or can cause clogged pores and dry, flaky patches of skin. Use makeup remover or a well-formulated toner to be sure every last trace is gone. Your skin will thank you in the morning!

It's also important to steer clear of alcohol-based, strongly fragranced makeup. Avoiding irritant-loaded formulas is just as critical for makeup as it is for skincare, and for all the same reasons we explain throughout this book. But you already knew that, didn't you?

TIPS FOR COMPLEXION PERFECTION

» **Regardless of your natural skin tone, opt for neutral foundation shades.** That means no obvious overtones of ash (grayish), copper, orange, peach, or pink. Those shades have an unflattering effect on skin and tend to look artificial or mask-like. Also be wary of overtly yellow-toned foundations, which can make skin look jaundiced.

» **Match your foundation shade to the skin on your neck, but also take your décolletage into consideration.** The skin tone on your face often is slightly lighter or darker than skin on your neck, so matching your foundation to the neck avoids the dreaded noticeable line of demarcation where your foundation starts and stops. If you're wearing a low-cut top, take the color of your décolletage into consideration as well. If your chest is darker than your face/neck, you may want to use a slightly darker foundation or strategically use bronzer around the edges of your face to complement the undertone of your décolletage without making your whole face look too dark.

» **Don't test foundation on the back of your hand.** The color of the back of your hand has nothing to do with the color of your face. Instead, test foundation on bare skin by swatching it on the side of your jaw and then checking it in daylight to make sure it looks right (store lighting just doesn't cut it).

» **If you have acne-prone skin, avoid thick or solid-form makeup products** like stick, pancake, cream, or cream to-powder compact foundations and concealers. The same goes for bronzers or blushes in stick, cream, or cream-to-powder form. The types of ingredients that keep these products in a solid form (often waxes) are iffy for those with breakout-prone skin because they can lead to clogged pores.

» **Resist the urge to cover your entire face in a blanket of full-coverage foundation to cover up minor flaws.** If you need to conceal breakouts or other imperfections, opt for a medium- to full-coverage foundation that is easily sheered out and strategically apply concealer only where you need it.

» **Apply foundation on your eyelids up to the brow.** Applying foundation on your eyelids will help eyeshadows go on smoothly and cover any redness, giving your entire face an even and smooth appearance.

» **Apply foundation as much as possible with downward strokes, especially if you have peach fuzz.** Applying with upward strokes will coat the peach fuzz with foundation, which can draw more attention to the hairs and create a thick cakey look.

» **After you've applied foundation**, use a clean makeup sponge and spot-check for blending along the hairline, near the temples, along the jaw line, and on the upper lip. All of these spots can "collect" foundation, so a quick spot check and blending out with the sponge can make a big difference.

» **Smooth out fine lines and large pores with a cosmetic wrinkle-filler before you apply foundation.** These types of products, which typically rely on silicone polymers for their smoothing effect, once applied, temporarily expand and "fill" in crevices (whether wrinkles or large pores). More to love, some wrinkle-filling products go the extra mile and include anti-aging ingredients that also help skin in the long run. Our professional favorites include: Mary Kay TimeWise Repair Volu-Fill Deep Wrinkle Filler ($45) and NARS Instant Line & Pore Perfector ($28).

» **Consider a foundation that contains sunscreen.** This is our favorite foundation recommendation. Even if you are wearing a moisturizing sunscreen, you can add a foundation with sunscreen; layering a foundation that's SPF-rated is a great way to get extra protection. If you have oily or blemish-prone skin and hate wearing a traditional moisturizing sunscreen, a foundation and pressed powder with sunscreen (assuming you're willing to apply it liberally and it is at least SPF 30) can be the only sunscreen you need.

» **Be cautious with powder foundations.** These can work, but they also can tend to look grainy and uneven. In addition, for dry skin they can be too absorbent, and therefore drying; if you have oily skin they can look choppy as the oil starts to pool during the day.

CONCEALER FIX-ITS

» **DO NOT use under-eye concealer that's two shades lighter than your skin color.** Despite what you might read in magazines, using lighter concealer under the eye can end up having a reverse-raccoon effect. A concealer that's half or one shade lighter than your foundation (or, if you don't wear foundation, your natural skin color) will brighten the under-eye area without creating a strong, distracting contrast.

» **When concealing under-eye bags or puffiness,** be sure to blend the concealer beyond the under-eye area, about ¼ inch to ½ inch below. If the concealer is applied only in the exact area where it is puffy, it will exaggerate the problem, not conceal it. You must blend it properly to avoid drawing attention to that area.

» **Under-eye concealer is NOT the same as spot-coverage concealer.** For spot coverage (think pimples, red marks from acne, brown spots) a higher level of coverage and matte finish is best to keep those areas tenaciously concealed. Under the eyes, however, a matte-finish concealer can be too drying and may enhance fine lines and wrinkles. A light- to medium-coverage concealer is the best way to go, with a slightly hydrating, satin finish. For a slight brightening effect, look for a concealer with a hint of luminosity, and the thinner the texture, the less likely you are to experience creasing.

» **What about covering dark spots?** A strategically applied full-coverage concealer can help cover dark spots, but in many cases, those spots are just too dark to cover convincingly; the more concealer or heavy-coverage foundation you apply, the less natural your skin looks. That's where good skin-lightening products and diligent sunscreen use comes into play. See Chapter 12, *How to Treat Special Skin Problems*, for recommended skin-lightening treatments.

» **Prevent under-eye concealer from creasing** by using a lightweight serum/moisturizer around the eyes during the day, as opposed to a rich eye cream, which can cause concealer to slip into lines. You want that area to be hydrated, but not slick!

» **If you have dry skin under your eyes and need to touch-up your concealer**, try dabbing a teeny amount of moisturizer under the eye area before reapplying your concealer.

BLUSH AND HIGHLIGHT TECHNIQUES

» **Lift and sculpt cheeks.** Apply matte bronzer in the hollow of your cheeks to sharpen your bone structure and add more definition to your face. Above that, apply a touch of blush on the apples of cheeks to create a lifting effect for the face.

» **DON'T smile as you apply blush to the apples of cheeks.** Doing so raises them, so when you stop smiling and cheeks return to their normal position, the blush color ends up being lower on the face and closer to the mouth.

» **If you happen to go a little too heavy with blush** or the color grabs too intensely in an area, try toning it down with a bit of extra pressed powder, and if that doesn't work blend it out using a foundation brush (or sponge) with a little bit of leftover foundation on it.... Voilà! Problem solved.

» **Strategically illuminate skin for a youthful glow.** Before applying makeup, prep your skin by layering lightweight hydrating products (toner, serum, fluid moisturizer) and then up the ante by adding a subtle glow. Enlivening skin can be as simple as infusing cheeks with a soft, luminous blush or restoring radiance in key areas (cheekbones, bridge of nose, cupid's bow) by applying highlighter, in powder, liquid, or cream form. It's a great way to add another dimension to enhance the benefits of the contouring step of your makeup application.

BETTER BROW KNOW-HOW

When filling in brows, match your natural color or go a shade *lighter*. Somewhere along the line, the idea that brows should be a shade darker became common advice, but it's actually more flattering to use a color that either matches or is slightly lighter than your brow color to avoid an unnatural color contrast. Even if you have black hair, you don't need a black brow color (which can look quite severe)—using a dark brown shade will give you fuller-looking, defined brows that look more natural and that don't make the brow look heavy or over-defined.

Pale blonde eyebrows are the exception. Try a color that's one or two shades darker to prevent brows from looking washed out or nonexistent. Consider using a brow tint. These products look like mascara, but they have a less stiff dry down and define the brow without looking drawn on.

For redheads, opt for an auburn undertone, which tends to be the most flattering, whether you're a natural redhead or not.

The most natural-looking-yet-defined brows are often created with a combination of brow products. For instance, a brow pencil is applied first, in between brow hairs to add shape and fullness, followed by brow powder to softly elongate/even out the brow's overall shape and/or add extra emphasis and depth to the arch of the brow. To create even more fullness, add a brow hair tint/mascara. Bonus: This combination also tends to hold up through almost anything!

» **Bolder brows.** Generally, when filling brows you want to use feathering strokes to mimic real brow hairs, but to thicken the shape, carefully and minimally add color to the top line of the brow, then brush the hairs upward to create lift and cover the line you have just drawn—the full density brow is born!

» **When trimming brow hairs, brush them in the direction that they grow.** Look for longer hairs that extend beyond your intended shape and use small brow-trimming scissors to avoid creating gaps and cutting too much hair.

» **If your over-tweezed brows have reached the point that they have trouble growing, consider Latisse.** Latisse is a prescription eyelash growth serum that also has research showing it can help stimulate brow hair growth. In the meantime, create more density and fill in sparse areas with an eyebrow powder, pencil, or cream.

» **When you don't know where to start, get professional help.** Experts at an eyebrow bar (including those in department stores) or a professional make-up artist can help you achieve a well-shaped brow.

PRO EYESHADOW TRICKS

» **Apply eyeshadow BEFORE face makeup.** Why? As you apply eyeshadow, you often end up with powdery fallout beneath your eyes, and if you're already wearing foundation or concealer it's tricky to wipe the flakes away without ruining your makeup. You can also end up making the under-eye area darker as you try to blend away the eyeshadow fallout if you're using deeper eyeshadow shades. Applying eye makeup first lets you easily clean up the fallout without any repercussions!

» **Plagued by creasing shadow, especially from oily eyelids?** Prep your lids with a mattifying concealer + powder OR try Urban Decay's Primer Potion ($20) to keep eyeshadow vibrant and crease-free.

» **Where wrinkles are present, stick to matte-finish eyeshadows.** Shimmering finishes highlight wrinkles and make them more noticeable. Matte textures, on the other hand, help diffuse the appearance of wrinkles, particularly when you use deeper shades.

» **Universally flattering eyeshadow secret.** An eyeshadow design that is darker on the outer third and then gradually transitions to a lighter shade toward the middle and the inner corner flatters just about any eye shape (at least it's worth a try).

» **Once your eyeshadow look is done, add a dab of a lighter and softly light-reflective shade to the center of your eyelid.** Use a small, flat eyeshadow brush, knock off the excess shadow, and lightly press/dab it in the middle of the eyelid. Even if you have already applied a dark shade there, this extra touch is the secret to looking bright-eyed.

EYELINER TRADE SECRETS

» **Visibly lift drooping eyes with eyeliner.** Swoop eyeliner up, beginning thinner at the inside corner of the eye and then slightly, or dramatically, thicker (depending on the effect you're going for) toward the outer third of your lash line. This will help visually reshape the eye, creating the optical illusion of thicker lashes while drawing attention to the high point of your eyeliner.

» **Eyeliner for hooded eyes.** Concentrate on lining the upper lash line with a very thin line that also goes in between the eyelashes (this is called tight-lining). You can focus on a thicker mascara application and be sure to use your highlighter at the inner corner of the eye. Your eyes will still be the focus—we promise!

» **For softer-looking results, line the lower lashes with a lighter shade than the upper lashes.** Black eyeliner is classic, but can look too severe if used all around the eyes; the same goes for dark brown. Instead, use your darker color to line the upper lash line and a softer variation of the same hue to line the lower lashes. For example, dark brown for the upper line, and light brown for the lower line.

» **If you want the intricacy of a liquid eyeliner for a cat-eye look**, but your hand isn't quite steady enough, use a combination of products. Use liquid eyeliner on the inner and outer corners of eyes, which is where you want the more precise detail, and combine it with a gel or pencil liner in the areas where you want a thicker line.

» **When it comes to gel/cream eyeliner, it's all about using the right brush.** Gel/cream eyeliners (the kind that come in a pot or jar) are a pro favorite due to their versatility, but if you aren't using the right brush for the type of design you're going for, it will be really hard to pull off. Here's what to look for:

  • **If you prefer a tight line**, go with a flat, thin brush to evenly distribute the eyeliner between lashes. Try: Laura Mercier Flat Liner Long Brush ($25)

  • **For a slight swoop at the outer corners**, a bent liner brush with a narrow tip allows you to easily control the fluidity for precise application. Try: Sonia Kashuk Bent Eye Liner Brush No. 107 ($5.99)

  • **For a dramatic cateye**, a small angled brush will help you guide the shape of the line. The slanted design allows you to easily maneuver precise angles as well as thicker edges. Try: M.A.C. 263 Small Angle Brush ($20)

- **Want one brush to do it all?** Opt for a precise, narrow, point-style brush so you have the option of creating a thin line or building color for a thicker line. Try: bareMinerals Essential Liner ($15)

MASCARA POINTERS

» **Use waterproof mascara to hold lash curl.** "Curling" mascaras rarely live up to their claims, leaving you with lackluster results. Instead, use an eyelash curler, followed by a generous application of waterproof mascara (it's like hairspray for your lashes). The tenacity of the formula will make it more difficult to remove, but if you have trouble keeping stick-straight lashes curled, this will do the trick. Just be sure to treat lashes gently when you're removing the waterproof mascara.

» **Prep eyelashes for touch-ups.** This probably sounds familiar: You go to apply another coat over the mascara you've already been wearing all day and end up fighting through dried mascara. The result? A flaky, clumpy mess. Resolve this issue with Urban Decay's Mascara Resurrection ($16), which softens already-mascara'd lashes so the next coat can glide on smoothly, plus it adds more volume! Another solution: Wet a clean spoolie brush and comb through lashes before applying the next coat of mascara. The results aren't quite as impressive as the Urban Decay solution, but it works in a pinch!

» **Is smudged mascara the bane of your makeup routine?** Here are three helpful hints:
  - **Avoid ultra-emollient products under your eyes during the day.** These can break down the mascara and lead to smeared "raccoon eyes."
  - **Use a mini fan brush to apply mascara to bottom lashes.** Simply dab the mascara wand on to the fan brush and use light strokes to precisely coat the tops of lashes (as opposed to getting mascara on the underside where it can end up smudging and smearing).
  - **Set mascara with a long-wearing topcoat that resists smearing.** We're big fans of Ulta's Raincoat Waterproof Mascara Topcoat ($10), which works well over any mascara.

LUST-WORTHY LIP TIPS

» **Make your lipstick last longer** by applying a matte-finish lipliner all over your lips (not just the edges) and put your lipstick on over that. Also, avoid greasy lipsticks and glosses because those will ensure your lipstick won't last. Matte-finish lipsticks in general have a better chance of lasting longer.

» **The secret to pulling off the perfect red lip?** Despite what you may have heard, picking out the perfect red lipstick doesn't have to be dictated by your skin's undertone. We've seen olive-skinned women pull of a blue-based red and pink-toned porcelain skin tones rock an orange-red lipstick. The thing you need to focus on is how your skin looks. If you are going to rock a red lip, then camouflage any red discolorations you have (blemishes, scars, red flushing...) with a neutral foundation or concealer (medium to full coverage depending on how dark the imperfection is).

» **Looking for the ideal shade of nude lipstick?** It isn't beige, which can actually look rather ghostly on certain skin tones! A true nude lip is the color of your lips without product on. Going either a shade lighter or darker is a surefire way to pull off an attractive nude lip.

» **Thin lips?** Avoid dark-hued lipsticks because they make already-small lips recede. Brighter, richer colors are a beautiful alternative to accentuate lips. Another trick? Highlighting the vermilion border of your upper lips will give the illusion of a fuller mouth without drastic overlining; any concealer or concealer pencil will work beautifully.

» **Prevent lipstick from feathering into lip lines with clear lipliner.** Simply apply the lipliner right along the outer lip line to create a tenacious, invisible border that blocks movement of the lipstick and prevents it from bleeding into lines. Try: Paula's Choice Long-Lasting Anti-Feather Lipliner ($10).

» **Apply concealer to the outer corners of your lips** to give your lips a lift, and then apply concealer or highlighter around the edge of the lower lip to enhance a pouty look.

MAKEUP APPLICATOR ADVICE

» **Invest in the right tools.** Mini applicators packaged with the makeup you buy are rarely worth using (other than in a pinch). You'll get far better results by investing in brushes that will last you for years. Pro favorites include brushes and other makeup tools from widely sold brands such as Sonia Kashuk, Laura Mercier, M.A.C., and Real Techniques.

» **You don't need a special "brush cleanser" to wash your brushes.** A normal facial cleanser works just as well. The exception is if your cleanser has an emollient-rich formula (milky or lotion-type cleansers)—those could create buildup on brush hairs. If that's the case, use your shampoo instead.

PAULA'S PERSONAL FAVORITE MAKEUP TIPS

» **Although I know this won't work for everyone, I strongly recommend checking or applying your makeup in a magnifying mirror.** This is especially true if you don't have the best vision. What you can't see, you can't fix; for example, makeup settling into the fine lines around your eye or perhaps into the folds around your mouth, or eyeshadow fallout on your cheeks. Any mirror of 4X magnification or greater (I personally use a 10X magnification) will do the trick, and these mirrors are widely available at most drugstores, Bed Bath and Beyond, Amazon.com, and beauty supply stores. Don't use these mirrors to be critical of flaws; this is just about applying a beautiful makeup, not becoming super critical of your skin.

» **Don't apply any part of your makeup that you don't have time to apply well.** If you're in a hurry, pick and choose what you can strategically apply for the best look without making a mess of it. For example, the typical thing I leave off when I'm in a hurry is my eye design. I simply apply foundation, blush, lipstick, brow color, and mascara and then head out the door. Apply only what you get on beautifully and leave off what you can't.

» **Buy sets of eyeshadow, blush and lipstick for an easy way to create new colors.** Rather than always buying a new eyeshadow or blush color, sets of colors allow mixing to create new shades.

» **Get your makeup done professionally at least once a year.** It never hurts to get someone else's viewpoint on how your makeup should look. At the very least, there is always something new you can learn or a bad habit you can change.

For more makeup advice, including step-by-step application tips, visit the companion site to this book, BeautyMythBusters.com.

A special thank you to the talented, world-famous makeup artists who shared their makeup tips and tricks:

» Wayne Goss (youtube.com/user/gossmakeupartist)
» Tiffany Lowry (Tiffany-colors.com)
» Trendee King (Instagram: @thetrendeemakeup)
» Sarah Tammer (sarahtammer.com)
» Michael Brown (michaelbrownbeauty.com.au)
» Max May (maxmade.com.au)

RECOMMENDED MAKEUP PRODUCTS

Similar to skincare, you can find amazing makeup products in all price points. These recommended products (both drugstore and higher-end brands) earn top honors based on performance, texture, finish, color selection and formulation.

FOUNDATIONS AND BB/CC CREAMS

For oily and/or acne-prone skin:
» Laura Mercier Smooth Finish Flawless Fluide ($48)
» M.A.C. Pro Longwear Nourishing Waterproof Foundation ($33)
» Rimmel London Stay Matte Liquid Mousse Foundation ($4.99)

For dry skin:
» bareMinerals Complexion Rescue Tinted Hydrating Gel Cream SPF 30 ($29)
» Make Up For Ever Ultra HD Invisible Cover Stick Foundation ($43)
» M.A.C. Mineralize Moisture SPF 15 Foundation ($36)

For anti-aging:
» Almay Smart Shade CC Cream Complexion Corrector SPF 35 ($9.99)
» Dolce & Gabbana Perfect Luminous Liquid Foundation ($61)
» Paula's Choice Resist Instant Smoothing Anti-Aging Foundation ($25)

CONCEALERS

For acne-prone skin/spot coverage:
» Kat Von D Lock-it Concealer ($25)
» Revlon ColorStay Concealer ($9.99)
» Smashbox 24 Hour CC Spot Concealer ($25)

Undereye concealers:
» Clinique All About Eyes Concealer ($18.50)
» L'Oreal Visible Lift Serum Absolute Advanced Age-Reversing Concealer ($12.95)
» philosophy hope for everywhere concealer ($26)

POWDERS, LOOSE
» Clinique Blended Face Powder and Brush ($25)
» NARS Light-Reflecting Loose Setting Powder ($36)
» Sonia Kashuk Undetectable Loose Powder ($9.99)

POWDERS, PRESSED
» Almay Line Smoothing Pressed Powder ($13.49)
» Lancome Translucence Mattifying Silky Pressed Powder ($31)
» Wet 'n Wild Coverall Pressed Powder ($2.99)

BLUSHES
- » Hourglass Ambient Lighting Blush ($35)
- » L'Oreal Visible Lift Color Lift Blush ($12.95)
- » Paula's Choice Blush It On Contour Palette ($36)

ILLUMINATORS
- » Becca Shimmering Skin Perfector ($41)
- » NARS Highlighting Blush ($30)
- » Sonia Kashuk Chic Luminosity Highlighter Stick ($10.99)

BROW FILLERS
- » Maybelline Define-a-Brow Eyebrow Pencil ($6.99)
- » Paula's Choice Brow-Defining Cream Duo ($20)
- » Stila Stay All Day Waterproof Brow Color ($21)

EYESHADOWS
- » Dolce & Gabbana Perfect Mono Intense Cream Eye Colour ($37)
- » Milani Bella Eyes Gel Powder Eyeshadow ($4.49)
- » Physicians Formula Matte Collection Quad Eye Shadow ($7.25)

EYELINERS
- » Flower Beauty On Your Mark Liquid Eyeliner ($6.98)
- » M.A.C. Fluidline ($16.50)
- » Smashbox Always Sharp Waterproof Kohl Liner ($20)

MASCARAS, REGULAR
- » Boots No7 Exceptional Definition Mascara ($8.99)
- » Clinique High Impact Mascara ($16.50)
- » Paula's Choice FANtastic Lash Mascara ($12)

MASCARAS, WATERPROOF
- » Bobbi Brown No Smudge Mascara ($26)
- » Maybelline Volum' Express The Falsies Waterproof Mascara ($7.99)
- » Revlon PhotoReady 3D Volume Waterproof Mascara ($8.99)

LIPSTICKS AND LIP PAINT
- » Laura Mercier Paint Wash Liquid Lip Colour ($28)
- » Maybelline Color Sensational Creamy Mattes ($7.99)
- » NARS Audacious Lipstick ($32)

LIP GLOSSES

» Lancome Lip Lover ($23.50)
» NYX Cosmetics Butter Gloss ($5)
» Paula's Choice Resist Anti-Aging Lip Gloss SPF 40 ($18)

LIP LINERS

» Mary Kay Lip Liner ($12)
» Revlon ColorStay Lipliner ($7.99)
» Smashbox Always Sharp Lip Liner ($20)

CHAPTER 16

Cosmetic Ingredient Dictionary

This chapter includes an A–Z list of the most common cosmetic ingredients you'll see in products today. Many of them will be familiar to you, some will not; some are beneficial and have much research supporting their benefits and use, others have documented evidence of their potential to harm skin; and some are controversial ones you're often told to avoid, but don't know or understand why. This chapter clears up much of the confusion about the different types of ingredients and about specific ingredients; for example, many natural ingredients we tend to think of as safer because, well, they're natural and the names are easy to pronounce! Our years of research, however, has shown time and time again that there are good and bad natural ingredients, just as there are good and bad synthetic ingredients.

Despite the scope of ingredients discussed in this chapter, it's just the tip of the iceberg, so to speak! There are hundreds more cosmetic ingredients discussed in our online Cosmetic Ingredient Dictionary at paulaschoice.com/cosmetic-ingredient-dictionary. We routinely add new ingredients to this online resource and regularly update the explanations and ratings as new research comes to light. It's one more step we take to ensure you're getting the most reliable information about cosmetic ingredients, knowledge that is essential for you to have and maintain the best skin of your life!

A

açai (BEST)

Pronounced "ah-sigh-ee," this small berry with a deep purple color is a potent source of antioxidants, including ferulic acid and epicatechin. According to in vitro research, açai has higher antioxidant content than cranberry, raspberry, blackberry, strawberry, or blueberry, but that doesn't necessarily mean it is the best antioxidant in comparison. Aside from its function as an antioxidant, there is limited research of it having benefits for health or skin.[331]

acetyl glucosamine (BEST)

Amino acid sugar and primary constituent of mucopolysaccharides and hyaluronic acid. Acetyl glucosamine can be considered a skin-identical and skin-repairing ingredient. In large concentrations, it can be effective for wound healing. There is research showing that chitosan (which is composed of acetyl glucosamine) can help wound healing in a complex physiological process.[332,333] However, the concentration used in those studies was significantly greater than the concentration used in cosmetics.

In terms of exfoliation, the research that does exist was performed by Procter & Gamble and by Estee Lauder, and both companies sell skincare products with acetyl glucosamine.[334,335] In terms of its antiwrinkle action, there is no research demonstrating that wrinkles are related to wounds.

Acetyl glucosamine also has research demonstrating that it has an inhibitory effect on melanin production; thus, it can be an important ingredient in skin-lightening products, particularly when combined with niacinamide. Most of the research concerning acetyl glucosamine's effect on hyperpigmentation is from Procter & Gamble, and their Olay brand uses acetyl glucosamine in many products. Still, the research is compelling and the protocols are sound.[336,337,338]

acetyl hexapeptide-8 (GOOD)

Synthetically derived peptide that is used in a wide range of skincare and makeup products, especially those claiming to have a muscle-relaxing effect similar to Botox injections. These claims typically have to do with relaxing muscle contractions when making facial expressions, thus reducing the appearance of expression lines.

If acetyl hexapeptide-8 really worked to relax facial muscles, it would work all over the face (assuming you're using the products as directed). If all the muscles in your face were relaxed you'd have sagging, not youthful, skin, not to mention that it would affect the hand and fingers you use to apply it, which would inhibit you from picking up a cup or holding the steering wheel of your car. For all the fear espoused by companies that feature this peptide in their "works-like-Botox" products, there is considerably more efficacy, usage, and safety documentation available for Botox.[339]

Despite claims being made for acetyl hexapeptide-8 (argireline), there is a clinical study revealing that this ingredient is not even remotely as effective as Botox in reducing wrinkles.[340]

It is also interesting to note that Botox, applied topically to skin, has no impact on skin or muscles in any way, shape, or form.[18] Still, like all peptides, acetyl hexapeptide-8 has water-binding properties and theoretical cell-communicating ability. It's not a throwaway ingredient, but neither is it as miraculous as the manufacturer would lead you to believe.

acetyl octapeptide-3 (GOOD)

Synthetic peptide that is based around octapeptide-3, a peptide complex composed of the amino acids aspartic acid, glutamic acid, glutamine, and methionine. Also known as SNAP-8, this peptide is said to reduce wrinkles formed from repetitive facial expressions, though there's no independent research supporting this claim.

Even if there were independent research, the concentrations used in the company-sponsored testing to support the improvement of deep wrinkles and expression lines was 3–10%, which is far greater than what's typically present in skincare products. Although this won't replace what Botox or dermal fillers can do for etched wrinkles, like all peptides it has water-binding properties and theoretical cell-communicating ability. It may play a role in helping skin look and act younger, and can help hydrate and smooth skin.

acrylates copolymer (GOOD)

See film-forming agent.

acrylates/C10-30 alkyl acrylate crosspolymer (GOOD)

See film-forming agent.

acrylates/dimethicone copolymer (GOOD)

Silicone-enhanced film-forming agent. Also functions as a binding agent so products adhere better to skin. *See* film-forming agent.

acrylates/steareth-20 methacrylate copolymer (GOOD)

Synthetic polymer that blends steareth-20 with one or more forms of methacrylic acid. Functions as a thickening agent. *See* thickening agent.

active ingredient (GOOD)

Ingredient in a cosmetic, drug, or pharmaceutical product considered to have a pharmacological effect. In the case of cosmetics, the effect on the skin must be documented by scientific evaluation, approved by the FDA, and adhere to FDA regulations. In addition, the amount and exact function of each active ingredient must be approved by the FDA. Active ingredients include such substances as sunscreen ingredients, skin-lightening agents, and anti-acne ingredients such as sulfur and benzoyl peroxide. The FDA also specifies that the active ingredient list must be first on a product label.

adenosine (BEST)

Yeast-derived ingredient that plays an important cell-signaling role in many bodily processes. Adenosine is a good anti-inflammatory ingredient. Adenosine is present in our cells and functions as a cell-communicating ingredient because it is a source of energy that supports healthy cellular activity.[341]

adenosine triphosphate (BEST)

Organic compound from adenosine, which is formed by the hydrolysis of yeast nucleic acids. All living things need a continual supply of energy to function. Animals obtain their energy by oxidizing foods, plants obtain their energy by photosynthesizing, using chlorophyll, to make energy from sunlight. However, before the energy can be used, it must first be changed into a form that the organism can readily use. This special form, or carrier, of energy, is the molecule adenosine triphosphate (ATP).

In humans, ATP serves as the major energy source within the cell to drive a number of biological processes such as protein synthesis. The cell breaks down ATP by hydrolysis to yield adenosine diphosphate (ADP), which is then further broken down to yield adenosine monophosphate (AMP).

Research has shown that ATP appears to have strong potential as a cell-communicating ingredient and as an inflammation modulator.[342,343]

AHA (BEST)

Acronym for alpha hydroxy acid. AHAs are derived naturally from various plant sources and from milk, but 99% of the AHAs used in cosmetics are synthetically derived. In low concentrations (less than 3%), AHAs work as water-binding agents. At concentrations greater than 4% and in a base with an acid pH of 3 to 4, these ingredients can exfoliate skin cells by breaking down the substance in skin that holds skin cells together.[31,32]

The most effective and well-researched AHAs are glycolic acid and lactic acid. Malic acid, citric acid, and tartaric acid may also be effective, but are considered less stable and less skin-friendly; there is little research showing them to have benefit for skin.[31,32]

AHAs may irritate mucous membranes and cause irritation. However, AHAs have been widely used for therapy of photodamaged skin, and also have been reported to normalize hyperkeratinization (over-thickened skin) and to increase viable epidermal thickness and dermal glycosaminoglycans content, all of which lead to younger-looking skin.[31,32]

There is a vast amount of research that substantially describes how the aging process affects skin and that demonstrates that many of the unwanted changes can be improved by topical application of AHAs, including glycolic and lactic acids. Because AHAs exfoliate sun-damaged cells from the surface of skin, and because this layer imparts some minimal sun protection for skin, there is a risk of increased sun sensitivity when using an AHA.[344] However, wearing a sunscreen daily eliminates this risk.[31,32]

Note: AHAs are of little benefit when added to rinse-off products, as their contact with skin is too brief for them to function as exfoliants or be absorbed into skin.[345]

alcohol (AVERAGE)

"Alcohol," the term, refers to a group of organic compounds with a vast range of forms and uses, in cosmetics and in other areas. For skin, there are good alcohols and bad alcohols, corresponding roughly to high-molecular-weight alcohols and low-molecular-weight alcohols, respectively, as we explain below. When fats and oils are chemically reduced, they become less dense fatty alcohols (like cetyl alcohol), which can have emollient properties or act as detergent cleansing agents. There also are benign forms, including glycols, which are used as humectants to help deliver ingredients into skin.

Alcohols with low molecular weights—the bad-for-skin alcohols—can be drying and irritating. The alcohols to be concerned about in skincare products are ethanol or ethyl alcohol, denatured alcohol, methanol, isopropyl alcohol, SD alcohol, and benzyl alcohol (when one or more of these are listed among the main ingredients; tiny amounts aren't a problem).

In addition to being drying and irritating, these alcohols can generate free-radical damage and disrupt skin's protective barrier. Alcohol helps ingredients like retinol and vitamin C penetrate into the skin more effectively, but it does that by breaking down the skin's barrier—destroying the very substances that keep your skin healthy over the long term.[276]

Alcohol immediately harms the skin and starts a chain reaction of damage that continues long after it has evaporated. A 2003 study published in the

Journal of Hospital Infection found that with regular exposure to alcohol-based products, cleansing becomes a damaging ordeal—skin is no longer able to keep water and cleansing agents from penetrating into it, thus further eroding the skin's barrier.[277]

There is actually a significant amount of research showing denatured alcohol (ethanol) causes free-radical damage in skin even at low levels. Small amounts of alcohol on skin cells in lab settings (about 3%, but keep in mind skincare products use amounts ranging from 5% to 60% or greater) over the course of two days increased cell death by 26%. It also destroyed the substances in cells that reduce inflammation and defend against free radicals, and actually caused more free-radical damage.[346]

If that weren't bad enough, exposure to alcohol causes skin cells to self-destruct. The research also showed that these destructive, aging effects on skin cells increased the longer the exposure to alcohol; that is, two days of exposure was dramatically more harmful than one day, and that is only a 3% concentration.[346]

When alcohol ingredients are at the top of an ingredient list, they are problematic for all skin types; when they are near the bottom of an ingredient list, they aren't present in a high enough concentration to be considered a problem for skin.

Algae/algae extract (GOOD)

Algae are very simple, chlorophyll-containing organisms in a family that includes more than 20,000 different known species. In cosmetics, algae act as thickening agents, water-binding agents, and antioxidants. Some algae are also potential skin irritants. For example, the phycocyanin present in blue-green algae has been suspected of allergenicity and of causing dermatitis on the basis of patch tests.[347]

Other forms of algae, such as Irish moss and carrageenan, contain proteins, vitamin A, sugar, starch, vitamin B1, iron, sodium, phosphorus, magnesium, copper, and calcium. Most of these are beneficial for skin, as emollients, anti-inflammatory agents, or antioxidants.[348,349] However, claims that algae can stop or eliminate wrinkling, heal skin, or provide other elaborate benefits are unsubstantiated.

Algae is not a critical ingredient in skin-care products. Although it does have a positive function, it isn't the miracle ingredient it's often made out to be.

allantoin (BEST)

By-product of uric acid extracted from urea and considered an effective anti-irritant.

allyl methacrylates crosspolymer (GOOD)

Synthetic, non-aqueous polymer whose chief function is as a film-forming agent. *See* film-forming agent.

almond oil (BEST)

Also known as sweet almond oil, this is a non-volatile, non-fragrant oil extracted from the seeds of almonds and used as an emollient. Almond oil is a rich source of skin-repairing ingredients including triglycerides and several fatty acids (oleic, linoleic, and myristic among them). It is not known to cause adverse reactions, although it's an ingredient to consider avoiding if you have nut allergies.

Almonds (*Prunus amygdalus*) can be sweet or bitter. Sweet almond is listed in Latin as *Prunus amygdalus dulcis* and does not contain toxic constituents. Bitter almond comes from another species, *Prunus amara*, and does contain toxic constituents.

aloe barbadensis leaf juice extract (GOOD)

May also be listed as aloe barbadensis leaf juice powder, aloe extract, or aloe juice. *See* aloe vera.

aloe vera (GOOD)

There is no real evidence that aloe vera (aloe barbadenis) helps the skin in any significant way, but it's not a throwaway ingredient. Some brands use aloe in place of water in their products, but aloe is actually 99.5% water.[350]

There is research indicating that isolated components of aloe vera, such as glycoprotein, can have some effectiveness for wound healing and as an anti-irritant.[351,352] However, when mixed into a cosmetic product, it is doubtful that those qualities remain, although it may still play a role in binding moisture to skin.[353] In pure form, aloe vera's benefits on skin are probably its lack of occlusion and the refreshing sensation it provides. Aloe serves as a water-binding agent for skin due to its polysaccharide (complex carbohydrate) and sterol content. (An example of a sterol that's beneficial for skin is cholesterol.) Although research has shown aloe also has anti-inflammatory, antioxidant, and antibacterial qualities, no study has proven it to be superior to other ingredients with similar properties, including such ingredients as vitamin C, green tea, pomegranate, and many other antioxidants.

alpha hydroxy acid (BEST)
See AHA.

alpha isomethyl ionone (POOR)
Volatile fragrance ingredient that must be listed on products that contain it due to its risk of causing a sensitized reaction. It's an ingredient to avoid if you have extra-sensitive skin, especially because it is almost always combined with other volatile fragrance components such as linalool and eugenol.[354,355,356]

alpha lipoic acid (BEST)
Enzyme that, when applied topically on skin, appears to be a very good antioxidant. Taken internally, alpha lipoic acid is a water- and fat-soluble antioxidant that is capable of regenerating other antioxidants, such as vitamins C and E. It is also believed to exert numerous anti-inflammatory effects.

While studies of alpha lipoic acid do exist, few of them were carried out on people, and none were double-blind in an attempt to evaluate its effects on wrinkling.[357,358]

The majority of alpha-lipoic-acid research was performed on human dermal fibroblasts in vitro (test tube) in cell-culture systems. In vitro results are interesting, but it's not known if the results translate to human skin. These models do mimic human skin, but something that mimics human skin is not the same as living skin.

It's clear from the research that alpha lipoic acid is a potent antioxidant, but it isn't the only one; there are lots of great antioxidants, whether in the form of food, supplements, or agents applied topically to skin. Note that alpha lipoic acid is extremely vulnerable to degradation by sunlight. Lastly, higher concentrations of alpha lipoic acid (5% or greater) are capable of causing a burning or stinging sensation and/or a mild rash on skin.[359]

alumina (GOOD)
Naturally occurring mineral used as an abrasive, a thickening agent, and an absorbent in cosmetics.

aluminum hydroxide (GOOD)
Synthetic ingredient that functions as an opacifying agent and skin pro-

tectant. Secondary uses include coloring agent and absorbent. Aluminum hydroxide has no known skin toxicity.

aluminum starch octenylsuccinate (GOOD)

Powdery thickening agent, absorbent, and anti-caking agent used in cosmetics. When listed among the first few ingredients in a product, chances are the product will have a powder-like matte finish.

aluminum stearate (GOOD)

Aluminum salt of stearic acid that functions as a thickening agent and helps stabilize products.

amino acid (GOOD)

Fundamental constituents of all proteins found in the body, such as: alanine, arginine, asparagine, aspartic acid, cysteine, glutamic acid, glutamine, glycine, histidine, isoleucine, leucine, lysine, methionine, phenylalanine, proline, serine, threonine, tryptophan, tyrosine, and valine. Some of these amino acids can be synthesized by the body; others (known as essential amino acids) must be obtained from protein in the diet.

In skincare products, amino acids act primarily as water-binding agents, but some have antioxidant properties and wound-healing abilities as well. However, amino acids cannot affect, change, or repair wrinkles.

aminomethyl propanol (GOOD)

Synthetic ingredient used in cosmetics at concentrations of 1% or less to adjust a product's pH.

ammonium hydroxide (AVERAGE)

Clear, colorless liquid used in cosmetics to adjust a product's pH. Ammonium hydroxide is synthetic and sometimes used instead of sodium hydroxide to maintain an acidic pH in AHA (alpha hydroxy acid) or similar exfoliant products. The small amounts used in cosmetics are not considered sensitizing on skin.

ammonium laureth sulfate (GOOD)

Used primarily as a detergent cleansing agent; considered gentle and effective. It can be derived from coconut.[360]

ammonium lauryl sulfate (GOOD)

Used primarily as a detergent cleansing agent; considered gentle and effective. It can be derived from coconut.

Angelica archangelica **root oil** (POOR)

Volatile oil obtained from the angelica plant. The oil contains chemical constituents that can be phototoxic, including bergapten, imperatorin, and xanthotoxin. Although some components of angelica oil have antioxidant ability, it is a risky ingredient to use on skin if it is exposed to sunlight.[361]

Anthemis nobilis **flower extract** (BEST)

See chamomile.

anti-irritant (BEST)

Any ingredient that reduces signs of inflammation, such as swelling, tenderness, pain, itching, or redness. Many ingredients perform the function of anti-irritants or anti-inflammatories, and better ones are being discovered all the time. The term "anti-irritant" is interchangeable with anti-inflammatory.

Interestingly, most antioxidants function as anti-irritants because one of the skin's responses to free-radical damage is irritation and inflammation. These ingredients go a long way toward helping the skin deal with its daily struggle against sun exposure, pollution, skincare routines (topical disinfectants, sunscreens, and exfoliants can be irritating to skin), and seasonal environmental extremes.[362,363]

antibacterial agent (GOOD)

Any ingredient that destroys or inhibits the growth of bacteria; in the case of skincare products, particularly the bacteria that cause acne. *See* benzoyl peroxide.

antioxidant (BEST)

General term for a large group of natural and synthetic ingredients that reduce free-radical damage and environmental stress on skin. For a detailed explanation of antioxidants, see our complete Cosmetic Ingredient Dictionary at paulaschoice.com/cosmetic-ingredient-dictionary.

apricot kernel oil (BEST)

Emollient plant oil pressed from the seeds of apricots, and similar to other non-fragrant plant oils in terms of its emollient, skin-smoothing, and antioxidant benefit.

arbutin (BEST)

Hydroquinone derivative isolated from the leaves of the bearberry shrub, cranberry, blueberry, some mushrooms, and most types of pear. Arbutin's hydroquinone content gives it melanin-inhibiting properties.

Although the research describing arbutin's effectiveness is persuasive, concentration protocols have not been established. That means we don't know how much arbutin it takes to have a skin-lightening effect and there is only limited research, mostly animal studies or in vitro, showing that the arbutin-containing plant extracts used in skincare products have any impact on skin. Whether or not these extracts are effective in the small amounts present in cosmetics has not been established.[364,365]

argan oil (*Argania spinosa*) (BEST)

Non-fragrant plant oil expressed from the kernels of argan trees. Argan oil contains several beneficial lipids and fatty acids for skin, including oleic acid, palmitic acid, and, especially, linoleic acid. It is also a good source of vitamin E (tocopherol) and, like several other plant oils, a source of antioxidant compounds.[366,367]

Much of the folklore surrounding the ingredient heralds argan oil as a restorative wonder, used by Moroccan women for years to tend to their hair, skin, and nails. Of course, this isn't truly relevant as not all Moroccan women have great skin, hair, and nails, or use argan oil; and different cultures use different oils, like olive or kukui oil, with mixed results.

Argan oil isn't a miraculous ingredient by any stretch of the imagination, but it's a good, emollient plant oil. It's a consideration if skin or hair is dry to very dry, but is no better than many other non-fragrant plant oils used in cosmetics.[366,367,368,369]

arginine (GOOD)

Amino acid that has antioxidant properties and can be helpful for wound healing.[370,371]

arnica extract/arnica oil (POOR)

Extract or oil obtained from the flowering plant *Arnica montana*. There is research showing that when arnica is taken orally before surgery it reduces inflammation and bruising.[372] However, in high amounts it is a risk for skin irritation, shown to kill keratinocytes (skin cells) and to have negative effects on naturally present antioxidants in skin.[373,374]

aroma/flavor (AVERAGE)

Seeing "aroma/flavor" on an ingredient list can be either good or bad. For example, if the aroma or flavor comes from mint or citrus, it can be irritating. But if the source is something more innocuous, like vanilla, then it shouldn't pose a risk of irritation.

According to the Personal Care Product Council's Ingredient Database, "Aroma is a term for ingredient labeling used to identify that a product contains a material or combination of materials normally added to a cosmetic to produce or to mask a particular flavor." The point to be aware of is what kind of flavor your lips (or skin) are being exposed to—and whether or not the exposure poses a risk of irritation. Lastly, be aware that highly flavored lip products can encourage lip-licking—after all, such products do tend to taste good—but they shouldn't be eaten, and licking your lips too often can cause or worsen dry, chapped lips.

ascorbic acid (BEST)

Form of vitamin C that has antioxidant properties.[375] Ascorbic acid is difficult to stabilize in formulations.[108,376] Its acid component can be a skin irritant, so formulary steps must be taken to reduce potential irritation, while ensuring the ingredient retains its considerable benefits for skin.

ascorbyl glucoside (BEST)

Form of vitamin C combined with glucose. It can function as an antioxidant, but only minimal research substantiates this activity, and its antioxidant potential is weaker than that of ascorbic acid.[377] The research that does exist involved a combination of ascorbyl glucoside with niacinamide, but it is possible the benefit resulted from only the niacinamide, and not the combination.[378]

ascorbyl palmitate (BEST)

Stable and nonacidic form of vitamin C that is effective as an antioxidant. Ascorbyl palmitate is particularly effective at reducing free radicals generated from UVB rays and, due to its palmitate portion, is also a moisturizing form of vitamin C.[379]

astaxanthin extract (BEST)

Carotenoid (carotene pigment) found in plants, algae, and fish, particularly salmon, that functions as a potent antioxidant.[380] Research also suggests that astaxanthin may be able to prevent the oxidative damage to skin after exposure to UVA radiation.[381]

Avena sativa (BEST)

See oatmeal and oat bran extract.

avobenzone (BEST)

Synthetic sunscreen ingredient (also known as Parsol 1789 and butyl methoxydibenzoylmethane) that can protect against the entire range of the sun's UVA rays. It has been used since 1981 and is the most-used sunscreen ingredient in the world. It is the number one sunscreen agent used in Australian, Canadian, and European sunscreen formulations. In the United States, the FDA approved avobenzone's use as a sunscreen agent only after more than seven years of study. Avobenzone had to meet scrupulous performance standards when Hoffman-LaRoche applied for it to receive new drug status from the FDA.[382,383]

New drug status is the most stringent FDA classification possible and requires more safety studies and efficacy substantiation than you can imagine.

avocado oil (BEST)

Emollient oil similar to other non-fragrant plant oils. It has antioxidant properties and is a good source of skin-repairing fatty acids.

azelaic acid (BEST)

Component of grains such as wheat, rye, and barley, azelaic acid is effective for a number of inflammatory skin conditions when applied topically. It's available by prescription (Azelex, Finacea) and in lower strengths in over-the-counter products.

For the most part, azelaic acid is recommended as an option for acne treatment, but there is also some research showing it to be effective for treatment of skin discolorations. Although the research hasn't shown exactly how azelaic acid works for lightening brown spots and other discolorations, it is believed to interrupt the pathway of melanin (skin pigment) formation; melanin is responsible for discolorations.[384]

Azelaic acid is also an antioxidant, and its pronounced anti-inflammatory effect may be what helps fade red marks from acne and why it can be so effective for reducing the redness that accompanies the skin disorder rosacea.[385,386]

B

balm mint extract (POOR)

Extract derived from a fragrant plant; it poses some risk of skin irritation. It also has some reported antiviral properties.[387] Claims that it can help heal wounds are not substantiated.

barley extract (AVERAGE)

Extract from barley plants. Can have antioxidant properties when ingested, but there is no research showing this to be the case when applied topically.[388] Barley and its extracts/derivatives are a source of gluten. When fermented (as it is when used to make beer or when combined with yeast in cosmetics), barley extract has been shown in animal studies to reduce topical inflammation that can lead to atopic dermatitis.[389]

bearberry extract (GOOD)

Bearberry extract (Latin name *Arctostaphylos-uva ursi*) has antibacterial and antioxidant properties, and there is a small amount of research showing it has skin-lightening properties.[390,391] Bearberry extract's potential efficacy is derived from its active components: hydroquinone and arbutin.[392]

Hydroquinone is well established as a melanin-inhibiting agent; arbutin has far less quantitative information available, but in high concentrations has been shown to inhibit melanin production.[393] However, the small amount of bearberry extract present in skincare products makes it unlikely that these products can affect melanin production. *See* hydroquinone and arbutin.

beeswax (GOOD)

Natural substance made by bees to build the walls of their honeycomb. It is a thickening agent that has some emollient properties, and is often used in lip balms.

bentonite (GOOD)

Type of clay that is used as an absorbent in cosmetics. It can be drying for skin, though its absorbent properties are helpful for those with oily skin.

benzalkonium chloride (AVERAGE)

Antimicrobial agent used as a preservative in skincare products. There is no research showing it has any effect against the acne-causing bacteria *Propionibacterium acnes*. It can be a skin irritant.[394]

benzoyl peroxide (BEST)

Considered the most effective over-the-counter choice for a topical antibacterial agent in the treatment of acne.[33]

The amount of research demonstrating the effectiveness of benzoyl peroxide is exhaustive and conclusive.[33,68,71] Among benzoyl peroxide's attributes is its ability to penetrate into the hair follicle to reach the bacteria that cause the problem, and then kill them—with a low risk of irritation. It also doesn't pose the problem of bacterial resistance that some prescription topical antibacterials (antibiotics) do.[72]

Research has also shown that benzoyl peroxide is more effective than some other prescription treatments for acne, such as oral antibiotics and topical antibiotics.[33,68,71]

Benzoyl peroxide solutions range in strength from 2.5% to 10%. It is best to start with lower concentrations because a 2.5% benzoyl peroxide presents a much lower risk of potential irritation product is much less irritating than a 5% or 10% concentration, and it can be just as effective.[33,68,71]

Although once thought to be a problem if applied at the same time as products with retinol or prescription retinoids (such as Renova, Retin-A, Differin, Tazorac, and generic tretinoin), recent research has shown that not to be the case.[75]

benzyl alcohol (GOOD)

Organic alcohol that occurs naturally in some fruits (apricots, cranberries) and teas. Its chief function in cosmetics is as a preservative, and it's among the least irritating preservatives in use.[395]

High amounts of benzyl alcohol can impart a noticeable floral-like scent to products, as it is part of the fragrance makeup of some essential oils such as jasmine.[361]

As a volatile alcohol, it can pose a risk of irritation when used in high amounts, but is considered safe as used in cosmetics.[396]

bergamot oil (POOR)

Volatile citrus oil that is a photosensitizer when used topically and also has photomutagenic properties, meaning it can induce malignant changes to cells.[397,398]

beta-glucan (BEST)

Polysaccharide sugar derived from yeast or oats. It has some antioxidant properties and is a strong anti-inflammatory agent.[399,400] It is considered an excellent ingredient for reducing redness and other signs of sensitive skin.

beta hydroxy acid (BEST)

See salicylic acid.

BHA (BEST)

See salicylic acid.

bisabolol (BEST)

Anti-irritant typically extracted from chamomile, but also derived synthetically. Bisabolol reduces pro-inflammatory cytokine production and ameliorates skin inflammation.[401]

bitter orange extract (POOR)

Frequently listed as *Citrus aurantium*, it can have antioxidant properties when eaten.[402] However, used topically its methanol content makes it potentially irritating for skin.[403]

black pepper extract and oil (POOR)

Used topically as a counter-irritant, which means it can cause significant skin irritation. May be listed by its Latin name *Capsicum*. *See* counter-irritant.

Boerhavia diffusa root extract (BEST)

Extract from a flowering plant. Studies on animals have shown that this plant has strong anti-inflammatory activity. Like all plant extracts, *Boerhavia diffusa* also has antioxidant ability.[402,404]

The leaves of this plant are a major source of the antioxidant quercetin.[405]

borage seed oil (BEST)

Non-fragrant, moisturizing plant oil that's a rich source of the essential fatty acid gamma linolenic acid.[406] Also listed as *Borago officinalis* extract or oil.

butyl methoxydibenzoylmethane (BEST)

See avobenzone.

butylene glycol (GOOD)

Commonly used slip agent that has multiple functions in cosmetics, depending on the formula. It's similar to propylene glycol, but has a lighter texture. The Cosmetic Ingredient Review Expert Panel has evaluated several toxicology tests and other research concerning butylene glycol and has determined it is safe as used in cosmetics products.[407]

butylparaben (GOOD)

See parabens.

butylphenyl methylpropional (POOR)

Synthetic fragrance ingredient with a strong floral scent. Its use in cosmetics is restricted due to concerns over irritation and allergic reactions. The presence of butylphenyl methylpropional must be indicated in the list of ingredients if the product contains more than 0.001% and is meant to be left on skin; it also must be listed if the product contains more than 0.01% and is meant to be rinsed, like cleansers and shampoos.[408]

C

C10-30 cholesterol/lanosterol esters (BEST)

Blend of cholesterol and fatty acid ester from lanolin. Functions as a skin-conditioning agent.

C12-15 alkyl benzoate (GOOD)

Used as an emollient and thickening agent in cosmetics. This common synthetic ingredient is soluble in oil and oil-like ingredients, and can impart a light, silky finish to products.

caffeine (GOOD)

Alkaloid found in coffee, tea, and kola nuts. Caffeine is the chief stimulant in beverages such as coffee and tea. It's often included in skincare products with claims that it will reduce cellulite or puffy eyes. Unfortunately, research into caffeine's effects in this regard are mixed.

Caffeine and its constituents are thought to convey antioxidant benefits when consumed orally. Studies have looked at oral consumption of caffeine-containing beverages followed by exposure to UVB light (the kind that causes sunburn and skin tumors) and found that, compared with those who drank decaffeinated beverages, the drinks with caffeine conveyed a protective benefit.[409,410,411]

Applied to skin, caffeine may have anti-inflammatory properties.[412] It can penetrate skin's barrier and has a constricting effect, which can help reduce redness but also may be irritating. Caffeine is not a slam dunk for reducing facial redness; in fact, it may worsen the problem, but it's worth experimenting with if you're curious.

Caffeine's popularity in products related to cellulite is due to its distant relationship to aminophylline (a pharmaceutical once thought to reduce cellulite), which is a modified form of theophylline, and caffeine contains theophylline.[413] There is no substantiated research proving theophylline can affect cellulite, but researchers have disproved aminophyilline's claimed impact on cellulite.

Research on caffeine's effect on cellulite when applied topically is mixed, and the more recent studies were performed on mice, not on humans with cellulite. Although caffeine may play a role in reducing the size or number of fat cells, the appearance of cellulite results from a combination of fat and changes in skin's structure, the latter of which caffeine cannot impact.[414,415]

When it comes to puffy eyes, there is no research indicating caffeine can have any benefit when applied topically. However, caffeine does have potential as an antioxidant, so it isn't a wasted ingredient in skincare products.[416,417]

calendula extract (GOOD)

Extract derived from the plant commonly known as pot marigold or *Calendula officinalis*, there is little research showing that it has any effect on skin, though it may have antibacterial, anti-inflammatory, and antioxidant properties. If you have ragweed (or similar plant) allergies, topical application of calendula is not recommended because of the risk of an eczematous allergic reaction.[418]

Camellia oleifera (BEST)

See green tea.

Camellia sinensis (BEST)

See green tea.

camphor (POOR)

Aromatic substance obtained from the wood of a tree common to Southeast Asia, *Cinnamomum camphora*, or manufactured synthetically. When applied to the skin, camphor produces a cooling effect and dilates blood vessels, which can cause skin irritation and dermatitis with repeated use. Inhaling camphor at concentrations of 2 ppm (parts per million) or more may cause irritation of the mucous membranes and respiratory depression. Camphor can also cause skin and eye irritation on contact. In fact, depending on the dose applied, acute poisoning can (and has) occurred.[419,420] Clearly, camphor is not an ingredient to take lightly, though it does have several medicinal applications.

candelilla wax (GOOD)

Extract derived from candelilla plants; used as a thickening agent and emollient to give products such as lipsticks or stick foundations their form.

caprylic/capric triglyceride (BEST)

Derived from coconut oil and glycerin, it's considered an excellent emollient and skin-repairing ingredient. It's included in cosmetics due to its mix of fatty acids that skin can use to repair its surface and resist moisture loss. Caprylic/capric triglyceride can also function as a thickener, but it's chief job is to moisturize and replenish skin. This ingredient's value for skin is made greater by the fact that it's considered non-sensitizing.

Due to its fatty acid content, caprylic/capric triglyceride may clog pores, but there is much debate about this because some researchers feel that the medium-chain fatty acids that comprise this ingredient have an anti-inflammatory effect that *reduces* the risk of breakouts. In addition, caprylic/capric triglyceride is not an oily or wax-like ingredient that can easily get stuck in the pore lining.

caprylyl glycol (GOOD)

Skin-conditioning agent that may be plant-derived or synthetic. Often used as part of a preservative blend with phenoxyethanol and chloroxylenol, two preservatives that meet current global regulations.

carbomers (GOOD)

Group of thickening agents used primarily to create gel-like formulations. High amounts of carbomers in a gel may result in the product rolling or balling up on skin, but this depends on other formulary steps taken to minimize this effect.

carnauba wax (GOOD)

Natural, hard wax obtained from the leaves of palm trees. Used primarily as a thickening agent, but also has film-forming and absorbent properties.

Carthamus tinctorius **oil** (BEST)

See safflower seed oil.

castor oil (GOOD)

Vegetable oil derived from the castor bean. It is used in cosmetics as an emollient, though its unique property is that when dry it forms a solid film that can have water-binding properties. It is rarely associated with skin irritation or allergic reactions, but can have a slightly sticky feel on skin.

cell-communicating ingredients (BEST)

Cell-communicating ingredients, theoretically, have the ability to tell a skin cell to look, act, and behave better, more like a normal healthy skin cell, or to stop other substances from telling the cell to behave badly or abnormally. They do this by either direct communication with the skin cell or by blocking damaging cellular pathways or other cell-communicating substances.

For all parts of our bodies to work properly, including skin cells, each cell must know how to perform the correct action at the correct time—and, hopefully, to ignore information (in the form of messenger substances) that tells cells to do the wrong thing. This takes place through constant communication, with many substances telling cells how and when to function properly, and the cells then relaying that information to each other. When cells have a miscommunication, or when substances relaying bad information get through to the cell, it can cause all sorts of problems. Every cell has a vast series of receptor sites for different substances; think of these receptor sites as the cell's communication hookup. When the right ingredient for a specific site shows up, it has the ability to attach itself to the cell and transmit information. In the case of skin, this means telling the cell to start doing the things a healthy skin cell should be doing. If the cell accepts the message, the cell can then share the same healthy message with other nearby cells and so on and so on.[421,422,423,424,425,426,427,428]

Theoretically, this area of investigation is incredibly exciting for skincare. For now, the skincare ingredients to look for in terms of cell-communicating ability include retinol, retinaldehyde, retinoic acid, epigallocatechin-3-gallate, eicosapentaenoic acid, niacinamide, lecithin, linolenic acid, linoleic acid, phospholipids, carnitine, carnosine, adenosine triphosphate, adenosine cyclic phosphate, most peptides, and *Pyrus malus* (apple) fruit extract.

Cera alba (GOOD)
See beeswax.

Cera microcristallina (GOOD)
See microcrystalline wax.

ceramides (BEST)
Naturally occurring, long chains of skin lipids (fats) that are major structural components of skin's outer layers. Skin as a barrier system inhibits water movement via its extracellular matrix, which has a unique composition of 50% ceramides, 25% cholesterol, and 15% free fatty acids. Together, these lipids form what researchers refer to as "crystalline lamellar structures."[429,430,431]

Ceramides are necessary for their water-retention capacity as well as for barrier repair and cell regulation. Adding ceramides to skincare products can help restore the skin's barrier.[432,433,434]

Nine different ceramides have been identified in skin, some of which are used in skincare products. On a skincare product ingredient label, you'll see those listed as ceramide AP, ceramide EOP, ceramide NG, ceramide NP, ceramide NS, phytosphingosine (which can produce numerous ceramides in skin), and sphingosine.[435]

The ceramides used in skincare products typically are derived from plants or are synthetic; there is no research showing that either form is preferred over the other. However, the chain length of synthetic ceramides can be controlled, while the chain length of plant or of animal-derived ceramides cannot be controlled. The benefit of controlling the chain length is that it can be made a "better fit" when the ceramide chain is applied to skin cells in need of help.[436]

cetearyl alcohol (GOOD)
Fatty alcohol used as an emollient, emulsifier, thickener, and carrying agent for other ingredients. Can be derived naturally, as in coconut fatty alcohol, or synthetically.

cetearyl ethylhexanoate (GOOD)
Oil-like liquid that functions as an emollient to prevent skin from losing moisture. Also adds an elegant slip to creams and lotions. *See* cetearyl alcohol.

cetyl alcohol (GOOD)

Fatty alcohol used as an emollient, emulsifier, thickener, and carrying agent for other ingredients. Can be derived naturally, as in coconut fatty alcohol, or synthetically. It is not an irritant and is not related to SD alcohol, denatured alcohol, or ethyl alcohol.

cetyl esters (GOOD)

Synthetic wax used in cosmetics as a thickening agent and emollient.

cetyl palmitate (GOOD)

Ester of cetyl alcohol and palmitic acid, this thickener and emollient helps smooth and condition dry skin while preventing moisture loss. The ingredients that comprise cetyl palmitate are naturally occurring fatty acids. It may be derived from animals, but also can (and usually is) derived from plants or manufactured synthetically.

chamomile (BEST)

Ingredient derived from plant species *Chamomilla recutita*, *Matricaria recutita*, and *Matricaria chamomilla*. Chamomile tea, brewed from dried flower heads, has been used traditionally for medicinal purposes. The main constituents of the flowers include phenolic compounds, primarily the flavonoids apigenin, quercetin, patuletin, luteolin, and their glucosides.

The principal components of the essential oil extracted from the flowers are the terpenoids α-bisabolol and its oxides and azulenes, including chamazulene. Chamomile has moderate antioxidant and antimicrobial activities, and significant anti-platelet activity in vitro. Animal model studies indicate it may have potent anti-inflammatory action, some antimutagenic and cholesterol-lowering action, as well as anxiolytic effects.[437,438]

Adverse reactions to chamomile, when consumed as a tisane or applied topically, have been reported among those with allergies to other plants in the daisy family.[439]

chlorphenesin (GOOD)

Type of alcohol used as a preservative in cosmetics. It is active against some types of bacteria, fungi, and yeast and is almost always combined with other preservatives.

cholesterol (BEST)

The barrier function of skin depends on the stratum corneum extracellular lipid matrix, which includes ceramides, cholesterol, and free fatty acids. Smaller amounts of cholesterol sulfate and cholesteryl oleate may be present. Applied topically, cholesterol in cosmetics can help maintain the skin's normal function. It is also a stabilizer, emollient, and water-binding agent.[440]

cinnamon (POOR)

Can have antimicrobial and antioxidant properties, but also can be a skin irritant.[441,442]

citric acid (GOOD)

Extract derived from citrus and used primarily in small amounts to adjust the pH of products to prevent them from being too alkaline.

Citrus medica limonum (POOR)

See lemon.

cocamide DEA and cocamide MEA (AVERAGE)

Both cocamide DEA (diethanolamine) and MEA (monoethanolamine) are widely used to thicken the water phase of cosmetics, keep ingredients blended, and boost foaming properties. Derived from plants (typically coconut oil) or made synthetically, these ingredients have been thoroughly evaluated for safety and are permitted for use in leave-on products in concentrations up to 10%. Cocamide DEA can react with other ingredients to form carcinogenic substances known as nitrosamines. According to the Cosmetic Ingredient Review (CIR) Expert Panel, "To prevent the formation of possibly carcinogenic nitrosamines, these ingredients should not be used in cosmetics and personal care products containing nitrosating agents." The CIR Expert Panel concluded that "Cocamide DEA was safe as used in rinse-off products and safe at concentrations of less than or equal to 10% in leave-on products."[443]

cocamidopropyl betaine (GOOD)

Gentle surfactant used in skincare products, almost always as a secondary cleansing agent and lather booster. When used alone as the sole cleansing agent, it is too mild to clean adult skin and hair.

coco-glucoside (GOOD)

Mixture of fatty alcohol from coconut and glucose. Functions chiefly as a cleansing agent. May be plant-derived or manufactured synthetically.

cocoa butter (BEST)

Oil extracted from cocoa beans, used as an emollient and with properties similar to those of other non-fragrant plant oils. Cocoa butter is a rich source of antioxidant polyphenols; in vitro research shows it helps improve skin elasticity and promotes healthy collagen production.[444]

Contrary to popular belief, topical application of cocoa butter during pregnancy does not prevent or reduce the number of stretch marks.[445,446]

coconut oil (BEST)

Non-volatile plant kernel oil whose high saturated fat content has emollient properties for skin. Coconut oil is a rich source of medium-chain fatty acids, also known as medium-chain triglycerides. Used by itself as a moisturizer, coconut oil's effectiveness is similar to that of mineral oil.[447,448]

All reports of using coconut oil (virgin, which means unrefined) to heal acne are anecdotal, which means you just have the claims of others, not solid research, to go on. However, there is one study showing that lauric acid, the major fatty acid in coconut oil, has antibacterial activity against acne-causing bacteria (Latin name *Propionibacterium acnes*, or *P. acnes*). Although one study isn't much to go on and the research did not demonstrate that the lauric acid reduced or eliminated acne, it's still intriguing. It seems that when lauric acid derived from coconut oil is applied to skin via liposomes (a type of delivery system), it fuses with the cell membrane of the acne-causing bacteria, where it then releases its fatty acid as the liposome dissolves, killing the acne-causing bacteria.[449] This isn't the same as applying pure coconut oil to skin; that is, the delivery systems varied and the study addressed topical application of only lauric acid, not of pure coconut oil, so we don't know if pure coconut oil would have similar results on acne bacteria.

Coconut oil has a growing reputation of being a viable "non-toxic" natural ingredient to use instead of your usual sunscreen—don't fall for it! Some health-themed websites are advising consumers to slather on extra-virgin (minimally processed) coconut oil instead of an SPF product, with the claim that it's been used by Pacific Islanders for "thousands of years." This is a dangerous idea, and demonstrates that folklore and anecdotal evidence can't hold a candle to what scientific research has shown to be factual.[450]

If you want to use coconut oil, whether extra-virgin, cold-pressed, or not, to improve dry skin or add a sexy glow to your legs, go for it; but, if your skin will be exposed to UV light, you must follow it with a well-formulated sunscreen rated SPF 30 or greater to ensure you're truly protecting your skin. To reiterate: There is no scientific evidence that coconut oil protects skin from sun damage. You can choose to follow the direction of some ostensibly well-meaning natural health sites, but we assure you that doing so will be to the detriment of your skin.

collagen (GOOD)

Type of fibrous protein arranged in a triple helix pattern and found extensively throughout the body, both in people and animals. It supports skin, internal organs, muscles, bone, joints, and cartilage.

There are at least 16 types of collagen that occur naturally in the body; the most abundant form in the human body is known as type I collagen. Collagen works in tandem with elastin to give skin its texture, structure, ability to stretch, and its smooth appearance.[5,6]

Sun damage (extrinsic aging) and chronologic aging (intrinsic aging) cause collagen in the skin to deteriorate.[5,6]

As a cosmetic ingredient, collagen is derived from animal sources, but plant derivatives that act like collagen (pseudo-collagen) and amino acid fragments of collagen such as hydroxyproline are also used. In any form, collagen is a good water-binding agent. Collagen in cosmetics, regardless of the source, has never been shown to have a direct effect on producing or building collagen in skin, even when it is manipulated to be small enough to penetrate past skin's uppermost layers.

comfrey extract (POOR)

Extract of a perennial herb that several studies have shown can have carcinogenic and/or toxic properties when taken orally. It is a major problem for the body when consumed orally because it contains pyrrolizidine alkaloids. These compounds occur naturally in every part of the comfrey plant, and are absorbed through the skin, where they cause problems when the liver attempts to metabolize them. It is these metabolites (referred to as pyrroles) that are highly toxic.[451]

Topical application of comfrey has anti-inflammatory properties, but it is recommended only for short-term use and only then if you can be sure the amount of pyrrolizidine alkaloids is less than 100 micrograms per application—something that is impossible to determine without sophisticated testing equipment—making comfrey an ingredient to avoid. The alkaloid content makes it a potential skin irritant.[452]

copper gluconate (GOOD)

Also known simply as copper, this mineral is an important trace element for human nutrition. The body needs copper to absorb and use iron, and copper is also a component of the powerful antioxidant enzyme superoxide dismutase.

The synthesis of collagen and elastin is in part related to the presence of copper in the body. Copper is also important for many other processes; for example, there is research showing that copper is effective for wound healing and for anti-aging due to its inhibitory effect on matrix metalloproteinases and stimulation of fibroblasts that build healthy collagen.[453] Copper gluconate is a potentially exciting anti-aging ingredient, but certainly not among the most well researched or proven when it comes to topical application.

counter-irritant (POOR)

Counter-irritants are used to induce local inflammation for the purpose of relieving inflammation in deeper or adjacent tissues. In other words, they substitute one kind of inflammation for another, which is never good for skin. Irritation or inflammation, no matter what causes it or how it happens, impairs the skin's immune and healing response.[454]

Ingredients such as menthol, peppermint, black pepper, camphor, and mint are counter-irritants.[455]

Although your skin may not show it or may not react in an irritated fashion, if you apply irritants to your skin the damage is still taking place and is ongoing, so its effects add up over time.[456]

cucumber extract (GOOD)

Non-irritating plant extract from the gourd family (think pumpkin) that's often reputed to be useful for puffy eyes. Claims of cucumber having anti-inflammatory or soothing properties are anecdotal, as there is no research to support this contention. However, there is research showing that the lutein component of cucumber can help suppress melanogenesis, the process that leads to skin discolorations. Also there is in vitro research showing that the constituents in cucumber can help protect skin against carcinogenic substances that cause tumors.[457,458]

Most types of cucumber are composed of 95% water; the other constituents are primarily ascorbic acid (vitamin C), caffeic acid (an antioxidant), the mineral silica, plus other trace minerals. Like most plants, cucumber contains chemical constituents that have some amount of antioxidant activity. Cucumber does not contain fragrant components known to be irritating to skin.[459,460]

Cucumis melo fruit extract (BEST)

More commonly known as cantaloupe or honeydew melon, *Cucumis melo* (melon) is a fruit rich in vitamins A and C and a wide range of various antioxidant compounds.[461,462]

curcumin (BEST)
Potent antioxidant and anti-inflammatory spice that can be effective in wound healing.[463,464]

cyclopentasiloxane (GOOD)
See silicone.

cyclotetrasiloxane (GOOD)
See silicone.

D

D&C (GOOD)
According to the U.S. Food and Drug Administration (FDA), D&C indicates that a coloring agent has been approved as safe in drug and cosmetics products, but it does not apply to food.

decyl glucoside (GOOD)
Sugar-derived ingredient used as a gentle detergent cleansing agent.

denatured alcohol (POOR)
See alcohol.

DHA (GOOD)
See dihydroxyacetone.

diazolidinyl urea (AVERAGE)
Water-soluble preservative that is very effective against a broad range of bacteria, while also having some antifungal ability. This preservative is considered safe for use at concentrations up to 0.5%, although it is usually present at lower concentrations because it is only one part of a blend with other preservatives (such as parabens).[465]
Diazolidinyl urea can be a formaldehyde-releasing preservative.[466] Although that sounds scary, the amount of formaldehyde released is well below the recommended limits of exposure. Moreover, other ingredients (such as

proteins) in a product cause the free formaldehyde to evaporate and become inactive before it could possibly harm skin.

dicaprylyl carbonate (GOOD)

Emollient ingredient that may be derived from synthetic or animal sources. It spreads easily and leaves a velvety feel on skin without seeming greasy or slick. It also helps other ingredients penetrate skin better.

diethanolamine (DEA) (AVERAGE)

Colorless liquid used as a solvent and pH adjuster. Also used as a lather agent in skincare and haircare products when coupled with a foaming or detergent cleansing agent, such as cocamide DEA (which is not the same as pure DEA).

In 1999, the National Toxicology Program (NTP) completed a study that found an association between cancer and tumors in laboratory animals and the application of diethanolamine (DEA) and certain DEA-related ingredients to their skin.[467]

The National Toxicology Program (NTP) tested potential effects of DEA when a pure concentration of this ingredient was directly applied to mouse skin for a period of 14 weeks (minimum) and 2 years (maximum). The study reported no evidence of carcinogenicity when low doses (50–100 mg per kilogram of body weight) were used. Internal changes to organs (liver, kidneys) and external signs (inflammation, ulcers) were found as the dosages of DEA increased (up to 800 mg was used).[467]

For the DEA-related ingredients, the NTP study suggested that the carcinogenic response is linked to possible residual levels of DEA. However, the NTP study did not establish a link between DEA and the risk of cancer in humans and, after evaluating the results of this study, the FDA ruled that there was no cause for concern with regards to DEA-related ingredients in cosmetics.[468]

Although the results of this study are interesting, it is still unrelated to how DEA is used in cosmetics products and how consumers use them. In most instances, our contact with DEA in any form is brief, as it is present in rinse-off products, and it is not proven to cause harm to people. In vitro research on human skin samples has shown that DEA penetration is low, even under the condition of constant skin contact over a 24-hour period.[469]

In 2013, DEA was reevaluated and was considered safe for use in cosmetics at current levels and when ingredients known to form nitrosamines are not included in the formula.[443]

dihydroxyacetone (GOOD)

Ingredient that affects the color of skin and that is present in most self-tanners. Derived from sugar, it reacts with amino acids found in the top layers of skin to create a shade of brown; the effect takes place within two to six hours and it can build color depth with every reapplication. It has a long history of safe use when applied topically to skin, where it affects only the uppermost layers.[470] Dihydroxyacetone doesn't pose a health risk to skin nor does it accelerate signs of aging.

dimethicone (GOOD)

See silicone.

dimethicone crosspolymer (GOOD)

Silicone derivative used as a stabilizing and suspending agent or as a thickener.

dipentaerythrityl hexacaprylate/hexacaprate (GOOD)

Mixture of fatty acids used as an emollient, emulsifier, and thickening agent.

dipropylene glycol (GOOD)

Synthetic slip agent and penetration enhancer.

disodium cocoamphodiacetate (GOOD)

Mild detergent cleansing agent derived from coconut; most often used in facial cleansers.

disodium EDTA (GOOD)

See EDTA.

disteardimonium hectorite (GOOD)

Used as a suspending agent, often with pigments.

DMDM hydantoin (AVERAGE)

Synthetic, formaldehyde-releasing preservative that has mixed research, some showing it can be more sensitizing AND some showing it can be less sensitizing than many other preservatives, although the majority of comparative studies indicate DMDM hydantoin is more sensitizing.[471,472,473]

Despite its connection to formaldehyde, the Cosmetic Ingredient Review Expert Panel has confirmed the safety of this preservative in three separate reviews, each spaced several years apart.[474]

In terms of effectiveness, DMDM hydantoin is strongly antibacterial, but rather weak against fungi. Therefore, it shouldn't be (and typically isn't) used as the sole preservative in a water-based product.

E

ecamsule (BEST)

See Mexoryl SX™.

EDTA (GOOD)

Acronym for ethylenediaminetetraacetic acid, a stabilizer used in cosmetics to prevent ingredients in a given formula from binding with trace elements (particularly minerals) that can be present in water. EDTA also keeps other ingredients from causing unwanted changes to a product's texture, odor, and/or consistency. Ingredients that perform this function are known as chelating agents. Common examples of EDTA ingredients are disodium EDTA and tetrasodium EDTA.

elastin (GOOD)

Major component of skin that gives it flexibility. There are different types of elastin, all of which bundle to form a complex, mesh-like network of support that interweaves with skin's other supportive element, collagen, as well as with skin-repairing substances such as hyaluronic acid.

Elastin in skincare products is derived from both plant and animal sources. It functions as a good water-binding agent, but that's it. Elastin in skincare products has never been shown to affect the elastin in skin or to have any other benefit, such as firming or lifting.

emollient (GOOD)

Supple, waxlike, lubricating, thickening agent that prevents water loss and has a softening and soothing effect on skin. Examples of emollients are ingredients like plant oils, mineral oil, shea butter, cocoa butter, petrolatum, and fatty acids (animal oils, including emu, mink, and lanolin, the latter probably the one ingredient that is most like our own skin's oil). More technical-sounding emollient ingredients, such as triglycerides, benzoates, myristates, palmi-

tates, and stearates, are generally waxy in texture and appearance but provide most moisturizers with their elegant texture and feel.

emulsifier (GOOD)

In cosmetics, any ingredient that helps keep unlike ingredients (such as oil and water) from separating in an emulsion. Examples of cosmetics ingredients that function as emulsifiers include polysorbates, laureth-4, and potassium cetyl sulfate. Emulsifiers are widely used throughout the cosmetics industry and are the unsung heroes of many cosmetics formulas that blend unlike ingredients together.

ensulizole (BEST)

Sunscreen agent that protects primarily against the sun's UVB rays, providing only minimal UVA protection. Ensulizole protects the skin from wavelengths of UV light in the range 290 to 340 nanometers, whereas the UVA range is 320 to 400 nanometers.[475] For complete protection, this ingredient (as well as many other UVB-protecting sunscreen ingredients) must be paired with the UVA-protecting ingredients avobenzone, titanium dioxide, zinc oxide, or Mexoryl SX™ (ecamsule); outside the United States, it can also be paired with Tinosorb.[9,475]

Because ensulizole is water-soluble, it has the unique characteristic of feeling relatively light on skin; thus, it is often used in sunscreen lotions or moisturizers whose aesthetic goal is a non-greasy finish.

enzymes (GOOD)

Vast group of protein molecules, produced by all living things, that act as catalysts in chemical and biological reactions, including photosynthesis, helping cells communicate, inhibiting free-radical damage, and many, many more. Enzymes are divided into six main categories: oxidoreductases, transferases, hydrolases, lyases, isomerases, and ligases. The names of most, but not all, enzymes end in –ase.[476,477]

Enzymes are used in skincare products to facilitate exfoliation, to help overall biological processes in skin that have slowed down because of age or sun damage, and to inhibit free-radical damage. Enzymes accelerate biochemical reactions in a cell that would proceed minimally or not at all if the enzymes weren't present. Most enzymes are finicky about how and under what conditions they will act. Sometimes several enzymes are required to carry out a particular chemical reaction, and their actions are affected by temperature and pH. Some enzymes depend on the presence of other enzymes, called coenzymes, to function, or they depend on a specific body temperature. It would require an exceptionally complicated process to stimulate enzyme activity via topical application to skin.[478]

erythrulose (GOOD)
Substance chemically similar to the self-tanning agent dihydroxyacetone. Depending on your skin color, there can be a difference in the color with erythrulose. Erythrulose needs about two to three days for the skin to show a color change, while dihydroxyacetone completely changes the color of skin within two to six hours. For this reason, most products that contain erythrulose also contain dihydroxyacetone.[479]

ethylhexyl palmitate (GOOD)
Mixture of a fatty alcohol and palmitic acid that functions as an emollient.

ethylhexyl stearate (GOOD)
See thickener and emollient.

ethylhexylglycerin (GOOD)
Synthetic skin-conditioning agent also used as a preservative or as a carrier or suspending agent for other preservatives such as phenoxyethanol.

ethylparaben (GOOD)
See parabens.

eucalyptus oil (POOR)
Fragrant plant oil whose active constituents are found in the leaves and in the oil obtained from them. The oil has antimicrobial and antifungal activity, but is also a potent skin irritant due to its chemical components, some of which are toxic and can be fatal if ingested. Truly a mixed bag, this oil, like rosemary oil, has benefits and risks. Low amounts of eucalyptus oil do not seem to pose a risk of allergic contact dermatitis in the general population, although its fragrance components are known irritants, and skin can be very good at concealing when it's being irritated.[480,481]

eugenol (POOR)
Volatile fragrance chemical that occurs naturally in cloves, basil, and bay leaves, among other plants. Eugenol is often part of the fragrance in cosmetics

products, and is known to cause irritation that may include redness, dryness, scaling, and swelling.[482,483,484]

A major component of clove oil, research has shown that the eugenol content of clove causes skin-cell death, even when low concentrations of clove (0.33%) were applied to cultured skin cells.[485] It is best to avoid leave-on products that contain eugenol.

evening primrose oil (BEST)

Non-fragrant plant oil that can have significant anti-inflammatory and emollient benefits for skin.

F

farnesol (AVERAGE)

Extract of plants that is used in cosmetics primarily for fragrance. A few animal studies and some in vitro research investigated farnesol's antibacterial and anti-cancer properties.[486,487] It may also have some antioxidant properties, but there is no research showing it has any benefit on skin.[488]

FD&C colors (GOOD)

General term for any color additive deemed safe and FDA-approved for use in foods, drugs, and cosmetics. When an FD&C color is followed by the word "lake," it means the color has been mixed with a mineral (most commonly calcium or aluminum) to make the color insoluble (not affected by water). For example, "FD&C Blue No. 1–Aluminum Lake" means that the color FD&C Blue No. 1 has been combined with aluminum. Lake colors are used for candies and for dyes used to color Easter eggs, among countless cosmetics applications.[489]

The current group of FD&C colors has been extensively studied, with many classified as "permanently approved" for use in drugs and foods. Some FD&C colors, such as Blue 1 and Blue 2, are derivatives of coal tar and can cause allergic reactions, although the amounts used in items such as lipsticks typically are lower than the amounts used in other types of coloring agents. No coal tar colors are permitted in products for use around the eyes, and every batch of coal tar color must be deemed safe before it can be used in foods, drugs, or cosmetics.[489]

Any coloring agent used in eye makeup must be specifically approved for that purpose by the FDA. The color of cosmetics products is often an emotional pull for many consumers. A soft pink lotion can denote a moisturizer

meant to calm or soothe skin, while a bright yellow balm may be deemed en-
ergizing. Whether natural or synthetic, coloring agents in skincare products
serve no purpose other than to create a perception or an emotional response
to the product. Coloring agents used in makeup are a different story, as they're
used to create an endless kaleidoscope of shades.[489]

ferric ferrocyanide (GOOD)
Coloring agent, also known as Iron Blue, used in cosmetics products, including those designed for use around the eye. Permanently listed (since 1978)
by the FDA as safe.[489]

ferulic acid (BEST)
Plant-based antioxidant that is found in bran, among other plants. Research suggests that it provides antioxidant and sun-protective benefits to
skin while enhancing the stability of topical applications of vitamin E.[490,491,492]

feverfew extract (AVERAGE)
Extract that can be very irritating to skin and can trigger allergic reactions
if a specific constituent of the feverfew plant known as parthenolide (technically, sesquiterpene lactone) is present. If the parthenolide is removed from feverfew, the ingredient is not a problem for skin and may actually be beneficial
because parthenolide-free feverfew has potent anti-inflammatory properties
and may reduce redness in skin.[493,494,495]

Interestingly, when parthenolide is present and feverfew is taken orally it
has been shown to relieve migraines and have anti-inflammatory properties,
including those related to pain reduction for certain types of arthritis.[495] If a
skincare product contains feverfew, you must contact the company to confirm
that the feverfew in their products is parthenolide-free. If they don't know or
won't tell you, do not use the product, especially if you have plant allergies.

film-forming agent (GOOD)
Large group of ingredients typically found in haircare products, but that
also are widely used in skincare products, particularly moisturizers. Film-forming agents include PVP, acrylates, acrylamides, and various copolymers. When
applied they leave a pliable, cohesive, and continuous covering over the hair or
skin. The film has water-binding properties and leaves a smooth feel on skin.
Film-forming agents can be weak skin sensitizers, but this almost always depends on the amount used; lower amounts generally are not problematic.[496]

fragrance (POOR)

One or a blend of volatile and/or fragrant plant oils (or synthetically derived oils) that impart aroma and odor to products. These are often skin irritants because they are composed of hundreds of individual chemical components. Fragrance is a leading source of allergic reactions to cosmetics.[11,403,497]

G

genistein (BEST)

Plant component (most often from soy) that is a rich source of antioxidants, although it can also be synthetically derived. Research has shown that topical application of genistein has several protective benefits for skin, including modulating the oxidative stress that skin endures in the presence of sunlight. Genistein is also effective at wound healing due to its anti-inflammatory action.[498,499,500]

geranium oil (POOR)

Fragrant oil that can have antimicrobial properties, but also can be a skin sensitizer or irritant.[501,502] Geranium extract is a very good antioxidant for skin, and the parts extracted are usually not fragrant, thus presenting minimal risk of irritation.[503]

ginger extract and oil (GOOD)

Extract from a plant in the *Zingiberaceae* family that has research showing it has anti-inflammatory and anti-carcinogenic activity when taken orally and when applied to skin.[504,505,506] When applied topically, however, the oil can be a skin irritant due to the fragrance compounds it contains.

Ginkgo biloba **leaf extract** (BEST)

Potent antioxidant that research shows can help improve blood flow. It also is often included in anticellulite products because of its relationship to circulation; however, there is no research showing that improved circulation affects cellulite.[507,508,509]

Applied topically, ginkgo leaf is a good antioxidant because it is a rich source of flavonoids. This plant extract also has antibacterial and antifungal effects. Other research has shown that ginkgo leaf can help protect skin from redness and inflammation during exposure to UVA/UVB light in a lab setting.

Ginkgo leaf also seems capable of increasing skin's moisture content and reducing factors in skin that lead to inflammation.[510,511,512]

gluten ingredients (GOOD)

Gluten is a protein that occurs naturally in many types of grains, including wheat, rye, and barley. Gluten ingredients include several grains or grain-derived ingredients that are potentially problematic for those diagnosed with the autoimmune disorder known as celiac disease. If you have celiac disease or a sensitivity to gluten, should you avoid cosmetics that contain gluten ingredients? The general advice is no, as gluten ingredients applied topically cannot penetrate skin and affect the small intestine. However, applying gluten products to lips means some amount of ingestion will occur, so you should avoid lip-care or lip color products with gluten ingredients.[513]

Some people with celiac disease are also allergic to wheat ingredients, including when they're applied to skin (via skincare) versus consumed as part of their diet. In such cases, it's advisable to avoid cosmetics with wheat or other gluten ingredients. According to a September 2012 analysis published in the *Journal of the Academy of Nutrition and Dietetics*, "individuals with celiac disease should not be concerned about products applied to the hair or skin, especially if the individual washes his or her hands after use. Individuals who are concerned about gluten in cosmetics that are applied to the lip or may be ingested should avoid products that contain "wheat," "barley," "malt," "rye," "oat," "triticum vulgare," "hordeum vulgare," "secale cereale," and "avena sativa.""[513]

glycereth-26 (GOOD)

Synthetic glycerin-based ingredient used as an emollient and thickening agent in cosmetics.

glycerin (BEST)

Also called glycerol or glycerine, glycerin is present in all natural lipids (fats), whether animal or vegetable. It can be derived from natural substances by hydrolysis of fats and by fermentation of sugars; it also can be synthetically manufactured.

Glycerin is a skin-identical and skin-repairing ingredient, meaning it is a substance found naturally in skin. In that respect, it is one of the many substances in skin that help maintain the outer barrier and prevent dryness or scaling.

Humectants such as glycerin have always raised the question as to whether or not they take too much water from skin. Pure glycerin (100% concentration) on skin is not helpful and can actually be drying, causing blisters if left on too long. So, a major drawback of any humectant (including glycerin) when used in pure form is that it can increase water loss by attracting water from the lower layers of skin (dermis) into the surface layers of skin (epidermis), where the water can easily be lost to the environment—that doesn't help dry skin or any skin type. For this reason, glycerin and humectants in general are always combined with other ingredients to soften skin. Glycerin combined with other emollients and/or oils is a fundamental cornerstone of most moisturizers.[514]

Research shows that a combination of ingredients, including glycerin, dimethicone, petrolatum, antixoxidants, fatty acids, lecithin, among many others, are excellent for helping skin heal, reducing associated dermatitis, and restoring normal barrier function if used on an ongoing basis.[515,516,517] Research also indicates that the presence of glycerin in the intercellular layer helps other skin lipids do their jobs better.[518]

glyceryl behenate (GOOD)
Simple mixture of glycerin and the naturally occurring fatty acid behenic acid. Glyceryl behenate has multiple functions in cosmetics products, including as an emollient, emulsifier, and surfactant.

glyceryl cocoate (GOOD)
Used as an emollient and thickening agent in cosmetics. May be plant-based or synthetic.

glyceryl dipalmitate (GOOD)
Mixture of portions of glycerin and palmitic acid used as an emollient and thickening agent in cosmetics. May be plant- or animal-derived or synthetic.

glyceryl distearate (GOOD)
Mixture of portions of glycerin and stearic acid used as an emollient and thickening agent in cosmetics. May be animal-derived or synthetic.

glyceryl isostearate (GOOD)
Mixture of portions of glycerin and isostearic acid used as an emollient and thickening agent in cosmetics. May be animal-derived or synthetic.

glyceryl myristate (GOOD)

Mixture of portions of glycerin and myristic acid used as an emollient, surfactant, emulsifier, and thickening agent in cosmetics. May be plant-derived or synthetic.

glyceryl oleate (GOOD)

Mixture of portions of glycerin and oleic acid used as an emollient, surfactant, emulsifier, and (less often) a fragrance ingredient in cosmetics. May be plant- or animal-derived or synthetic.

glyceryl palmitate (GOOD)

Mixture of portions of glycerin and palmitic acid used as an emollient, surfactant, and emulsifier. May be plant- or animal-derived or synthetic.

glyceryl polymethacrylate (GOOD)

Blend of glycerin and polymethacrylic acid that functions as a film-forming agent. It has a smooth finish and is used to enhance the texture and application of many skincare products. *See* film-forming agent.

glyceryl stearate (GOOD)

Mixture of portions of glycerin and stearic acid used as an emollient, surfactant, and emulsifier. May be animal-derived or synthetic.

glyceryl stearate SE (GOOD)

Widely used ingredient that is a self-emulsifying (that's what the "SE" stands for) form of glyceryl stearate. *See* glyceryl stearate.

Glycine soja **oil** (BEST)

See soybean oil.

Glycine soja **sterols** (BEST)

Sterol derived from the *Glycine soja* (soy) plant. A sterol is a solid complex alcohol derived from animals and plants. Despite the alcohol origin, sterols are not drying or irritating on skin; rather, they serve to lubricate dry skin and have an emollient texture.

glycolic acid (BEST)

See AHA.

glycosaminoglycans (BEST)

Also known as mucopolysaccharides, these are a fundamental component of skin tissue, essentially a group of complex proteins. Chondroitin sulfate and hyaluronic acid are part of this ingredient group, all of which function as skin-identical or skin-repairing ingredients.

glycyrrhetic acid (BEST)

One of the active, anti-inflammatory components of licorice extract. *See* licorice extract.

Glycyrrhiza glabra (BEST)

See licorice extract.

gold (POOR)

Common allergen that can induce dermatitis on skin, especially on the face and eyelids and gold particles present a risk of oxidative damage and toxicity. [519,520,521] In fact, gold won the dubious title of Allergen of the Year in 2001 from The American Contact Dermatitis Society.[522] Claims of gold helping to create electric charges in skin to trigger wrinkle repair are completely unproven.

Another form of gold used in skincare products is "colloidal gold," which means that the gold particles have been reduced in size (usually to 1–15 nanometers) so that it remains dispersed evenly throughout a solution.[523] Although gold is a heavy metal, and heavy metals are subject to regulations, colloidal gold preparations are not regulated, so the risks are unknown. Initial research shows that it is fairly safe because it seems to be eliminated through urine.

Colloidal gold also is used in the world of medicine, where there is a minor amount of research that it might benefit rheumatoid arthritis because of assumed anti-inflammatory properties. Most of that research, however, is either very old or was performed on only a very small group of people, not enough to prove efficacy.

Even if gold were a good anti-inflammatory agent, its effects have never been compared with the effects of the numerous potent and stable anti-inflammatory ingredients that are commonly used in skincare products and that have a great deal of research proving their benefit and safety. What is for certain: There is no published research proving that gold, normal or colloidal in size, has any anti-aging or wrinkle-fighting benefits.

grape seed extract (BEST)

Contains chemical constituents such as proanthocyanidins, polyphenols, flavonoids, and anthocyanins, all of which are very potent antioxidants that help to diminish the sun's damaging effects and reduce free-radical damage. [524,525] Grape extract has also been shown to have wound-healing properties. [526,527] When combined with other antioxidants, topical application reduces the biomarkers in skin responsible for skin cancer.[528] Red grapes contain resveratrol, considered a very potent antioxidant and believed to be chiefly responsible for the health benefits of red wine (and grape juice).[529]

grape seed oil (BEST)
Emollient, non-fragrant plant oil that also has strong antioxidant properties. *See* grape seed extract.

grapefruit oil (POOR)
Citrus oil whose volatile components (chiefly substances known as furocoumarins) are irritating to skin. Topical application of grapefruit oil may cause contact dermatitis from its chief fragrance chemical, limonene.[530,531,532] *See* limonene.

grapefruit peel extract (POOR)
Typically listed as *Citrus X paradisi* (grapefruit) peel extract on ingredient lists, the peel from this fruit is loaded with a class of ingredients known as furanocoumarins and coumarins, which are primarily responsible for what's known as a phototoxic reaction that occurs when skin is exposed to the sun—the result can leave skin discolored.[530,531,532,533] Low amounts of these ingredients aren't likely to be problematic, but watch out if it's listed toward the beginning to middle of an ingredient list, especially if the product in question has a telltale grapefruit scent.

grapefruit seed extract (AVERAGE)
Labelled as *Citrus paradisi* (grapefruit) seed extract, this is often claimed as a natural preservative when added to cosmetics. However, research has demonstrated that it is not a broad-spectrum preservative agent, which means it cannot protect against both mold and bacterial growth—even in sealed, pump-style packaging.[534,535,536] Yes, citrus extracts can have antibacterial benefits, but they're simply not strong enough to defend a product like this from a broad range of pathogens.

green tea (BEST)

Significant amounts of research have established that tea, including black, green, and white tea, has many intriguing health benefits, including anti-aging. Dozens of studies point to tea's potent antioxidant as well as anticarcinogenic properties.[537]

The *Journal of Photochemistry and Photobiology* (December 31, 2001) stated that polyphenols "are the active ingredients in green tea and possess antioxidant, anti-inflammatory and anticarcinogenic properties.[538]

Green tea and the other teas (e.g., white tea, which is what green tea begins as) show a good deal of promise for skin, but they are not the miracle that cosmetics and health food companies make them out to be. Most researchers agree that tea (black, green, or white) has potent anti-inflammatory properties and that it is a potent antioxidant whether consumed orally or applied topically.[539,540,541] Current research also indicates that epigallocatechin-3-gallate (EGCG), green tea's active component, can prevent collagen breakdown and reduce UV damage to skin, which is a very good reason to use skincare products that contain one or more forms of tea.[542]

gums (GOOD)

Substances that have water-binding properties, but that are used primarily as thickening agents in cosmetics. Some gums have a sticky feel and are used as film-forming agents in hairsprays, while others can constrict skin and have irritancy potential. Natural thickeners such as acacia, tragacanth, and locust bean are types of gums used in cosmetics.

H

Hamamelis virginiana (POOR)

See witch hazel.

Helianthus annuus **seed oil** (BEST)

See sunflower seed oil.

hexyl cinnamal (POOR)

Fragrance ingredient used in many perfumes and often seen in fragranced skincare products. Hexyl cinnamal imparts a jasmine-like scent. It's considered a fragrance allergen, which is why it must be called out on an ingredient statement, whereas in the past a cosmetics company could lump ingredients like hexyl cinnamal into the catchall term "fragrance."[354,543,544]]

homosalate (BEST)

FDA-approved sunscreen active ingredient that provides primarily UVB protection. Its UVA range is very narrow, and so it is not used alone in sunscreens. Homosalate is internationally approved for use in sunscreens, up to a maximum concentration of 15%. It's considered non-sensitizing and non-toxic, and is most often seen in sunscreens rated SPF 30 and greater.[51,382,383]

honey (BEST)

Substance produced by bees from the nectar of flowering plants. Composed primarily of the sugars fructose and glucose and consumed as food, honey also has applications when it comes to skincare. This is due to its amino acid, peptide, and vitamin content.[545]

The primary research on honey and skin has to do with its multi-faceted role in wound healing: it protects the wound and its sugars serve as an alternative food source for bacteria that may otherwise prolong healing or cause infection. For general skincare that does not involve wounds (and remember, wrinkles are not wounds), honey has anti-inflammatory properties and also functions as an antioxidant. Dark honeys have a stronger antioxidant effect than light honeys. Regular honey is also known as clarified honey or purified honey.[545]

Manuka honey shows up in some skincare products, and is hyped as a special kind of honey. It's produced in New Zealand from bees that pollinate the country's native manuka bush. Manuka honey is similar to "regular" clover honey except it's said to contain more of a chemical called methylglyoxal, which might give manuka honey an antibacterial and, potentially, antiviral advantage. Some research, however, shows that it doesn't necessarily have an edge; it depends on the type of bacteria present.[546,547,548]

horse chestnut extract (GOOD)

May have anti-inflammatory properties for skin. Taken orally, it has been shown to reduce edema in the lower leg by improving the elastic tissue surrounding the veins.[549,550]

horsetail extract (AVERAGE)

Plant extract that has antioxidant and anti-inflammatory properties, but there's no solid research showing it can exert these effects when applied to skin.[551] Horsetail may be listed by its Latin name *Equisetum arvense*.

hyaluronic acid (BEST)

Component of skin tissue. Synthetic variations are used in skincare products to function as a superior skin-identical ingredient. Hyaluronic acid has cell-communicating abilities and can boost skin's moisture content, reduce inflammation, and help prevent moisture loss.[552,553]

hydrogenated lecithin (BEST)

Hydrogenated form of the cell-communicating ingredient lecithin. It may be derived from animals or plants (egg yolk is a source) or manufactured synthetically. *See* lecithin and hydrogenated olive oil.

hydrogenated olive oil (BEST)

When a plant oil is hydrogenated, it is chemically converted from a liquid to a semi-solid or solid form using a process that involves hydrogen gas under high pressure. Hydrogenation allows an oily liquid to remain in a solid state at room temperature. Hydrogenated olive oil is a rich source of antioxidants, and, as described, hydrogenating the oil changes it from its natural liquid state into a solid state.

hydrogenated palm glycerides (GOOD)

Palm glycerides are the fatty acid component of palm oil. Hydrogenation allows the oily liquid to remain in a solid state at room temperature. *See* hydrogenated olive oil.

hydrogenated polydecene (GOOD)

Synthetic polymer that functions as an emollient and skin-conditioning agent. *See* hydrogenated olive oil.

hydrogenated polyisobutene (GOOD)

Synthetic polymer used as a skin-conditioning agent and emollient. It has a rich, thick texture. *See* hydrogenated olive oil.

hydrolyzed vegetable protein (GOOD)

Composed of various protein substances derived from vegetables and broken down by water and hydrochloric acid to form a new complex with properties different from the original source. Used as a water-binding agent.

hydrolyzed wheat protein (GOOD)

Protein fraction from wheat that has been hydrolyzed, which is a chemical process involving the reaction of a substance with water and hydrochloric acid to form a modified substance. Functions as a hair conditioning and film-forming agent.

hydroquinone (BEST)

Strong inhibitor of melanin (skin pigment) production that has long been established as the most effective ingredient for reducing and potentially eliminating brown spots and hyperpigmentation from melasma, because it prevents skin from producing melanin, the substance responsible for skin color. [554] Hydroquinone does not bleach the skin, which is why "bleaching agent" is a misnomer; it can't remove pigment from the skin cell, but it can limit melanin production.

Over-the-counter hydroquinone products can contain 0.5% to 2% concentrations of hydroquinone; 4% (and sometimes higher) concentrations are available only from physicians. In medical literature, hydroquinone is the primary topical ingredient for inhibiting melanin production. Using it in combination with other ingredients—especially tretinoin—can greatly reduce and even eliminate skin discolorations.[555,556]

Some concerns about hydroquinone's safety on skin have been expressed, but the research regarding topical application indicates that negative reactions are minor, are the result of using extremely high concentrations, or result from using it in combination with other agents such as glucocorticoids or mercury iodine. This is particularly true in Africa, where adulterated skin-lightening products are commonplace. According to Howard I. Maibach, M.D., professor of dermatology at the University of California School of Medicine, San Francisco, "Overall, adverse events reported with the use of hydroquinone ... have been relatively few and minor in nature.... To date there is no evidence of adverse systemic reactions following the use of hydroquinone, and it has been around for over 30 years in skincare products." Maibach also stated that "hydroquinone is undoubtedly the most active and safest skin-depigmenting substance...."[557]

Despite the controversy, abundant research from reputable sources shows hydroquinone to be safe and effective. Surprisingly, there is even research showing that workers who handle pure hydroquinone actually have a lower incidence of cancer than the population as a whole.[558,559,560,561]

You may have read that hydroquinone is linked to leukemia. That connection has to do with the chemical benzene, which can be metabolized into hydroquinone. It's the benzene at the starting point that raises that concern, it's not the hydroquinone as used in topical skin-lightening products. Other research examining this connection was carried out on cultured internal (inside the body) cells or via oral consumption of pure hydroquinone, which is not at all related to how hydroquinone is used in skincare products. More to the point, the amount of hydroquinone used in the studies that suggest an association with leukemia are considerably higher amounts than what people are exposed to via skincare products that contain hydroquinone. Research also has shown that humans metabolize hydroquinone completely, whereas rats (the most common animal used in toxicity studies for hydroquinone) metabolize hydroquinone much differently, which is likely why oral administration or injection of hydroquinone causes the problems noted in the research. [558,559,560,561,562]

Bottom line: Hydroquinone is not carcinogenic (cancer-causing). Considerable analysis of the animal research that raised this concern has shown that hydroquinone is not and cannot be classified as a human carcinogen. If you're struggling with brown spots or sun-induced skin discolorations, hydroquinone remains among the best ingredient to treat them.[558,559,560,561,562]

hydroxyethyl acrylate/sodium acryloyldimethyl taurate copolymer (GOOD)
Synthetic polymer that functions as a stabilizer, thickening agent, and opacifying agent.

Hydroxyethylcellulose (GOOD)
Plant-derived thickening agent typically used as a binding agent or emulsifier. Also used (most often in hairstyling products) as a film-forming agent.

I

imidazolidinyl urea (AVERAGE)
Preservative considered weaker than its "cousin" diazolidinyl urea because it is active against bacteria but does not have the antifungal action of diazolidinyl urea. Most often used with parabens because they work well together. Imidazolidinyl urea is considered a formaldehyde-releasing preservative. Although that sounds scary, the amount of formaldehyde released is well below

the limits for safe exposure. Still, some regulatory experts caution against using products with imidazolidinyl urea on infants.[466]

inactive ingredient (GOOD)

The list of inactive ingredients is the part of an ingredient label that is not regulated by the FDA, other than the requirement that it be a complete list of the contents in descending order of concentration; that is, the ingredient with the largest concentration is listed first, then the next largest, and so forth. If it's an over-the-counter drug product made in the United States, an alphabetical list of inactive ingredients is acceptable. Thousands and thousands of inactive ingredients are used in cosmetics, and there is controversy about how truly inactive some of these substances are in regard to safety as well as about their long-term and short-term effects on skin or the human body.

iodopropynyl butylcarbamate (GOOD)

Synthetic preservative typically used in concentrations of 0.1% or less. It's very active against fungi, but has weak antibacterial activity, which is why it should always be used with other preservatives in water-based products.[563]

iron oxides (GOOD)

Compounds of iron that are used as coloring agents in some cosmetics. They also are used as a metal polish called jewelers rouge, and are well-known in their crude form as rust. Although iron oxides occur naturally, the forms used in cosmetics are synthetic. Iron oxides are closely regulated by the U.S. Food and Drug Administration. According to the website CosmeticsInfo.org (which links to the FDA's Code of Federal Regulations for iron oxides), "Synthetic iron oxides are produced in various ways, including thermal decomposition of iron salts, such as ferrous sulfate, to produce reds; precipitation to produce yellows, reds, browns, and blacks; and reduction of organic compounds by iron to produce yellows and blacks."

isobutylparaben (GOOD)

See parabens.

isododecane (GOOD)

Synthetic hydrocarbon ingredient used as a solvent. Isododecane enhances the spreadability of products and has a weightless feel on skin. All hydrocarbons used in cosmetics help prevent the evaporation of water from skin.

isohexadecane (GOOD)

Synthetic, dry-finish ingredient with a powder-like finish. Used as a detergent cleansing agent, emulsifier, and thickening agent in cosmetics, particularly those for oily skin.

isononyl isononanoate (GOOD)

Synthetic ester that functions as an emollient skin-conditioning agent. Occurs naturally in cocoa oil and lavender oil.

isopropyl alcohol (POOR)

Also known as rubbing alcohol. *See* alcohol.

isopropyl myristate (GOOD)

Thickening agent and emollient as used in cosmetics. Historically, animal testing has shown it causes clogged pores.[564] However, the results derived from the animal testing were eventually considered unreliable, and there has been no subsequent research showing this ingredient is any more of a problem for skin than other emollient, waxy, thickening ingredients used in cosmetics.[565]

isopropyl palmitate (GOOD)

Thickening agent and emollient as used in cosmetics. As is true for any emollient or thickening agents, it can potentially clog pores, depending on the amount in the product and your skin's response.[565]

ivy extract (POOR)

Plant extract that can be a skin irritant due to its stimulant and astringent (skin-constricting) properties, especially if the person has allergies, asthma, or atopic dermatitis.[566,567] Despite this, there's no research demonstrating that tiny amounts of ivy extract applied via skincare products are harmful; however, there also is no reliable information on ivy's benefits when applied to skin.

J

jasmine oil (POOR)

Fragrant oil, often used as a source of perfume, whose volatile fragrance chemicals (chiefly linalool) can be skin irritants or sensitizers. Jasmine oil may have antifungal properties.[501,568,569,570]

jojoba esters (BEST)

Complex mixture of esters from jojoba oil and hydrogenated jojoba oil. The result is an ingredient with a wax-like texture that functions as an excellent emollient and occlusive agent for skin, especially when used with glycerin.[571] *See* hydrogenated olive oil.

jojoba oil (BEST)

Emollient, non-fragrant oil similar to other non-fragrant plant oils. Jojoba oil has been shown to enhance skin's barrier-repair properties and ability to heal from damage.[572,573] As a plant oil that's a rich source of fatty acids skin recognizes and can use, jojoba oil also seems to stimulate collagen production and help skin better defend itself against UV light damage. Jojoba oil can also provide topical anti-inflammatory benefits.[574]

juniper berry (POOR)

Plant (Latin name *Juniperus communis*) that can have anti-inflammatory properties for skin, although with repeated application (due to its methanol content) can result in skin irritation.[575] Juniper lacks sufficient data proving it is safe for use on skin, and is chiefly added, in oil or extract form, to impart fragrance.[576]

K

kaolin (GOOD)

Naturally occurring clay mineral (silicate of aluminum) used in cosmetics for its absorbent properties. Kaolin's absorbent properties make it a popular ingredient in clay masks for oily skin. Used too often in high amounts, it can be drying, but is otherwise a benign ingredient.

kojic acid (GOOD)

By-product of the fermentation process of malting rice for use in the manufacture of sake, Japanese rice wine. In vitro and in vivo research and animal studies have shown that kojic acid is effective for inhibiting melanin production.[171,577]

Kojic acid's downside is that it's an extremely unstable ingredient in cosmetic formulations. On exposure to air or sunlight, it turns a strange shade of brown and loses its efficacy. Many cosmetics companies use kojic dipalmitate as an alternative because it is more stable in formulations. However, there's no research showing that kojic dipalmitate is as effective as kojic acid, although it's a good antioxidant.[578]

kojic dipalmitate (GOOD)

Mixture of kojic acid and palmitic acid that functions as a skin-conditioning agent and a fat-soluble antioxidant.[579] Although it's more stable than the similar-sounding kojic acid, there's no research showing kojic dipalmitate is as effective as kojic acid.

kukui nut oil (BEST)

Also known as candlenut or candleberry oil, this non-fragrant plant oil is found throughout Hawaii, India and Indonesia. Research has shown it has anti-inflammatory, pain-reducing, and wound-healing benefits.[580,581,582]

L

L-ascorbic acid (BEST)

Form of vitamin C that is a potent antioxidant and anti-inflammatory agent and can improve the appearance of wrinkles, uneven skin tone, and brown spots.[108,172,583] L-ascorbic acid is often labelled as the INCI compliant "ascorbic acid" on ingredient lists, but there is no difference between the two—they refer to the same ingredient.[584,585]

lactic acid (BEST)

Alpha hydroxy acid (AHA) extracted from milk, although most forms used in cosmetics are synthetic because that form is easier to formulate with and stabilize. In a pH-correct formula, lactic acid exfoliates cells on the surface of skin by breaking down the material that holds skin cells together. It may irritate mucous membranes and cause irritation, although this isn't common. Lactic acid also has water-binding properties and, like glycolic acid (another AHA), may help lighten skin discolorations.[32,586]

lanolin (GOOD)

Emollient, very thick substance derived from the sebaceous glands of sheep. Lanolin has long been burdened with a reputation for being an allergen or sensitizing agent, which has always been a disappointment to formulators because lanolin is such an effective moisturizing ingredient. A study in the *British Journal of Dermatology* concluded "that lanolin sensitization has remained at a relatively low and constant rate even in a high-risk population (i.e., patients with recent or active eczema)." Based on a review of 24,449 patients who were tested with varying forms of lanolin, it turned out that "The mean annual rate of sensitivity to this allergen was 1.7%"—and it was lower than that for a 50% concentration of lanolin. It looks like it's time to restore lanolin's good reputation.[587]

That's a very good thing for someone with dry skin, though it can be a problem for someone with oily skin, because lanolin closely resembles the oil from human oil glands. Also, as an animal-derived ingredient, lanolin is sometimes viewed as less favorable in comparison to synthetic or plant-derived alternatives.

lanolin alcohol (GOOD)

Emollient derived from lanolin. Despite the "alcohol" in the name, this ingredient is not a skin irritant. Instead, it's a fatty alcohol that can greatly benefit dry skin because it helps prevent moisture loss and maintain a supple feel on skin.

laureth-23 (GOOD)

Derived from lauryl alcohol and used either as a surfactant or emulsifier (or, in many cases, as both). *See* surfactant; emulsifier.

laureth-4 (GOOD)

Derived from lauryl alcohol and used either as a surfactant or emulsifier (or, in many cases, as both). *See* surfactant; emulsifier.

laureth-7 (GOOD)

Form of lauryl alcohol (a non-irritating fatty alcohol derived from coconut oil) that can function as an emulsifier or as a surfactant. Despite information found on the Internet, there's no substantiated evidence that this ingredient is comedogenic.

lauric acid (BEST)

One of several fatty acids found in coconut oil and other natural fats, lauric acid has multiple uses in cosmetics. Its natural bay leaf-like scent can be used in high amounts to add fragrance to products, but it's more often used as a base for detergent cleansing agents, and, increasingly, for its antibacterial and anti-inflammatory actions.

Research has shown that lauric acid on skin can help control acne-causing bacteria. The lauric acid fuses to the bacterial membrane of *P. acnes* bacteria, keeping it from proliferating. Lauric acid can also reduce inflammation from acne.[83,449]

lauroyl lysine (GOOD)

Amino acid derivative that functions as a skin- and hair-conditioning agent. It also contributes to a product's texture by helping to gel the solvents, while also remaining stable under high heat conditions.[588]

lavender extract and oil (POOR)

Widely used plant that's a member of the mint family. May be listed by its Latin names *Lavandula angustifolia* or *Lavandula officinalis*. Primarily a fragrance ingredient, although it may have antibacterial properties. In-vitro research indicates that components of lavender, specifically linalool and linalyl acetate, can be cytotoxic, which means that topical application of as little a concentration as 0.25% causes cell death.[589] This study was conducted on endothelial cells, which are cells that line blood pathways in the body and play a critical role in the inflammatory process of skin.

As linalool and linalyl acetate are both rapidly absorbed by skin and can be detected within blood cells in less than 20 minutes, endothelial cells are an ideal choice for such a test.[590] The results of this research also demonstrated that lavender has a damaging effect on fibroblasts, which are cells that produce collagen.

The fragrance constituents in lavender oil, linalool and linalyl acetate, oxidize when exposed to air, and in this process their potential for causing an allergic reaction is increased.[591] If you're wondering why lavender oil doesn't appear to be problematic for you, it's because research has demonstrated that you don't always need to see it or feel it happening for your skin to suffer damage.[2]

lecithin (BEST)

Phospholipid found in egg yolks and the membranes of plant and animal cells. Widely used in cosmetics as an emollient and water-binding agent. Lecithin also has cell-communicating ability.[592]

lemon (POOR)

Citrus fruit that's a potent skin sensitizer and irritant. Although it can have antibacterial properties, the irritation can hurt skin's immune response.[593]

The juice from lemon is often touted as being a natural option for lightening brown spots or "bleaching" skin. The truth is that lemon juice is highly acidic (has a very low pH of 2) and exceedingly irritating to skin. Lemon juice applied to skin can cause what's known as a phytophotodermatitis (PPD) on exposure to sunlight. The symptoms can range from a red rash to brown discolorations, which is ironic given that many people, mistakenly, turn to lemon juice to lighten brown spots. The PPD is due to a volatile fragrance chemical known as limonene, which is abundant in lemon juice. Lemon, whether in juice or oil form, is a must to avoid in cosmetics.[593] *See* limonene.

lemon oil (POOR)

Commonly used citrus oil that can be a skin irritant, especially on abraded skin.[139,594] Lemon oil has limited research proving any benefits for skin, although there is plenty of anecdotal information with claims that it purifies oily skin, purges clogs from pores, and improves acne-prone skin. As with many fragrant oils, lemon oil has antioxidant components that can be beneficial, but there's no valid reason to tolerate the bad to get the good.

Lemon oil contains numerous fragrance chemicals that make it phototoxic, which means it can cause a reaction when on skin that's subsequently exposed to sunlight. Examples of the fragrance chemicals in lemon oil include limonene, bergapten, and oxypeucedanin.[139,601] Although it smells great, fragrance is not skincare! The major fragrance chemical in lemon oil is limonene. *See* limonene.

lemongrass oil (POOR)

This fragrant oil can be effective as a mosquito repellent.[595] As a volatile fragrant oil, it contains compounds (including limonene and citral) that can cause irritation when applied to skin.

licorice extract (BEST)

Plant extract that has anti-inflammatory properties.[596] In addition, licorice root contains constituents that interrupt the stimulation of an enzyme that activates melanin production, so this part of the plant can be effective for improving dark spots and hyperpigmentation.[597,88]

Licorice has been shown to have efficacy against acne-causing bacteria.[598] One of its components, known as glabridin, is a potent antioxidant and anti-inflammatory ingredient, which is why licorice often shows up in products meant for sensitive, reddened skin.[599,600]

lime oil and extract (POOR)

Citrus fruit whose volatile compounds are skin irritants and photosensitizers. Lime oil is a known fragrance allergen that contains the fragrance chemicals bergapten and limonene, both of which can cause what's known as a phototoxic reaction when applied to skin that's subsequently exposed to sunlight. A phototoxic reaction can result in a patchy, long-lasting tan-to-brown skin discoloration.[139,594,601,602] Although lime extract and oil may have some antibacterial activity on skin (as well as antioxidant activity), their irritant potential outweighs any benefit.

limonene (POOR)

Chemical constituent of many natural fragrant ingredients, notably citrus oils such as lemon (d-limonene) and pine trees or species of the mint family (l-limonene). Early research suggests that limonene may be a potential anti-cancer ingredient and immune stimulant when consumed orally, but other research suggests that limonene may promote the growth of tumors.

Topically, limonene can cause contact dermatitis and is best avoided unless its presence in skincare products is minuscule. Also, because of its penetration-enhancing effects on skin, it's particularly important to avoid products that contain limonene plus other skin irritants like alcohol.[603,604]

Research has shown that another form of limonene (R-limonene) forms "allergenic oxidation products on contact with air." A concentration as low as 0.5% was shown to produce a negative reaction, proving that limonene and its components can be a contact allergen.[605]

linalool (POOR)

Fragrant component of lavender and coriander that can be a potent skin irritant, allergen, or sensitizer when exposed to air.[591] Research also indicates that this component of lavender can be cytotoxic (meaning toxic to skin cells).[589]

linoleic acid (BEST)

Unsaturated omega-6 fatty acid found in corn, safflower, and sunflower oils and used as an emollient and thickening agent in cosmetics. There is some research showing it to be effective in cell regulation and skin-barrier repair, as well as being an antioxidant and an anti-inflammatory agent.[606,607,608]

linolenic acid (BEST)

Naturally occurring, colorless polyunsaturated fatty acid liquid that functions as a skin-conditioning agent and cell-communicating ingredient. Also known as alpha-linolenic acid, this ingredient is a plant-based omega-3 fatty acid that occurs in vegetable oil and flax seed oil as well as canola and soy oils. Walnuts are a top dietary source of this fatty acid. Linolenic acid has research showing topical application helps improve many skin concerns, including eczema, psoriasis, acne, and non-melanoma skin cancers.[609]

Linolenic acid can help repair skin's barrier function and reduce pro-inflammatory substances that would otherwise cause damage. It's believed to communicate with cells that comprise skin's immune system, as evidenced by research showing that topical linolenic (and similar) fatty acids improve wound healing.[610]

M

magnesium aluminum silicate (GOOD)
Powdery, dry-feeling, white solid that is used as a thickening agent and powder in cosmetics.

magnesium ascorbyl palmitate (GOOD)
Fatty acid–based derivative of vitamin C that can be an effective antioxidant. Research shows this form of vitamin C is less stable than others such as magnesium ascorbyl phosphate, which is why we don't rate it as highly as other forms of vitamin C.[611]

magnesium ascorbyl phosphate (BEST)
Form of vitamin C that is considered stable and is an effective antioxidant for skin.[108,612] This form of vitamin C is also known to increase skin's hydration levels and improve its elasticity.[117] Like most forms of vitamin C, magnesium ascorbyl phosphate (in amounts of 5% or greater) has been shown to improve hyperpigmentation.[613,614]

mandelic acid (AVERAGE)
Alpha hydroxy acid (AHA), also known as amygdalic acid. There's scant research showing this to be an effective alternative to other AHAs, although it does have germicidal activity. Unlike glycolic acid, mandelic acid is light-sensitive and must be packaged in an opaque container to remain effective.[615]

manganese violet (GOOD)
Coloring agent/additive permanently listed in 1976 by the FDA as safe for

use in cosmetics products, including those for use around the eye.[489]

Mangifera indica (mango) seed butter (BEST)
Plant-based emollient as it is a rich source of fatty acids and anti-inflammatory ingredients.[616,617]

matricaria flower extract and oil (BEST)
See chamomile.

Melaleuca alternifolia (GOOD)
See tea tree oil.

Mentha piperita (POOR)
See peppermint.

menthol (POOR)
Derived from peppermint, menthol can have the same irritating effect as peppermint on skin.[455,618] Despite its documented ability to irritate skin, menthol is included in a surprisingly large number of products, particularly those claiming to help oily or acne-prone skin. Unfortunately, the cooling, refreshing sensation menthol causes is direct evidence that your skin is being irritated, not soothed.

menthoxypropanediol (POOR)
Synthetic derivative of menthol. Can result in allergic dermatitis and carries the same potential for irritation as menthol.[455,618,619] Menthoxypropanediol is most often used in lip-plumping products.

menthyl lactate (POOR)
Used as a cooling agent and fragrance in cosmetics. This derivative of menthol is supposed to be less irritating than menthol, but less irritating doesn't mean no irritation at all.

methyl gluceth-20 (GOOD)
Synthetic liquid that functions as a water-binding and skin-conditioning agent.

methylchloroisothiazolinone (POOR)
In combination with methylisothiazolinone, it goes by the trade name

Kathon CG (among others). Introduced into cosmetics in the mid-1970s, it elicited a great number of sensitizations in consumers. This led to it not being included in cosmetics other than rinse-off products.[620,621] When combined with methylisothiazolinone, methylchloroisothiazolinone offers broad-spectrum activity against microorganisms. This blend is used in many products instead of parabens, despite the fact that parabens have a better safety track record and lower incidence of causing a sensitizing reaction. It has maintained its reputation as a frequent allergen in leave-on products, particularly hair care and feminine hygiene.[622]

methylisothiazolinone (POOR)

Preservative that's generally recommended for use only in rinse-off products such as cleansers or shampoos. Although used in leave-on products, methylisothiazolinone is known to be sensitizing when used in leave-on products. In fact, the American Contact Dermatitis Society named methylisothiazolinone its Allergen of the Year in 2013![623]

As with most ingredients with problematic potential, much depends on the amount used, but, as a general rule, if you see methylisothiazolinone in the middle of an ingredient list for a leave-on product, you should avoid it, particularly if you have sensitive skin or if this preservative is used in conjunction with sunscreen actives like octinoxate or avobenzone.

Methylisothiazolinone is active against bacteria, but has weak antifungal properties. Its use in both rinse-off and leave-on cosmetics products is restricted to low amounts as a means to avoid irritation while maintaining its efficacy as a preservative; however, but even in the low amount permitted (0.01%) it has raised questions about it being more sensitizing than most other preservatives.[624]

In combination with methylchloroisothiazolinone, this preservative becomes a more frequent allergen in leave-on products, particularly for hair care, baby care, and feminine hygiene.[622,625] To be clear: Neither of these preservatives is considered problematic when used in rinse-off products such as cleansers or body washes; it's the leave-on products, especially those meant for use around the eyes.

methylparaben (GOOD)

See parabens.

methylpropanediol (GOOD)

Glycol that functions as a solvent. Methylpropanediol can enhance the penetration of ingredients (such as salicylic acid) into skin. It also has hydrating properties and can leave a smooth, moist finish on skin

Mexoryl SX™ (BEST)

Also called ecamsule (technical name terephthalylidine dicamphor sulfonic acid), Mexoryl SX is a synthetic sunscreen agent developed and patented by L'Oreal and used in the company's sunscreen products sold outside the United States since 1993 (approved for use in Europe in 1991).[626]

In July 2006, the FDA approved the use of Mexoryl SX in the United States, but only in a single sunscreen product, La Roche-Posay's Anthelios SX SPF 15 (L'Oreal owns La Roche-Posay). The FDA did not approve Mexoryl SX for use in any other sunscreen; only in that one specific product. Anthelios SX will list Mexoryl SX as ecamsule on the label along with the other actives avobenzone and octocrylene (both of these sunscreen ingredients have been approved for use in the United States for years). L'Oreal blitzed the media with press releases about this approval, touting Mexoryl SX's improved stability when compared with avobenzone, or intimating that it is the best UVA sunscreen available.[626]

According to sunscreen expert Ken Klein, former president of Cosmetech Labs and teacher of sunscreen formulation classes for the Society of Cosmetic Chemists, although Mexoryl SX doesn't degrade after hours of sun exposure at the same rate as avobenzone, it does indeed break down, losing 40% of its protective properties. Studies have shown that after controlled doses of UV exposure, avobenzone breaks down at a rate of 65%, so Mexoryl SX does have a slight stability edge. However, avobenzone can be, and often is, made more stable by combining it with other active ingredients, specifically octocrylene. [626] Outside the United States, Tinosorb (another sunscreen active) is often used to enhance the stability of avobenzone.[627]

It's important to note that all sunscreen ingredients break down to some extent when exposed to sunlight, which is why reapplication of sunscreen is critical to maintaining protection. Regarding protection, UVA rays have a range of 320–400 nanometers. Although Mexoryl SX protects within this range, titanium dioxide and zinc oxide protect across the entire UVA and UVB spectrum, from 230 to 700 nanometers. Mexoryl SX is an effective UVA sunscreen agent, but it is by no means the only or absolute best one.

mica (GOOD)

Earth mineral included in products to give them sparkle and shine. The level and look of the shine mica provides depends on the color and how finely it's milled for use in liquid, cream, or powder products.

microcrystalline wax (GOOD)

Plastic-type, highly refined wax derived from petroleum and purified for use in cosmetics. Used as a thickener and to give products a semi-solid to solid smooth texture.

mineral oil (GOOD)

Clear, odorless oil derived from petroleum that is widely used in cosmetics because it rarely causes allergic reactions. It cannot become a solid and clog pores. Despite mineral oil's association with petroleum and the hype that it's bad for or ages skin, keep in mind that petroleum is a natural ingredient derived from the earth. Once it's purified to become mineral oil USP (cosmetics- and pharmaceutical-grade mineral oil), it has no resemblance to the original petroleum and isn't a source of contaminants or carcinogens.[628,629]

Cosmetics-grade mineral oil and petrolatum are considered the safest, most nonirritating moisturizing ingredients ever found. Mineral oil and petrolatum are known to be efficacious in wound healing, and are also among the most effective, established moisturizing ingredients available.[628,629]

Mineral oil is not an ingredient to avoid unless you have oily skin, in which case the somewhat greasy texture of mineral oil won't feel good. But again, mineral oil doesn't clog pores, cause acne, or suffocate skin.

The mineral oil in skincare products is certified as either USP (United States Pharmacopeia) or BP (British Pharmacopoeia). It's completely safe, soothing, non-irritating, and perfectly healthy for skin.[628,630,631,632,633]

montmorillonite (GOOD)

Type of clay that's a mix of bentonite (another clay) and fuller's earth, the latter being a white to brown substance found in sediment. Like all clays, montmorillonite has absorbent properties and can be a helpful ingredient for oily skin and breakouts. It also functions as a thickener.

mulberry extract (GOOD)

Non-fragrant plant extract that, due to its naturally occurring components known as mulberroside A and F, has shown potential to prevent excess melanin production.[577,634,635] Concentration protocols have not been established, so it's best to look for mulberry extract in combination with other proven skin-lightening ingredients.

myristic acid (GOOD)

Detergent cleansing agent that also creates foam and, due to its relation to soap, can be drying.

myristyl myristate (GOOD)

Used in cosmetics as a thickening agent and emollient. It has a wetter feel and is best for dry skin.

N

natural ingredient (AVERAGE)

The FDA tried to establish official definitions and guidelines for the use of such terms as "natural" and "hypoallergenic," but its regulations were overturned in court. That means that cosmetics companies can use these terms on ingredient labels to mean anything they want, which in turn means that they almost always mean nothing at all. The term natural has considerable market value in promoting cosmetics products to consumers, but a close look at most ingredient labels on such products reveals that the plant extracts make up only a small percentage of the product. Plus, when a plant is added to a cosmetic, preserved, and stabilized with other ingredients, it loses much of its natural quality.[636]

neopentyl glycol dicaprylate/dicaprate (GOOD)

Used as an emollient and thickening agent.

neopentyl glycol diheptanoate (GOOD)

Mixture of film-forming and solvent ingredient neopentyl glycol and grape-derived fatty acid heptanoic acid. The compound functions as a non-aqueous skin-conditioning agent and thickener.

neroli oil (POOR)

Fragrant plant oil (Latin name *Citrus aurantium*) whose fragrance component, which has an orange blossom scent, can be a skin irritant and sensitizer. It can also be a potent antioxidant.[637,638]

See limonene and linalool.

niacinamide (BEST)

Also known as vitamin B3 and nicotinic acid, niacinamide is a potent cell-communicating ingredient that offers multiple benefits for aging skin. Assuming skin is being protected from sun exposure, niacinamide can improve skin's elasticity, dramatically enhance its barrier function, help erase discolorations, and revive skin's healthy tone and texture.[79,182,653,654,655,656]

Topically applied niacinamide has been shown to increase ceramide and free fatty acid levels in skin, prevent skin from losing water content, and stimulate microcirculation in the dermis. It also has a growing reputation for being able to treat an uneven skin tone and to mitigate acne and the red marks it leaves behind (known as post-inflammatory hyperpigmentation). Niacinamide, an excellent ingredient for those struggling with wrinkles and breakouts, is stable in the presence of heat and light.[79,182,653,654,655,656]

nylon-12 (GOOD)
Powder substance used as an absorbent and thickening agent. When present in high amounts in skincare or makeup products, nylon-12 tends to have mattifying properties.

O

oat bran extract (BEST)
Portion of the oat plant that contains antioxidant and anti-inflammatory properties. Research has shown that topical application to skin can protect fibroblasts (collagen- and elastin-producing cells in skin) from the oxidation that results from free-radical damage, which means the collagen isn't harmed.[639]

oatmeal (BEST)
Natural ingredient that has anti-irritant and anti-inflammatory properties on skin.[640]

octinoxate (BEST)
Also known as octyl methoxycinnamate and ethylhexyl methoxycinnamate, octinoxate is the oldest and most common sunscreen active used to protect skin, primarily against UVB rays. Although octinoxate does provide some UVA protection, it does not protect against the entire range of UVA wavelengths; therefore, there should be another UVA-protecting active present in any sunscreen you use.

Octinoxate has a solid record of safety (decades of research and thousands of studies establishing its safety in sunscreens as indisputable). Unfortunately, unfounded claims that this staple of SPF formulas causes cancer have made many afraid to use sunscreens that contain it. There are no studies that demonstrate octinoxate, when and as used in SPF products, causes or increases the risk of developing cancer. In the sole studies cited when the "octinoxate = cancer" claim is made, the conditions are completely inapplicable to how sunscreen ingredients are used in skincare products. For example, such "studies" use extremely high concentrations of octinoxate (much higher than would ever be used in sunscreens) applied directly to isolated skin cells (rather than intact skin), or even fed to lab animals.[641,296]

Octinoxate is safe as long as you don't drink it! There simply isn't any research backing the claim that octinoxate has any link to causing cancer or other illnesses when used in sunscreen formulas. In fact, the European Union's permitted usage level for octinoxate in sunscreens is higher than the maximum amount permitted in the United States (7.5% in the United States, 10% in the EU).[296,641]

octisalate (BEST)

Technical name for active sunscreen ingredient octyl salicylate (also known as ethylhexyl salicylate). *See* octyl salicylate.

octocrylene (BEST)

Sunscreen agent that protects skin from the UVB range of sunlight.[643] It also helps stabilize the UVA sunscreen avobenzone. Like all synthetic (or "chemical") sunscreen actives, octocrylene can be sensitizing for some people, particularly those who take the oral arthritis drug ketoprofen.[622,644]

octyl palmitate (GOOD)

Derived from palm oil, widely used in cosmetics as a thickening agent and emollient.

octyl salicylate (BEST)

Sunscreen agent also known as ethylhexyl salicylate. It's used to protect skin primarily from UVB rays.[643] Research into whether or not this sunscreen disrupts hormones (the endocrine system) did not find conclusive evidence of this happening, nor was octyl salicylate found to have estrogenic activity.[645]

octyl stearate (GOOD)

Used in cosmetics as a thickening agent and emollient. *See* stearic acid.

octyldodecanol (GOOD)

Emulsifier and opacifying agent, used primarily as a thickener in moisturizers because of its lubricating and emollient properties.

octyldodecyl myristate (GOOD)

Mixture of octyldodecanol (thickener) and myristic acid that forms a new compound that is used as a skin-conditioning agent and emollient.

octyldodecyl neopentanoate (GOOD)

Skin-conditioning agent and emollient.

Olea europaea (GOOD)

See olive oil.

oleth-10 (GOOD)

Form of fatty (non-irritating) oleyl alcohol that functions as an emulsifier and surfactant. Oleyl alcohol occurs naturally in fish oils, but a synthetic form is typically used in cosmetics.

olive oil/olive fruit oil (GOOD)

Emollient plant oil (Latin name *Olea europaea*) with benefits similar to those of several other non-fragrant plant oils. Olive oil is beneficial for dry skin because of its fatty acid content, some of which comes from the emollient squalene. Olive oil contains essential fatty acids dry skin needs, including oleic, palmitic, and linoleic acids. It also contains phenolic compounds that provide antioxidant benefit. A small number of animal tests show that topically applied olive oil can protect against UVB damage.[646,647,648]

Used alone, olive oil has been shown to be problematic for skin because it seems to reduce skin's barrier integrity and delay healing of injured skin, especially when compared with sunflower seed oil, a plant oil whose fatty acid profile is markedly different from that of olive oil. It's believed that olive oil's high oleic acid content may be responsible for this. This plant oil maintains a low potential for irritancy or allergic reaction.[448,649,650] To be very clear: When olive oil is mixed in a formula in small amounts with other beneficial ingredients, you get the benefit of its slip and emollient properties along with some antioxidant benefit. The negative effects of olive oil are apparent only when used alone on skin, particularly infant skin.

oxybenzone (BEST)

Sunscreen agent (also known as benzophenone-3) that protects primarily from UVB rays, and some, but not all, UVA rays. It is part of the benzophenone group of chemicals. Oxybenzone is approved for use in specific concentrations for sunscreens sold in all major countries, including the United States, Canada, European Union countries, Japan, Australia, China, and South Korea. [289,295]

As a group, the benzophenones are used not only for sun protection but also as photostabilizers in cosmetics products. They keep products from turning color or from degrading in the presence of sunlight. They also have other uses, including flavor enhancers in food.

Like many sunscreen ingredients, oxybenzone has been subject to controversies and scare-tactic stories. We discuss these in Chapter 14, under the question "Can I Get Cancer from Sunscreen?"

ozokerite (GOOD)

Mineral wax used as a thickening agent in cosmetics, especially to add stability to lipsticks and stick foundations and keep them blended.

P

palmitic acid (GOOD)

Fatty acid found naturally in skin and used as the basis for many palmitate ingredients, such as isopropyl palmitate. Palmitic acid has many functions in cosmetics, from detergent cleansing agent to emollient. In a cleanser, it has the potential to be drying depending on what it's combined with and the cleanser's pH level. In moisturizers, palmitic acid is a very good emollient. It helps reinforce skin's healthy barrier function for a smoother surface. [651,652]

palmitoyl oligopeptide (BEST)

See palmitoyl hexapeptide-12.

palmitoyl hexapeptide-12 (BEST)

Blend of the fatty acid palmitic acid with several amino acids, including alanine, arginine, aspartic acid, glycine, histidine, lysine, proline, serine, and/or valine. Also known as pal-KTTKS. Theoretically, many peptides have cell-communicating ability and can help skin cells function in a more normal, healthy manner. Although the research is far from conclusive and formulary protocols need to be followed to ensure the peptide remains stable during use, this peptide may stimulate collagen production and encourage the production of intercellular matrix substances such as hyaluronic acid.[653]

palmitoyl tetrapeptide-7 (BEST)
Synthetic peptide (trade name Matrixyl 3000) believed to work by muting the effect of chemical messengers known as interleukins in the skin that trigger an inflammatory response. Also seems to play a role in thickening skin that has become thinner due to age.[654]

palmitoyl tripeptide-5 (BEST)
Synthetic peptide that's believed to play a role in collagen synthesis and in preventing the breakdown of collagen within skin.[655]

***Panax ginseng* root extract** (BEST)
Plant extract that may have potent antioxidant properties (potentially anti-cancer) and may promote wound healing. Whether or not it can have an impact on cellulite is unknown.[656,657]

panthenol (GOOD)
Alcohol form of the B vitamin pantothenic acid. Panthenol is used in skincare products as a humectant because of its ability to attract and hold moisture. Sometimes called pro-vitamin B5, panthenol mixes readily with many different types of ingredients, making it a versatile ingredient to be used in formulas because it improves skin's barrier function and maintains the proliferation of fibroblasts, the cells that create collagen.[658]

papain (POOR)
Enzyme extracted from papaya. Topically, papaya latex can cause severe irritation and blisters. Severe allergic reactions have been reported in sensitive individuals. Other research has confirmed that papain is a strong allergen on skin.[659]

papaya extract (AVERAGE)
Plant extract that is the source of the enzyme papain, which theoretically can have exfoliating properties on skin, although the majority of the research was not performed on skin. Papaya can be a skin irritant, but it's not as potentially risky as pure papain.[660] Still, it's not an ingredient to apply daily; there

are better options for leave-on exfoliants, including glycolic acid and salicylic acid. *See* glycolic acid; salicylic acid.

parabens (GOOD)

Group of preservatives, including butylparaben, propylparaben, methylparaben, and ethylparaben, that at one time were among the most widely used group of preservatives in cosmetics. Parabens are believed to cause less irritation than some preservatives and they also have broad antifungal and good antibacterial activity. They have become stigmatized as preservatives due to their alleged relation to breast cancer. After researching this issue extensively, we have come to the conclusion that parabens are not harmful ingredients that consumers should avoid. For more information on this topic, see Chapter 14.

paraffin (GOOD)

Waxy, petroleum-based substance used as a thickener in cosmetics.

Parsol 1789 (BEST)

See avobenzone.

PEG compounds (GOOD)

PEG is an acronym for polyethylene glycol. Various forms of PEG compounds are mixed with fatty acids and fatty alcohols to create a variety of ingredients that have diverse functions in cosmetics, including surfactants, binding agents (which keep ingredients blended), stabilizers, and emollients. Common PEG ingredients include the thickening and emulsifying agent PEG-100 stearate, and many PEG compounds combined with hydrogenated oils, which function as emollients or binding agents. PEG compounds may also function as cleansing agents; for example, PEG-7 glyceryl cocoate, PEG-80 sorbitan laurate, and PEG-40 stearate are mild cleansing agents.[661,662]

The greater the number following the PEG designation, the "heavier" and more complex the molecule. For example, PEG-200 palm glyceride is a heavier ingredient than PEG-100 stearate. PEG compounds are widely used throughout the cosmetics industry. They've been extensively tested and are considered safe for use in cosmetics products.[661,662]

pentaerythrityl tetraisostearate (GOOD)

Non-aqueous ester that functions as a thickener and binding agent, derived from the ingredient isostearic acid.

peppermint (POOR)

Both the oil and the extract can have antimicrobial properties, but they can also have an irritating, sensitizing effect on skin.[663] Peppermint oil is a more potent irritant than peppermint water. Peppermint is a common cause of allergic contact dermatitis on the face, particularly around the mouth, as it's frequently used as flavoring in toothpastes.[664,665]

peptide (BEST)

Portions of proteins that are long (or sometimes short) chains of amino acids. In the body, peptides regulate the activity of many systems by interacting with target cells. Some peptides have hormonal activity, some have immune activity, some are cell-communicating ingredients that tell cells how to react and what to do, some are believed to play a role in wound healing, and still others are believed to affect the pathology of skin conditions such as atopic dermatitis.[18]

In theory, all peptides have cell-communicating ability, assuming the formulation supports the type of peptide used and is packaged to protect it from degrading during use (no jars!).

Whether peptides have benefit when applied topically to skin for wound healing, skin-barrier repair, or as disinfectants is difficult to ascertain because they generally cannot penetrate skin and at the same time remain stable because they are too hydrophilic, or water-loving. Ironically, peptides can become unstable in water-based formulas.[666] Further, because peptides are vulnerable to enzymes, the abundant enzymes present in skin can break the peptides down to the point where they have no effect at all.

The latest research is examining how different types of synthesized peptides can enter the living membrane of cells and, more interestingly, transport biologically active ingredients to these cells without them breaking down en route. Some peptides have demonstrated a remarkable anti-inflammatory effect. Creating specific peptide chains in the lab and then attaching a fatty acid component to them allows peptides to overcome their inherent limitations when it comes to being absorbed and remaining stable. Lab-engineered peptides appear to have the kind of efficacy and benefit that go beyond skin's surface, which is exciting, but there's still more to learn.[18,666]

For specialized peptides to exert a benefit beyond that of a water-binding agent, three criteria must be met: the peptides must be stable in their base formula; they must be paired with a carrier that enhances their absorption into skin; and they must be able to reach their target cell groups without breaking down.

Final note: Despite claims to the contrary, there are no peptides being used in skincare products that work like Botox, lasers, or dermal fillers. Peptides also cannot plump lips (at least not to a noticeable extent), lift sagging skin, lighten dark circles, or eliminate puffy eyes. You'll see all of these claims and more on products with peptides, but such claims are not supported by published, peer-reviewed research.

persicaria hydropiper extract (BEST)

Persicaria hydropiper (water pepper) extract is the extract of the whole plant, *Persicaria hydropiper polygonaceae*. It is rich in flavonoids (as quercetin) and sesquiterpenes, showing antioxidants and anti-inflammatory properties, and has have been shown in vitro to inhibit the expression of collagen-depleting MMP-1 when applied to human fibroblast cells.[667,668]

It has been demonstrated to exhibit bactericidal activity against *Staphylococcus aureus* and other skin pathogens. It is used in cosmetics to improve skin hydration and to reduce inflammation.[669,670]

petrolatum (GOOD)

Vaseline is pure petrolatum, and pure petrolatum is a rich emollient and FDA-approved skin protectant. For some unknown and unsubstantiated reason, petrolatum has attained a negative image in regard to skin, despite solid research to the contrary. Topical application of petrolatum can help skin's outer layer recover from damage, reduce inflammation, and generally heal skin.[671,672] It's widely considered safe and highly effective.

phenoxyethanol (GOOD)

Common cosmetics preservative that's considered one of the least irritating for use in formulations. It does not release formaldehyde. Phenoxyethanol is approved worldwide for use in all types of water-based cosmetics, up to a 1% concentration.[673]

The safety of phenoxyethanol has been assessed by the Cosmetic Ingredient Review (CIR) Expert Panel several times. This group evaluated the foundational scientific data plus the newer relevant data, and concluded that phenoxyethanol is safe as a cosmetic ingredient. Interestingly, although the phenoxyethanol used in skincare products is almost always synthetic, this chemical occurs naturally in green tea.[673]

Further studies and accumulated safety data have shown that phenoxyethanol is practically nontoxic via oral and dermal (skin) administration. In a study examining oral intake, increased weights of some organs were noted when high doses of phenoxyethanol were swallowed. The doses in this study were considered much higher than those that would result from using cosmetics and personal care products that contain phenoxyethanol (plus cosmetics aren't meant to be eaten). In short, phenoxyethanol is considered a safe and effective preservative when used in amounts approved for use in leave-on or rinse-off cosmetics products.[673]

phenyl trimethicone (GOOD)

Silicone with a drier finish than dimethicone. In skincare, it functions as an occlusive and conditioning agent, contributing to a product's silky texture and feel on skin. It's one of the better silicone ingredients for those with dry skin due to its higher viscosity.

phenylethyl resorcinol (AVERAGE)

Synthetic antioxidant often seen in skin-lightening products. Compared to proven skin-lightening agents, such as hydroquinone and forms of vitamin C, phenylethyl resorcinol has scant research behind it. The most compelling research looked at the results of a cream with phenylethyl resorcinol plus three other skin-lightening agents. The product was applied over a period of three months by 20 women, all of whom also used sunscreen. At the end of the study, it was determined that the women's dark spots decreased by 43%.[674,675]

The problem is we don't know how much of this improvement is due to phenylethyl resorcinol, as it wasn't used alone, which is the case with most products using this ingredient as a means to lighten brown spots. Until more research comes to light, this isn't an ingredient to bank on for great results if dark spots are your concern; however, it's fine to use in products that also contain other skin-lightening ingredients with established track records of success.[674,675]

phospholipid (BEST)

Type of lipid (fat) composed of glycerol, fatty acids, and phosphate. Phospholipids are essential to the function of cell membranes by providing a stable surrounding structure. Lecithin is an example of a phospholipid. *See* lecithin.

phytosterol (BEST)

Naturally occurring, cholesterol-like molecule found in all plant foods; the highest concentrations are found in vegetable oils such as canola, peanut, safflower, and sesame. Overall, nuts, seeds, and legumes are excellent sources of phytosterols, both for the body and for skin. Applied to skin, research has shown that phytosterols can stop the formation of substances in skin that break down collagen. These degrading substances are more prevalent in sun-damaged skin, so phytosterols can be a good addition to skincare when the goal is to reduce signs of sun damage. Soy phytosterols can help repair a damaged skin barrier, while a common type of phytosterol known as beta-sitosterol has been shown to reduce symptoms of atopic dermatitis.[676,677,678]

pineapple extract (AVERAGE)

Contains the enzyme bromelain, which can break down the connecting layers between skin cells to prompt exfoliation. However, bromelain used alone is a more effective source of exfoliation, and does not have the irritating properties of the pineapple fruit.[679,680]

poloxamer 184 (GOOD)

Synthetic polymer that functions as a cleansing agent.

polybutene (GOOD)

Synthetic polymer derived from mineral oil and used as a thickener and lubricant. *See* polymer.

polyethylene (GOOD)

Form of plastic (synthetic polymer) that has numerous functions in cosmetics products. Rounded polyethylene beads serve as an abrasive agent in many facial scrubs, often used instead of overly abrasive alternatives like walnut shells and ground fruit pits. Also used as a stabilizer, binding agent, thickener, and film-forming agent in moisturizers.

In December 2013, research published in the peer-reviewed journal, *Marine Pollution Bulletin*, demonstrated that although polyurethane beads are non-toxic to humans, they are not filtered during sewage treatment, so are accumulating in waterways, which may have a negative effect on animals that consume them.[681]

Additional research published in December 2013 demonstrated that polyurethane beads have the potential to absorb pollutants while in waterways. This research was conducted to establish the potential of absorption; however, it was not conducted using samples from actual waterways.[682]

Personal care brands, like Johnson & Johnson and Unilever, have announced plans to phase out the ingredient from their product lines throughout 2015.[683,684]

polyethylene glycol (GOOD)

Also listed as PEG on ingredient labels, polyethylene glycol is an ingredient that self-proclaimed "natural" websites have attempted to make notoriously evil. They gain a great deal of attention by attributing horror stories to PEG, associating it with antifreeze (however, antifreeze is ethylene glycol, not polyethylene glycol), but there's no research indicating that it poses any problem for skin. In the minuscule amounts used in cosmetics, it helps keep products stable and performs functions similar to those of glycerin. Because polyethylene glycol can penetrate skin, it is also a vehicle that helps deliver other ingredients deeper into skin. It is also used internally in medical procedures to flush and cleanse the intestinal tract. *See* PEG compound.

polyhydroxystearic acid (GOOD)

Synthetic polymer related to stearic acid that functions as a suspending agent. *See* polymer.

polyisobutene (GOOD)

Polymer of the hydrocarbon isobutylene obtained from petroleum oil. It functions as a thickening and film-forming agent and does not penetrate skin due to its large molecular size.

polymer (GOOD)

Word that literally means "many parts." Any of numerous compounds having a high molecular weight, either from being composed of many smaller molecules or by condensing many small molecules into larger molecules that can take on new forms and perform different functions. Plastic is an example of polymer technology, as is nylon. Polymers do not have a defined formula because they consist of various chains of different lengths. Natural polymers exist, too; examples are polysaccharides, rubber, and cellulose. The human body contains many polymers in the form of various proteins, nucleic acids, and the energy source glycogen. Hundreds, if not thousands, of cosmetic ingredients with various functions have been created based on the evolving science of polymers.

polymethyl methacrylate (GOOD)

Polymer that's commonly used as a synthetic film-forming agent. According to the website CosmeticsInfo.org, "The Food and Drug Administration (FDA) has approved Polymethyl Methacrylate for use in medical devices including intraocular lenses, bone cement, dental fillers and dermal fillers. These devices are placed directly into the body and are intended to remain in the body for long periods of time. The FDA also permits Polymethyl Methacrylate to be used as an indirect food additive in adhesives and polymers that come into contact with food."[685]

The safety of polymethyl methacrylate has been assessed by the Cosmetic Ingredient Review (CIR) Expert Panel. After evaluating the scientific data, experts concluded that this ingredient is safe as used in cosmetics. *See* polymer.

polymethylsilsesquioxane (GOOD)

Polymer formed from the condensation and hydrolysis of the silicone methyltrimethoxysilane. *See* polymer.

polysilicone-11 (GOOD)

Specialized, synthetic cross-linked siloxane that functions as a film-forming agent and polymer. *See* polymer.

polysorbates (GOOD)

Large group of ingredients (including the common polysorbate 20) most often derived from lauric acid, which is derived from coconuts. Polysorbates function as emulsifiers and also have mild surfactant properties; some polysorbates are derived from the food ingredient sorbitol, which occurs naturally in many fruits, while others have a fatty acid component. Polysorbates are considered non-toxic and safe as used in the concentrations found in cosmetics and food products (in food products, polysorbates function as stabilizers).

pomegranate extract (BEST)

Pomegranate and its extracts have antioxidant and anticancer properties that, while not conclusively demonstrated on human skin, show promise in animal and in vitro studies. Topical application of products containing pomegranate may improve the appearance of wrinkled skin by reducing inflammation and forestalling further damage. Research also shows that an extract from pomegranate peel has an inhibitory effect on the collagen-depleting substance MMP-1.[686,687,688]

potassium hydroxide (AVERAGE)

Highly alkaline ingredient (also known as lye) used in small amounts in cosmetics to modulate the pH of a product. It's also used as a cleansing agent. In higher concentrations, it's a significant skin irritant.

potassium myristate (AVERAGE)

Detergent cleansing agent that's a constituent of soap; it can be drying and sensitizing for some people.

potassium sorbate (GOOD)

Used as a preservative due to its ability to inhibit mold and yeast growth in cosmetics products once it breaks down into sorbic acid. It has weak activity against bacteria, which is why it is almost always used in conjunction with other preservatives.[689]

preservative (GOOD)

Substance used in cosmetics to prevent bacterial and microbial contamination of products, particularly water-based formulas. Although there's definitely a risk of irritation from these types of ingredients, the risk to skin and eyes from using a contaminated product is considered by many scientists to be even greater.[690]

propylene glycol (GOOD)

Along with other glycols and glycerol, this is a humectant or humidifying and delivery ingredient used in cosmetics. There are websites and spam e-mails stating that propylene glycol is really industrial antifreeze and that it is the major ingredient in brake and hydraulic fluids. These sites also state that tests show it's a strong skin irritant. They further point out that the Material Safety Data Sheet (MSDS) on propylene glycol warns users to avoid skin contact because systemically (in the body) it can cause liver abnormalities and kidney damage. As ominous as this sounds, it's so far from the reality of cosmetics formulations that almost none of it holds any water or poses any real concern. In fact, research from toxicologists has shown that propylene glycol and similar ingredients don't present a health risk for people when used in cosmetics.[691]

It's important to realize that the MSDS refers to a 100% concentration of a substance. Even water and salt have frightening comments regarding their safety according to their MSDS reports. In cosmetics, propylene glycol is used only in the smallest amounts to keep products from melting in high heat or from freezing. It also helps active ingredients penetrate skin. In the minute amounts in cosmetics, it's not a concern in the least. People aren't suffering from liver problems because of propylene glycol in cosmetics.

And, finally, according to the U.S. Department of Health and Human Services, within the Public Health Services Agency for Toxic Substances and Disease Registry, "studies have not shown these chemicals (propylene or the other glycols as used in cosmetics) to be carcinogens."[692] The Cosmetic Ingredient Review Expert Panel and other groups have analyzed all of the toxicology data and exposure studies concerning topical application of propylene glycol as commonly used in cosmetics products. Their conclusion was that it is safe and does not pose a health risk to consumers.

propylene glycol dicaprylate/dicaprate (GOOD)
Gel-textured ingredient used in many lightweight moisturizers. It's a mix of propylene glycol and capric acid, a fatty acid derived from plants.

propylene glycol isostearate (GOOD)
Mixture of propylene glycol and isostearic acid used as an emollient and emulsifier.

propylene glycol laurate (GOOD)
Ester of propylene glycol and lauric acid, which is a constituent of many vegetable fats.

propylene glycol stearate (GOOD)
Mixture of propylene glycol and stearic acid used as a skin-conditioning agent and emulsifier.

propylparaben (GOOD)
See parabens.

Pyrus malus (GOOD)
Species of apple; the pectin derived from it is used as a thickener in cosmetics. Apple stem cells do not have special anti-aging properties for skin. *See* stem cells.

Q

quaternium-15 (AVERAGE)
Formaldehyde-releasing preservative used in cosmetics. It can be a skin sensitizer, as can all preservatives, although quaternium-15's ability to sensitize skin is very low if the amount in a product is less than 0.2%.[693]

quercetin (BEST)

Bioflavonoid ingredient from plants. Quercetin occurs naturally in red wine, tea, onions, kale, tomatoes, berries, and many other fruits and vegetables, with the highest concentrations found in the leaves and skins. It functions as an antioxidant, anti-inflammatory agent, and skin-healing ingredient, likely owing to the stimulating effect it has on the immune system, of which skin is our body's first line of defense. Quercetin is present in some herbal ingredients, too, including St. John's wort and *Ginkgo biloba*.

In terms of skincare, research has shown that a lipid-based delivery system is optimal for quercetin to exert antioxidant benefits.[694] Even more exciting, this type of formula provides an initial burst of quercetin followed by sustained release over a 24-hour period. When quercetin is mixed with silicone and lipids, the intake is greater, as confirmed by testing on human skin.[695]

More good news on the skincare front: Quercetin can help defend skin from UVB-related damage, reduce the production of an elastin-degrading enzyme, and help heal and improve the appearance of scars.[696,697,698]

R

resveratrol (BEST)

Potent polyphenolic antioxidant abundant in red grapes and, therefore, in red wine. Resveratrol has been reported in numerous studies to be one of the most potent natural chemopreventive agents for inhibiting the cellular processes associated with tumor development, including initiation, promotion, and progression. It also has significant anti-inflammatory properties and seems to have a stimulating and protective effect on glutathione, the body's master antioxidant.[699,700,701,702] Conversely, there's also research showing it to be associated with cell death when applied in pure doses directly to skin cells that are then exposed to UV radiation. Of course, this has nothing to do with how resveratrol is used in skincare products, but it's an interesting example of how more is not necessarily better when it comes to skincare ingredients!

retinoids (BEST)

Large group of over 2,500 chemicals related to vitamin A. Topical, over-the-counter retinoids include retinol, retinyl palmitate, retinaldehyde, and retinyl linoleate, among others. Prescription retinoids include tretinoin (Renova, Retin-A), adapalene (Differin), and tazarotene (Tazorac). Other retinoid chemicals include beta-carotene and various carotenoids found in brightly colored and dark green fruits and vegetables.[19,92,95,96]

When applied topically, retinoids function in multiple ways. Primarily, they work as cell-communicating ingredients, essentially connecting with a receptor site on a skin cell and "telling" it to behave in a more normal and healthier manner. Retinoids have benefits for more than 125 different skin issues, from acne to psoriasis to wrinkles and other signs of sun damage. They can improve, to some extent, how new skin cells are formed and how they behave as they mature (differentiate) and make their way to the skin surface.

Tolerability can be an issue with all retinoids, with the prescription forms more likely to cause side effects than over-the-counter retinol products. The most common side effects from topical application of retinoids include irritation, flaking skin, and redness (sometimes resembling and/or feeling like sunburn, with skin being tender to the touch).[95,96] The side effects tend to appear within 2–4 days from the time you apply the retinoid. In most cases, they subside within a few weeks as your skin adjusts; however, there will always be some people whose skin is simply intolerant of retinoids.

It's important to avoid applying too much of any retinoid product; more isn't necessarily better and can often make the potential side effects an unwelcome reality. For example, the directions for prescription retinoid creams state to apply a pea-size amount, which is plenty. Applying more per use won't get you better or faster results, but it can increase the chances of unwanted side effects.

Research has shown that varying strengths of retinol and prescription retinoids are beneficial; with any type of retinoid, the "if a little is good, more must be better" mentality can backfire. Some people's skin can tolerate higher amounts of retinoids, but it's always best to begin with the lower strength to see how your skin responds and then increase the concentration if results are positive. It's also fine to alternate between lower- and higher-strength retinoid products; for example, one night you can apply an over-the-counter retinol product, and the next evening apply a prescription retinoid.[19,92,95,96]

retinol (BEST)

Name for the entire vitamin A molecule. Retinol has value for skin on several fronts: It's a cell-communicating ingredient and an antioxidant. Skin cells have a receptor site that's very accepting of retinoic acid, which is a component of retinol. This relationship between retinoic acid and skin cells allows for a type of communication in which the cell is told to function normally (that is, not like a damaged or older cell), and it can, to some extent, conform to that request. That's one of the reasons retinol is an exciting anti-aging ingredient. Retinol cannot communicate with a cell until the retinol is broken down into retinoic acid.[5,19,20]

Retinol helps skin cells create better, healthier skin cells, provides antioxidant support, and increases the amount of substances that enhance skin's structural elements. Packaging is still a key issue, so any container that lets in air (like jar packaging) or sunlight (clear containers) just won't cut it, which applies to most state-of-the-art skincare ingredients. Lots of retinol products come in unacceptable packaging; these should be avoided because the retinol will most likely be (or quickly become) ineffective.[5,19,20]

Many consumers are concerned about the percentage of retinol in anti-aging products such as serums or moisturizers. Although the percentage can make a difference (especially if it's too low), it is not helpful in understanding how a retinol product will benefit your skin. Far more important is the delivery system, packaging, and the other ingredients present with the retinol. Using a product with a range of anti-aging ingredients plus retinol is far more valuable for skin than using a product with only a supposedly high percentage of retinol. Skin is the largest organ of the body and needs far more than any one ingredient can provide. It doesn't make sense to fixate on the percentage of retinol when so many other elements are also important.[5,19,20]

Because retinol is one of the ingredients known to help improve skin structure, it has some value in anti-cellulite products. Of all the ingredients to look for in a cellulite product, this should be at the top of the list. However, most cellulite products contain only teeny amounts of retinol (at best) and they are often in packaging that won't keep this air-sensitive ingredient stable.

retinyl palmitate (BEST)
Combination of retinol (pure vitamin A) and palmitic acid. Research has shown it to be effective as an antioxidant and skin-cell regulator.[703] Is retinyl palmitate safe for skin? We discuss this in depth in Chapter 14, under the question of whether or not sunscreen ingredients cause cancer.

retinyl retinoate (BEST)
Synthetic, "new generation" retinoid with research showing its usefulness for wrinkles, acne, and hyaluronic acid synthesis in skin. Retinyl retinoate has been shown, in limited but promising research (most coming from the same team of Korea-based researchers), to be less irritating than retinoic acid (prescription-strength) and over-the-counter retinol. Retinyl retinoate may be less irritating than pure retinol because of its slower conversion in skin to retinoic acid. However, when it comes to irritation from retinol, there's much that

can be done using time-release delivery systems and ingredient additions to maximize its benefits to skin while minimizing, if not eliminating, its risk of irritation (so-called "retinol dermatitis").[723,724,725]

Although there's reason to consider retinyl retinoate if your skin seems intolerant of retinol and prescription retinoids, it shouldn't be construed as better or safer for skin than over-the-counter products that contain retinol or other types of cosmetic retinoids.[704,705,706]

rice bran oil (GOOD)

Emollient oil similar to other non-fragrant plant oils. Research has not shown that it has any superior benefit for skin.

Rosa damascena oil (POOR)

Oil of a very fragrant pink rose used as fragrance in cosmetics. Extensive research has shown it has mixed benefits. In the pro column, inhaling this flower's scent seems to have relaxing, blood pressure–lowering benefits and the plant's petals contain anti-inflammatory and antioxidant compounds that can benefit skin.[707]

On the flipside, the numerous chemicals that create this rose's distinctive fragrance pose a risk of irritation and allergic contact dermatitis.[707]

rose flower oil (POOR)

Fragrant, volatile oil that can be a skin irritant and sensitizer. There's no research showing this has any benefit for skin, although components of rose can have anti-inflammatory and antioxidant effects on skin.[707] The trick is to get those ingredients onto your skin without exposing your skin to the fragrant components that other research has shown can be irritating to skin.

rosehip oil (GOOD)

Non-fragrant emollient plant oil that has antioxidant properties.[708,709]

rosemary extract (AVERAGE)

Extract that can have antioxidant benefit for skin, but its aromatic components can cause irritation or sensitizing reactions.[452,710] However, in most skincare products the amount of rosemary extract is unlikely to be a risk, and rosemary extract is much less of a problem for skin than rosemary oil because the extract usually doesn't contain much, if any, of rosemary oil's fragrance components.

rosemary oil (POOR)

Fragrant plant oil derived from rosemary (Latin name *Rosmarinus offici-nalis*). This ingredient is used primarily as a fragrance in cosmetics, but the volatile chemicals that give it its fragrance (camphor is among them) are also capable of causing irritation when applied to skin. Research has shown that rosemary has antifungal, antibacterial, and antioxidant benefits; however, because many other ingredients provide these benefits without the risk of irritation presented by rosemary oil, there's no compelling reason to apply it. If you enjoy the scent, it's fine to inhale, such as from scented candles.[711,712,713]

rosewood oil (POOR)

Fragrant plant oil with a spicy-sweet scent, also known as bois de rose. Extracted from wood chips from a species of evergreen tree, rosewood oil contains several volatile fragrance chemicals, including camphene, geranial, geraniol, limonene, linalool, myrcene, and neral. Rosewood oil is used chiefly as a fragrance and flavoring ingredient; there's no research pertaining to its benefit for skin, although it does not appear to have toxic properties. Still, it can kill healthy skin cells, even though this effect seems greater on cancerous cells that would otherwise continue to spread.[714,715]

S

saccharide isomerate (GOOD)

Good water-binding agent and emollient for skin, and particularly helpful for dry skin because it seems to have the ability to bind to skin's proteins and to stick around longer than other emollients, which are more easily washed away.

safflower seed oil (BEST)

Emollient plant oil similar to all non-fragrant plant oils. Safflower seed oil contains beneficial fatty acids, primarily linolenic acid, that can help repair skin's barrier and that are of particular value to those with dry skin.

salicylic acid (BEST)

Also called beta hydroxy acid (BHA), this multifunctional ingredient addresses many of the systemic causes of acne.[716] For decades, dermatologists have been prescribing salicylic acid as an exceedingly effective keratolytic (exfoliant), but it's also an anti-irritant because it is a derivative of aspirin (both are salicylates—aspirin's technical name is acetylsalicylic acid), and so it also functions as an anti-inflammatory.[31,33]

Another notable aspect of salicylic acid for treating breakouts is that it has antimicrobial properties.[69] It has the ability to penetrate into the pore lining and exfoliate inside the pore as well as on the surface of skin, which makes it effective for reducing breakouts, including blackheads and whiteheads.[31,33]

It is also well that documented that salicylic acid can improve skin thickness, barrier function, and collagen production.[16,31,33] As an exfoliant, in concentrations of 8% to 12%, it is effective in medications to remove warts. In concentrations of 0.5% to 2%, it is far gentler, and, much like AHAs, can exfoliate the surface of skin.

sandalwood oil (POOR)

Fragrant oil (Latin name *Santalum album*) that can cause skin irritation or allergic reactions. One animal study showed it to have antitumor properties. [717] Sandalwood oil is a must to avoid if you have extra-sensitive skin or if you normally react to fragrance.

SD alcohol (POOR)

See alcohol.

sea buckthorn (GOOD)

Berry extract that grows on a shrub-like tree. The fruit of this plant contains malic and acetic acids (AHA-like ingredients that give the fruit an astringent, acidic taste) as well as beneficial compounds known as flavonoids, plus fatty oils. Sea buckthorn is a rich source of vitamin C, but most of it is lost when the fruit is processed for production (which includes manufacture for use in cosmetics products).

Sea buckthorn is believed to have several topical benefits, including for acne, but the research to support such claims is lacking. More convincing is the research pertaining to sea buckthorn's ability to help skin heal when applied to wounds, and it does appear to have some antioxidant ability.[718,719]

Research has also shown that oral consumption of sea buckthorn can help reduce topical symptoms of UV damage by controlling the rate of collagen degradation and by increasing the activity of superoxide dismutase, a naturally occurring antioxidant that helps skin repair damage.[720]

sesame oil (GOOD)

Emollient oil (Latin name *Sesamum indicum*) similar to other non-fragrant plant oils. Despite the similarity to other plant oils, sesame oil isn't quite as impressive as some others we've rated higher.

shea butter (BEST)

Plant lipid, extracted from the karite tree, that is used as an emollient in cosmetics. Shea butter is a rich source of antioxidants, including epicatechin gallate, gallocatechin, epigallocatechin, gallocatechin gallate, and epigallocatechin gallate, as well as quercetin.[721]

silica (GOOD)

Mineral found abundantly in sandstone, clay, and granite, as well as in parts of plants and animals. It's the principal ingredient of glass. In cosmetics it is used as an absorbent powder and thickening agent.

silica dimethyl silylate (GOOD)

Used as a slip and suspending agent in cosmetics.

silicone (GOOD)

Substance derived from silica (sand is a silica). The unique fluid properties of silicone give it a great deal of slip, and in its various forms it can feel like silk on skin, impart emollience, and be a water-binding agent that holds up well, even when skin becomes wet. In other forms, it's used extensively for wound healing and for improving the appearance of scars.[722]

There are numerous forms of silicones used in cosmetic products, particularly leave-on skincare products and all manner of hair-care products. Common forms of silicone are cyclopentasiloxane and cyclohexasiloxane; other forms include various types of dimethicone and phenyl trimethicone.

Claims that silicones in any form cause or worsen acne have not been substantiated in published research, nor have reports that silicones are irritating to or "suffocate" skin. Almost all of these claims are either myths or based on anecdotal evidence, which isn't the best way to determine the safety or efficacy of any cosmetic ingredient. How do we know that silicones don't suffocate skin? Because of their molecular properties they are at the same time porous and resistant to air. Think of silicones in a skincare formula like the covering of a tea bag. When you steep the tea bag in water; the tea and all of its antioxidant properties are released.

Silicones remain on the surface of your skin and the other ingredients it's mixed with "steep" through. All ingredients must be suspended in some base formula; some of the ingredients remain on the surface, some are absorbed. The intent is for the "actives" to get through. Think of how many topical medications are suspended in petrolatum or mineral oil and the active ingredients absolutely get through, and petrolatum is far more effective at preventing moisture loss than silicones are.

Moreover, the molecular structure of commonly used silicones makes it impossible for them to suffocate skin (not to mention skin doesn't breathe). The unique molecular structure of silicones (large molecules with wide spaces between each molecule) allows them to form a permeable barrier and also explains why silicones rarely feel heavy or occlusive, although they offer protection against moisture loss.[723]

Interestingly, silicone has been shown to be helpful for offsetting dryness and flaking from common anti-acne active ingredients such as benzoyl peroxide and topical antibiotics.[724] Also, silicones are sometimes used as fillers to improve the appearance of acne scars, which certainly wouldn't be the case if silicone were a pore-clogging ingredient.[725] Perhaps the most telling reason why silicones do not clog pores and cause acne (or blackheads) is because, from a chemistry standpoint, most silicones are volatile. That means their initially viscous (thick) texture evaporates quickly and does not penetrate the pore lining where acne is formed. Instead, they help ensure the even application of other ingredients and leave behind a silky, almost imperceptible feel that noticeably enhances skin's texture and appearance—without irritation.

slip agent (GOOD)

Term used to describe a range of ingredients that help other ingredients spread over skin and penetrate into it. Slip agents also have humectant properties. Slip agents include butylene glycol, glycerin, polysorbates, and propylene glycol, to name a few. They are as basic to the world of skincare as water.

sodium acrylate acryloyldimethyl taurate copolymer (GOOD)

Synthetic polymer used as a stabilizing and suspending agent and as a thickening agent. *See* polymer.

sodium ascorbyl phosphate (BEST)

Stable, water-soluble form of vitamin C that functions as an antioxidant. [379,611] There's limited, but promising, research demonstrating that concentrations above 1% have antibacterial action against acne-causing bacteria, while concentrations of 5% reduce the inflammatory response related to acne.[111,726]

This form of vitamin C is also potentially effective for lightening skin discolorations, although there isn't much research supporting its use for this purpose over other forms of vitamin C.

sodium benzoate (GOOD)

Salt of benzoic acid used as a preservative. The benzoic acid portion of this ingredient conveys some amount of preservative benefit, most notably against fungi.

sodium C14-16 olefin sulfonate (POOR)

Used primarily as a detergent cleansing agent, but is potentially drying and irritating for skin. Can be derived from coconut. It's tricky to include in formulas due to stability issues, but it does produce copious foam. Secondary surfactants can be used with this cleansing agent to minimize its negative impact on skin, but why not just use a cleanser that contains gentler cleansing agents? All skin types do better with gentle cleansing agents, and there are plenty of options in that regard, so no need to settle for one that contains this potentially problematic cleansing agent.

sodium chloride (GOOD)

More popularly known as common table salt. Used primarily as a binding agent in skincare products and occasionally as an abrasive in scrub products. Perhaps the most common use of sodium chloride in cosmetics is as a thickening agent. Salt is commonly used to thicken the water (also known as aqueous) phase of shampoos, body washes, and non-soap facial cleansers.

sodium cocoamphoacetate (GOOD)

Gentle cleansing agent derived from coconut fatty acids. It functions as a cleansing agent and can also have mild conditioning properties. It has a slight tendency to foam during use.

sodium cocoate (POOR)

Cleansing agent used primarily in soaps and bar cleansers. It can be drying and irritating for skin.

sodium cocoyl glutamate (GOOD)

Cleansing agent derived from coconut oil. This ingredient is also used to help soften (remove excess minerals from) hard water.

sodium cocoyl isethionate (GOOD)

Derived from coconut, a mild detergent cleansing agent and the chief ingredient in non-soap Dove Beauty Bar.

sodium dehydroacetate (GOOD)

Organic salt used as a preservative.

sodium hyaluronate (BEST)

Salt form of skin-identical ingredient hyaluronic acid; considered more bioavailable to skin than pure hyaluronic acid. *See* hyaluronic acid.

sodium hydroxide (AVERAGE)

Also known as lye, sodium hydroxide is a highly alkaline ingredient used in small amounts in cosmetics to establish and hold the pH of a product. Also used as a cleansing agent in some cleansers. In high concentrations, it's a significant skin irritant.[727]

sodium laureth sulfate (GOOD)

Used primarily as a detergent cleansing agent. Can be derived from coconut. It's considered gentle and effective as typically used in cosmetics products (typically facial or body cleansers and shampoos). Despite the name similarity, sodium laureth sulfate is NOT the same as sodium lauryl sulfate. The former is a milder cleansing agent due to a higher amount and different chemical structure of the fatty alcohols required to manufacture this cleansing agent. The safety of sodium laureth sulfate has been reviewed by numerous industry experts and deemed safe as used.[360,728]

sodium lauroamphoacetate (GOOD)

Mild surfactant (cleansing agent) also used as a lather agent.

sodium lauryl sulfate (POOR)

Versatile ingredient composed of several non-volatile alcohols. Functions primarily as a surfactant, but can also be used as a skin-conditioning agent, emulsifier, and solvent. Sodium lauryl sulfate (SLS) is one of the most irritating cleansing agents used in skincare products. In fact, it's considered a standard comparison substance for measuring the skin irritancy of other ingredients. Thus, in scientific studies, when they want to establish whether or not an ingredient is problematic for skin, they compare its effect to the effect of SLS.[360]

In amounts of 2% to 5%, sodium lauryl sulfate can cause allergic or sensitizing reactions for many people.[729,730] Despite the irritancy issue, it is not the same as the dire and erroneous warnings floating around the web about this ingredient.

sodium methyl cocoyl taurate (GOOD)
Mild surfactant derived from coconut; often used in cleansers when the desired effect is a creamy foam.

sodium palmate (POOR)
Soap ingredient created by the salts of acids derived from palm oil. May be naturally derived or synthetic. As a soap ingredient, it can be drying and is typically formulated at an alkaline pH, which disrupts skin's barrier function and can increase harmful bacteria on skin.

sodium PCA (BEST)
Natural component of skin, PCA (pyrrolidone carboxylic acid) is also a very good water-binding agent. Sodium PCA also functions as a skin-repairing ingredient.[155]

sodium polyacrylate (GOOD)
Versatile, synthetic polymer used as a film-forming agent, stabilizer, absorbent, thickening agent, and emollient.

solvent (GOOD)
Large group of ingredients, including water, that are used to dissolve or break down other ingredients. Solvents are also used to degrease skin and to remove sebum.

sorbic acid (GOOD)
Preservative derived from mountain ash berries or manufactured synthetically. Sorbic acid is used in many products, including several foods and even in contact lens solutions. A study of contact sensitization to preservatives among 514 volunteers with eczema showed that sorbic acid caused a reaction in only 0.6% of participants. In contrast, many other preservatives had much higher rates of negative reactions, upwards of 13.6%.[731]

sorbitan stearate (GOOD)

Emulsifier used to thicken and stabilize cosmetics formulations. *See* emulsifier.

soy extract (BEST)

Potent antioxidant and anti-inflammatory agent for skin.[732] Soy is one of many phytochemicals (phyto = plant) that are biologically active against free radicals. Soy extract's increasing use in anti-aging products is largely due to studies showing that its antioxidant genistein (a component of soy) has a collagen-stimulating effect and that various compounds in soy influence skin thickness and elasticity.[733,734]

Researchers have also looked at *Bifidobacterium*-fermented soy milk extracts. On mouse skin and in human skin fibroblasts (lab cultured), this bacteria-modified form of soy was shown to stimulate the production of hyaluronic acid in skin. This was due to the amount of genistein released during the fermentation process.[734,735]

Soy extract has been shown to help reduce the effects of UVB exposure on human skin cells.[736,737]

Research hasn't shown that soy extract or soy oil has estrogenic effects when applied to skin, as it can when taken orally.[738]

soy oil (BEST)

Emollient oil similar to all non-fragrant plant oils.

squalene (BEST)

Oil derived from shark liver or from plants (usually olives) and sebum. Its derivative squalane is a natural component of skin and a good emollient that has antioxidant and immune-stimulating properties.[739,740]

St. John's wort (GOOD)

Plant that contains several components that can cause a negative reaction on skin in the presence of sunlight. Any product that contains St. John's wort should be followed by application of a broad-spectrum sunscreen.[741]

St. John's wort's association with improving depression when taken as an oral supplement is unrelated to its topical impact on skin. However, it does have potent antioxidant properties.[742]

In terms of skin healing, research has shown that St. John's wort enhances the process while minimizing pain, making it a suitable option for helping to minimize the formation and ultimate appearance of scars. St. John's wort also has antifungal and antibacterial activity.[743]

stearic acid (GOOD)

Fatty acid used as an emollient and emulsifier. *See* emollient; emulsifier.

stearyl alcohol (GOOD)

Fatty alcohol used as an emollient and to help keep other ingredients intact in a formulation. Not to be confused with the drying, irritating types of alcohol such as SD alcohol or denatured alcohol.

stem cells (AVERAGE)

Cells in animals and in plants that are capable of becoming any other type of cell in that organism and then reproducing more of those cells. Despite the fact that stem cell research is in its infancy, many cosmetics companies claim they are successfully using plant-based or human-derived stem cells in their anti-aging products. The claims run the gamut, from reducing wrinkles to repairing elastin to regenerating cells, so the temptation for consumers to try these products is intense.

The truth is that stem cells in skincare products do not work as claimed; they simply cannot deliver the promised results. In fact, they likely have no effect at all because stem cells must be alive to function as stem cells, and by the time these delicate cells are added to skincare products, they are long since dead and, therefore, useless. Actually, it's a good thing that stem cells in skincare products can't work as claimed, given that studies have revealed that they pose a potential risk of cancer.

Plant stem cells, such as those derived from apples, melons, and rice, cannot stimulate stem cells in human skin; however, because they are derived from plants they likely have antioxidant properties. That's good, but it's not worth the extra cost that often accompanies products that contain plant stem cells. It's also a plus that plant stem cells can't work as stem cells in skincare products; after all, you don't want your skin to absorb cells that can grow into apples or watermelons!

There are also claims that because a plant's stem cells allow a plant to repair itself or to survive in harsh climates, these benefits can be passed on to human skin. How a plant functions in nature is completely unrelated to how human skin functions, and these claims are completely without substantiation. It doesn't matter how well the plant survives in the desert, no matter how you slather such products on your skin, you still won't survive long without ample water, shade, clothing, and other skin-protective elements.

Another twist on the stem cell issue is that cosmetics companies are claiming they have taken components (such as peptides) out of the plant stem cells and made them stable so they will work as stem cells would or that they will influence the adult stem cells naturally present in skin. In terms of these modified ingredients working like stem cells, this theory doesn't make any sense because stem cells must be complete and intact to function normally. Using peptides or other ingredients to influence adult stem cells in skin is something that's being explored, but to date scientists are still trying to determine how that would work and how it could be done safely. For now, companies claiming they've isolated substances or extracts from stem cells and made them stable are most likely not telling the whole story. Currently, there's no published, peer-reviewed research showing these stem cell extracts can affect stem cells in human skin.

sulfates (GOOD)

In cosmetics, used mainly as cleansing agents in skincare and hair-care products; they include sodium lauryl sulfate, ammonium lauryl sulfate, and sodium laureth sulfate. Many consumers are scared of sulfates in their cosmetics products because of widespread misinformation. Sulfates are not a problem, but once organizations and companies build up fears among consumers about certain cosmetics ingredients there's almost no going back, the damage is done.[360,744,745,746]

In reality there's absolutely no research showing that sulfates are a problem in skincare or hair-care products, other than causing irritation, but that is also true for the sulfate-free cleansing agents that some cosmetics companies advertise and sell. And, whether or not a cleansing agent will cause irritation depends on the amount of sulfate and on other ingredients present in a specific formula.[360,744,745,746]

Following are some of the most typical unsupported comments about sulfates:

"Sulfate-free shampoos and cleansers are better for hair and skin." No research has shown that to be even remotely the case. Sulfates are supposed to be terribly drying and damaging to hair, when in fact they function no differently from the cleansing agents in sulfate-free shampoos. Almost every company that touts the fact that they don't contain sulfates do use detergent cleansing agents such as sodium lauryl sulfoacetate, disodium laureth sulfosuccinate, sodium lauroyl sarcosinate, cocamidopropyl hydroxysultaine, sodium cocoyl isethionate, cocamidopropylamine oxide, and sodium methyl 2-sulfolaurate.

Why those are supposedly any better for skin is never explained, and no research is ever cited—because none exists. Sometimes these companies list those ingredients as being derived from or coming from coconut to make them sound natural and, by association, better for skin—but they all end up being primarily synthetic. That doesn't make them bad in any way; it's just that the claims are completely disingenuous. What you need to know is that both the sulfate-free cleansing agents and the sulfate versions can be drying and irritating depending on the formulation and/or your skin's own reaction. All of these cleansing agents remove oil, built-up skin cells, and the gunk from styling products, which is exactly what a shampoo should do.

"Sulfates cause cancer, cataracts, and kidney and liver failure." These are perhaps the most frightening of the misguided comments you may have heard, but none of these are supported by research. Even the websites that love to scare you about ingredients conclude there's no research showing that sulfates in shampoos or cleansers can cause these health problems.

Another website includes a study from the 1980s where a pure sulfate cleansing agent was used in the eyes of rabbits. Not surprisingly, putting a pure sulfate into a rabbit's eyes caused irritation, but these kinds of studies showed the same thing for mascara (which most women use every day) and would show the same thing for lemon or peppermint. How any of that relates to the amount present in shampoos and to how shampoos are used is just inexplicable thinking. Even more to the point, those who work in the manufacture of pure sulfates have no increased risk of cancer, cataracts, or anything else.

Despite the fact that there is no research showing any association between sulfates and these grave health problems, it still gets mentioned because some sulfates have been found to contain a minute amount of 1,4-Dioxane, which is classified as a probable human carcinogen because of results from animal studies where rats were fed this substance. But ingesting pure 1,4-Dioxane is not the same thing as using it on skin or hair. Keep in mind, not all products containing sulfates contain 1,4-Dioxane and the alternative sulfate-free cleansing products could easily contain 1,4-Dioxane, but that issue is never addressed. Of course, it wouldn't be because these companies don't want to scare you away from using their products. They simply want to reinforce the "sulfates are bad, our products are safe" message.

"Sulfates clog pores." Simply ridiculous! If anything, there's research showing that when used in appropriate amounts, these cleansing agents clean hair and skin gently and reduce breakouts!

"Sulfates in cleansers are cheap." This one is true, but so what? Lots of ingredients, both natural and synthetic, are cheap, others are expensive, which has absolutely nothing to do with quality or efficacy. The first ingredient in sulfate-free shampoos is water (about 90% water) and no other cosmetic ingredient is cheaper than that!

"Sulfates are used in floor cleaners and are corrosive." This can be true, when used in large amounts and when left on surfaces over time, but so what? Salt is used to melt ice on the roadway, but it also rusts cars, which doesn't make salt bad; it just depends on how much you use and how long you leave it on something. This is also true for the alternative sulfate-free shampoos and cleansers as well; they can also be corrosive over time depending on how much is used and how long it is left on.

"Sulfates can be irritating." This can absolutely be true, but again, so what? As a general category, sulfates are not irritating when used in appropriate amounts in shampoos and cleansers and the same is true for sulfate-free alternative cleansing agents. All of the research about sulfates being irritating are from patch tests where a concentration is left on skin under a bandage for 24 hours, which is not how a cleanser or shampoo is used. Sodium lauryl sulfate is considered one of the more irritating cleansing agents and we recommend avoiding it when it is high up on the ingredient list, but that's NOT because it's a sulfate; rather, it's because of its interaction with skin.

In summary, not all sulfates are the same, and there are plenty of them that are completely safe and beneficial in skincare and hair-care formulations. More to the point, sulfate-free alternatives can also be extremely drying and irritating when left on skin for long periods of time under occlusion, but that's not how they are used, either.

sunflower seed oil (BEST)

Non-volatile, non-fragrant plant oil used as an emollient in cosmetics. Sunflower seed oil has the ability to help repair skin's barrier and reduce inflammation. It's a rich source of fatty acids skin can use, including linoleic acid, and is excellent for dry skin.[649]

superoxide dismutase (BEST)

Enzyme considered a potent antioxidant in humans.[747,748,749]

surfactant (GOOD)

Short term for surface active agent. Surfactants degrease and emulsify oils and fats and suspend soil, allowing them to be washed away. Surfactants are used in most forms of cleansers and many are considered gentle and effective for most skin types. There are several types of surfactants that can be sensitizing, drying, and irritating for skin. When those are the main ingredients in a facial cleanser, body wash, or shampoo, they should be avoided; the most common among drying, irritating surfactants is sodium lauryl sulfate. The similar-sounding ingredient sodium laureth sulfate is fine.[360,744,745,746]

T

talc (GOOD)

Naturally occurring silicate mineral that is typically the main ingredient in face powders and is also used as an absorbent in skincare products. Extensive research indicates there's no increased risk of lung cancer when using talc-based products or for those involved in the manufacture of talc products.[750] Although there's epidemiological evidence that frequent use of pure talc over the female genital area may increase the risk of ovarian cancer.[751,752] However, a study reviewed in *Regulatory Toxicology and Pharmacology* stated that "Talc is not genotoxic, it is not carcinogenic when injected into ovaries of rats…. There's no credible evidence of a cancer risk from inhalation of cosmetic talc by humans."[753]

tangerine oil (POOR)

Fragrant, volatile citrus oil that can be a skin irritant (Latin name *Citrus tangerina*). Tangerine's chief irritant potential comes from the fragrance chemical limonene.[754] *See* limonene.

tea tree oil (GOOD)

Also known as melaleuca, from the name of its native Australian plant source, *Melaleuca alternifolia*. It has disinfecting properties that have been shown to be effective against the bacteria that cause acne. Tea tree oil also has anti-inflammatory properties and is an antioxidant.[755]

Tea tree oil has some interesting research demonstrating it to be an effective antimicrobial agent. *The Journal of Applied Microbiology* stated, "The essential oil of Melaleuca alternifolia (tea tree) exhibits broad-spectrum antimicrobial activity. Its mode of action against the Gram-negative bacterium *Escherichia coli AG100* , the Gram-positive bacterium *Staphylococcus aureus* NCTC 8325, and the yeast *Candida albicans* has been investigated using a range of methods. The ability of tea tree oil to disrupt the permeability barrier of cell membrane structures and the accompanying loss of chemiosmotic control is the most likely source of its lethal action at minimum inhibitory levels."[756]

In addition, in a randomized, placebo-controlled pilot study of tea tree oil in the treatment of herpes cold sores, tea tree oil was found to have similar degree of activity as 5% acyclovir.[757]

For acne there's also some credible published information showing it to be effective as a topical disinfectant for killing the bacteria that can cause pimples.[758] However, the crux of the matter for tea tree oil is: How much is needed to have an effect?

The Medical Journal of Australia compared the efficacy of tea tree oil to the efficacy of benzoyl peroxide for the treatment of acne. A study of 119 patients using 5% tea tree oil in a gel base versus 5% benzoyl peroxide lotion was discussed. There were 61 subjects in the benzoyl peroxide group and 58 in the tea tree oil group. The conclusion was that "both treatments were effective in reducing the number of inflamed lesions throughout the trial, with a significantly better result for benzoyl peroxide when compared to the tea tree oil. Skin oiliness was lessened significantly in the benzoyl peroxide group versus the tea tree oil group." However, while the reduction of breakouts was greater for the benzoyl peroxide group, the side effects of dryness, stinging, and burning were also greater—"79% of the benzoyl peroxide group versus 49% of the tea tree oil group."[759]

For acne, tea tree oil concentrations of 5% to 10% are recommended. However, the amount present in most skincare products is usually less than 1%; therefore, it is not considered effective for disinfecting. Note that tea tree oil is a fragrant oil whose volatile components of limonene and eucalyptol can cause contact dermatitis on exposure to oxygen. Careful use and storage of tea tree oil is advised.[760,761]

TEA-lauryl sulfate (POOR)

Detergent cleansing agent that's considered too drying, particularly when it's the primary cleansing ingredient. While there's abundant research showing that sodium lauryl sulfate is a sensitizing cleansing agent, there's no similar supporting research for TEA-lauryl sulfate. However, because the relationship between the two is so close, we recommend against using either of them. The basis for this is a judgment call, made from a desire to protect skin from sensitization; however, there are no specific studies we can cite for this recommendation, although there are those who will understandably disagree with our conclusion.

tetrahexyldecyl ascorbate (BEST)

Stable form of vitamin C that is considered an analogue of L-ascorbic acid.

Unlike pure vitamin C (ascorbic acid), tetrahexyldecyl ascorbate is lipid (fat) soluble. Some researchers believe this form of vitamin C has a greater affinity for skin because its fatty acid component helps aid penetration and protect the vitamin C component from rapid oxidation. This form of vitamin C has been shown to stimulate healthy collagen production and reduce wrinkle depth.[112]

tetrasodium EDTA (GOOD)

Chelating agent used to prevent minerals present in formulations from bonding to other ingredients.

thickening agents (GOOD)

Substances that can have a soft to hard wax-like texture or a creamy, emollient feel, and that can be great lubricants. There are literally thousands of ingredients in this category that give each and every lotion, cream, lipstick, foundation, and mascara, as well as other cosmetics products, their distinctive feel and form. The various combinations of thickeners play a large role in whether or not you prefer one product over another.

thyme extract (AVERAGE)

Extract derived from the leaf or flower of the thyme plant. It can have potent antioxidant properties. Its fragrant component can also cause skin irritation, but thyme extract's beneficial components can benefit skin.[762] Generally speaking, thyme extract should not be one of the chief antioxidants in skincare products; however, in lower amounts and mixed with other antioxidants, it can be a beneficial addition.

thyme oil (POOR)

Plant oil (Latin name *Thymus vulgaris*) that is a source of potent antioxidants, but its fragrant components (which are part of the oil itself) pose a risk of irritation. For this reason, products with thyme extract are a safer bet in terms of getting the "good" antioxidants from thyme without the volatile fragrance components that, while also being antioxidants, also may cause irritation.[442]

Thyme oil does have medicinal uses because, in concentrations of 3% and above, it has antifungal and antibacterial properties.[763,764] However, in these instances the oil was used short-term to eliminate the fungus and/or kill the problematic bacteria, not every day for (potentially) years as would be the case with a skincare product that contains thyme oil.

Tinosorb (BEST)

In Europe there are two sunscreen ingredients—Tinosorb S (bis-ethylhexyloxyphenol methoxyphenyl triazine) and Tinosorb M (methylene bis-benzotriazolyl tetramethylbutylphenol)—that are approved for sun protection across the entire range of UVA radiation.[627] Whether they are preferred over the other UVA-protecting ingredients used in sunscreens has not been established. At the time this book went to print, neither Tinosorb S nor Tinosorb M had been approved for use in the United States or Canada.

titanium dioxide (BEST)

Inert earth mineral used as a thickening, whitening, lubricating, and sunscreen ingredient in cosmetics. It protects skin from UVA and UVB radiation and is considered to have no risk of skin irritation.[643] Because of its gentleness, titanium dioxide is an excellent sunscreen active for use on sensitive or rosacea-affected skin. It's also great for use around the eyes, as it is highly unlikely to cause stinging.

Although titanium dioxide is a natural ingredient, pure titanium dioxide in nature is almost always adulterated with potentially harmful contaminants such as lead and iron. Therefore, titanium dioxide is purified via synthetic processes for use in cosmetics and sunscreens.

Titanium dioxide is typically micronized and coated for use in cosmetics products. The micronizing makes this somewhat heavy-feeling ingredient easier to spread on skin, plus a bit more cosmetically elegant. Micronized titanium dioxide also is much more stable and can provide better sun protection than non-micronized titanium dioxide. Micronized titanium dioxide does not penetrate skin so there's no need to be concerned about it getting into your body. Even when titanium dioxide nanoparticles are used, the molecular size of the substance used to coat the nanoparticles is large enough to prevent them from penetrating beyond the uppermost layers of skin.[289,765] This means you're getting the sun protection titanium dioxide provides without any risk of it causing harm to skin cells.

The coating process improves application, enhances sun protection, and also prevents the titanium dioxide from interacting with other ingredients in the presence of sunlight, thus enhancing its stability. It not only makes this ingredient much more pleasant to use for sunscreen, but also improves efficacy and eliminates safety concerns. Common examples of ingredients used to coat titanium dioxide are alumina, dimethicone, silica, and trimethoxy capryl silane.

Titanium dioxide as used in sunscreens is commonly modified with other ingredients to ensure efficacy and stability. Examples of what are known as surface modifier ingredients used for titanium dioxide include stearic acid, isostearic acid, polyhydroxystearic acid, and dimethicone/methicone copolymer.

Some websites and doctors maintain that titanium dioxide is inferior to zinc oxide, another mineral sunscreen whose core characteristics are similar to those of titanium dioxide. We're not sure where the information about titanium dioxide not being a great active sunscreen ingredient came from, but the reality is titanium dioxide is a great broad-spectrum SPF ingredient and is widely used in all manner of sun-protection products. What gets confusing for some consumers is trying to decipher research that ranks sunscreen ingredients by a UV spectrum graph. By most standards, broad-spectrum coverage for any sunscreen ingredient is defined as one that surpasses 360 nanometers (abbreviated as "nm," this is how the sun's rays are measured). Titanium dioxide exceeds this range of protection, but depending on whose research you look at, it either performs as well as or slightly below zinc oxide.

Although it's true that titanium dioxide does not rank as high for UVA protection as zinc oxide, it ends up being a small measurement of difference (think about it like being 10 years old versus 10 years and 3 months old). This is not easily understood in terms of other factors affecting how sunscreen actives perform (such as the base formula), so many, including some dermatologists, assume that zinc oxide is superior to titanium dioxide for UVA protection. When carefully formulated, titanium dioxide provides excellent UVA protection. Its UVA protection peak is lower than that of zinc oxide, but both continue to provide protection throughout the UVA range for the same amount of time.[290,789]

tocopherol (BEST)
See vitamin E.

tocopherol acetate, tocopheryl acetate (BEST)
See vitamin E.

trehalose (GOOD)
Plant sugar that has water-binding properties for skin.

tribehenin (GOOD)

Skin-conditioning agent that's a mixture of glycerin and behenic acid. Also known as glyceryl tribehenate.

tridecyl stearate (GOOD)

Used in cosmetics as a thickening agent and emollient. *See* thickening agents; emollient.

tridecyl trimellitate (GOOD)

Used as a skin-conditioning agent and thickening agent. *See* thickening agents.

triethanolamine (GOOD)

Used in cosmetics as a pH balancer. Like all amines, it has the potential for creating nitrosamines. There's controversy as to whether or not this poses a real problem for skin, given the low concentrations used in cosmetics and the theory that nitrosamines cannot penetrate skin.[766]

triethoxycaprylylsilane (GOOD)

Silicone that functions as a binding agent and emulsifier.

U

ubiquinone (BEST)

Also known as coenzyme Q10, ubiquinone is a very good antioxidant and anti-inflammatory ingredient when applied topically or consumed orally. In cosmetics, ubiquinone is usually synthetic.

ultramarines (GOOD)

Inorganic pigments (of various colors) permanently listed by the FDA for external use only, including around the eye area.

urea (GOOD)

Component of urine, although synthetic versions are used in cosmetics. In small amounts urea has good water-binding and exfoliating properties for skin; in larger concentrations it can cause inflammation.[767]

V

***Vanilla planifolia* fruit extract** (GOOD)

Extract used primarily as a fragrance and flavoring agent. The vanilla plant is a source of catechins (also known as polyphenols), which have antioxidant activity and serve as anti-inflammatory agents.[768]

vinyl dimethicone/methicone silsesquioxane crosspolymer (GOOD)

Blend of silicone polymers that functions as a thickening agent and texture enhancer. *See* thickening agents.

vitamin A (BEST)

See retinol.

vitamin B3 (BEST)

See niacinamide.

vitamin B5 (BEST)

See panthenol.

vitamin C (BEST)

See ascorbic acid.

vitamin E (BEST)

One of the most well-known and researched antioxidants, both when taken orally and when used in skincare products. If there were an antioxidant hall of fame, vitamin E would likely be its inaugural member (though do not take that to mean it is the "best" antioxidant—there is no single best, just lots of great options). It's fat-soluble and available in various forms; the most biologically active form is alpha-tocopherol.

There are eight basic forms of the entire vitamin E molecule, which are either synthetically or naturally derived. The most typical forms are d-alpha-tocopherol, d-alpha-tocopheryl acetate, dl-alpha tocopherol, and dl-alpha tocopheryl acetate. The "d" prefix in front of the "alpha" indicates that the product was derived from natural sources, such as vegetable oils or wheat germ; the "dl" prefix indicates that the vitamin was created from a synthetic base. Research has shown that natural forms of vitamin E are more potent and have a higher retention rate in skin than their synthetic counterparts, but both definitely have antioxidant activity.[769]

What about using pure vitamin E for scars? Low amounts of pure vitamin E can be a helpful addition when mixed with other skin-healing ingredients, but high amounts can be a problem. Research published in *Dermatologic Surgery* concluded that the "... study shows that there's no benefit to the cosmetic outcome of scars by applying (pure) vitamin E after skin surgery and that the application of topical vitamin E (such as what you may squeeze from a vitamin E pill) may actually be detrimental to the cosmetic appearance of a scar." In 90% of the cases in this study, topical vitamin E either had no effect on, or actually worsened the cosmetic appearance of scars.[770] However, as many dermatologists will attest, many patients believe vitamin E prevents or reduces the appearance of scars, thus its usage and anecdotal results continue.[771]

Small amounts of vitamin E can have antioxidant effects without the risk of the contact dermatitis that high amounts present. In that sense, vitamin E can be a helpful addition to skin-healing products.

VP/eicosene copolymer (GOOD)

Film-forming agent often used in water-resistant sunscreen products. It helps the sunscreen adhere better to skin and resist breaking down in water. It does not, however, last for hours, which is why you must reapply even water-resistant sunscreens at regular intervals.

VP/hexadecene copolymer (GOOD)

Synthetic polymer that functions as a binding agent, thickener, and dispersing agent in cosmetics. *See* polymer.

W

walnut-shell powder (AVERAGE)

Abrasive used in scrub products. Walnut shell powder is not preferred to polyethylene beads in a scrub because it's impossible to make walnut shell particles smooth, which means the sharp edges can cause microscopic scrapes and tears in skin, damaging its barrier.

water (GOOD)

Most widely used cosmetic ingredient; water is almost always listed first on an ingredient label because it is usually the ingredient with the highest concentration. Yet, despite claims of skin's need for hydration and claims regarding special types of water, it turns out that water may not be an important ingredient for skin. Only a 10% concentration of water in the outer layer of skin is necessary for softness and pliability in this part of the epidermis.[772] Studies that have compared the water content of dry skin with that of normal or oily skin do not find a statistically significant difference in moisture levels between them.[773]

Further, too much water can be a problem for skin because it can disrupt skin's intercellular matrix, the substances that keep skin cells bonded to each other. The most significant aspect of skin health is the structural organization of the intercellular lipids and the related materials that keep skin intact and prevent water loss.[774,775,776]

willow bark (GOOD)

Plant extract that contains salicin, a substance that when taken orally is converted by the digestive process to salicylic acid (beta hydroxy acid). The process of converting the salicin in willow bark into salicylic acid requires the presence of enzymes, and is complex. Further, salicin, much like salicylic acid, is stable only under acidic conditions. The likelihood that willow bark in the tiny amount used in cosmetics can mimic the effect of salicylic acid is at best questionable, and in all likelihood impossible. However, willow bark may indeed have some anti-inflammatory benefits for skin because, in this form, it appears to retain its aspirin-like composition.[777]

witch hazel (POOR)

Commonly used plant extract that can have potent antioxidant properties and some anti-irritant properties. However, witch hazel's high tannin content (tannin is a potent antioxidant) can also make it irritating if used repeatedly on skin because it constricts blood flow. The bark of the witch hazel plant has a higher tannin content than the leaves. Producing witch hazel water by steam distillation removes the tannins, but the plant's astringent qualities are what most believe give it benefit.[778,779,780]

Alcohol is added during the distillation process, the amount typically being 14–15%.[781] Witch hazel water is distilled from all parts of the plant; therefore, you never know exactly what you're getting, although the alcohol content remains.

Depending on the form of witch hazel, you're exposing your skin either to an irritating amount of alcohol (which causes free-radical damage and collagen breakdown) or to tannins, or both. Moreover, witch hazel contains the fragrance chemical eugenol, which is another source of irritation.[782]

See eugenol.

X

xanthan gum (GOOD)

Natural ingredient used as a thickening agent and to stabilize emulsions, which is a general term for mixtures of unlike substances such as oil and water.

Y

yeast (GOOD)

Group of fungi that ferment sugars. Yeast is a source of beta-glucan, which is a good antioxidant. Yeasts are basically fungi that grow as single cells, producing new cells either by budding or fission (splitting). Because it reproduces readily, *Saccharomyces cerevisiae* is the organism that is most widely used in biotechnology. Nevertheless, some forms of yeast are human pathogens, such as *Cryptococcus* and *Candida albicans*.

In relation to skin, there is limited information about how *S. cerevisiae* may provide a benefit. Live yeast-cell derivatives have been shown to stimulate wound healing, but research about this is scant.[783] Much of what is known about yeast's effects on skin is theoretical, and concerns yeast's tissue-repair and protective properties or yeast's antioxidant properties.[784] As a skincare ingredient yeast has potential, but what its function may be or how it would affect skin is not fully understood.

ylang-ylang (POOR)

Fragrant, volatile oil that can also be a skin irritant and has been a known skin sensitizer since 1971. It presents a bigger risk when used daily rather than intermittently.[785,786]

yogurt (AVERAGE)

There's no research showing that yogurt is effective when applied topically.

Z

zinc (BEST)

Element that has growing evidence that it can be a significant anti-irritant and antioxidant. It also can have anti-acne benefits when combined with a topical antibiotic such as erythromycin. Taken orally, zinc may have positive effects for wound healing and other health benefits.[787,788,789]

zinc oxide (BEST)

Inert earth mineral used as a thickening, whitening, lubricating, and sunscreen ingredient in cosmetics. Along with titanium dioxide, zinc oxide is considered to have no risk of skin irritation. It can also be an anti-irritant and, potentially, an antioxidant.[790,791]

Nano-sized zinc oxide is not believed to be a safety concern for skin.[289]

Cited References

1   Thornfeldt C. Chronic inflammation is etiology of extrinsic aging. J Cosmet Dermatol. 2008;7(1):8-82.

2   Basketter D, Darlenski R, Fluhr J. Skin irritation and sensitization: mechanisms and new approaches for risk assessment. Skin Pharmacol Physiol. 2008.;21(4):191-202.

3   Jeremy A, Holland D, Roberts S, Thomson K, Cunliffe W. Inflammatory events are involved in acne lesion initiation. J Invest Dermatol. 2003;121(1):20-7.

4   Tanghetti E. The role of inflammation in the pathology of acne. J Clin Aesthet Dermatol. 2013;6(9):27-35.

5   Baumann L. Skin ageing and its treatment. J Pathol. 2007;211(2):241-51.

6   Puizina-Ivić N. Skin aging. Acta Dermatovenerol Alp Pannonica Adriat. 2008;17(2):47-54.

7   Rabe J, Mamelak A, McElgunn P, Morison W, Sauder D. Photoaging: Mechanisms and repair. J Am Acad Dermato. 2006;55(1):1-19.

8   Green A, Williams G, Logan V, Strutton G. Reduced melanoma after regular sunscreen use: Randomized trial follow-up. J Clin Oncol. 2011;29:257-263.

9   Kullavanijaya P, Lim H. Photoprotection. J Am Acad Dermatol. 2005;52:937-958.

10 Bakkalia F, Averbeck S, Averbeck D, Idaomar M. Biological effects of essential oils - A review. Food Chem Toxicol. 2008;46(2):446-475.

11 Johansen J. Fragrance contact allergy: a clinical review. 2003. Am J Clin Dermatol.;4(11):798-98.

12 Jack A, Norris P, Storrs F. Allergic contact dermatitis to plant extracts in cosmetics. Semin Cutan Med Surg. 2013;32(3):140-6.

13 Edlich R, Winters K, Lim H, Cox M, Becker D, Horowitz J, Nichter L, Britt L, Long W. Photoprotection by sunscreens with topical antioxidants and systemic antioxidants to reduce sun exposure. J Long Term Eff Med Implants. 2004;14(4):317-40.

14 Chen L, Hu J, Wang S. The role of antioxidants in photoprotection: A critical review. J Am Acad Dermatol. 2012;67(5):1013-24.

15 Poljsak B, Dahmane R. Free radicals and extrinsic skin aging. Dermatol Res Pract. 2012;2012:135206.

16 Harding C, Watkinson A, Rawlings A, Scott I. Dry skin, moisturization and corneodesmolysis. Int J Cosmet Sci. 2000;22(1):21-52.

17 Rawlings A. Trends in stratum corneum research and the management of dry skin conditions. Int J Cosmet Sci. 2003;25(1-2):63-95.

18 Lupo M, Cole A. Cosmeceutical peptides. Dermatol Ther. 2007;20(5):343-9.

19 Rossetti D, Kielmanowicz M, Vigodman S, Hu Y, Chen N, Nkengne AOT, Fischer D, Seiberg M, Lin C. A novel anti-ageing mechanism for retinol: induction of dermal elastin synthesis and elastin fibre formation. Int J Cosmet Sci. 2011;33(1):62-9.

20 Ganceviciene R, Liakou A, Theodoridis A, Makrantonaki E ZC. Skin anti-aging strategies. Dermatoendocrinol. 2012;4(3):308-319.

21 Gabard B, Chatelain E, Bieli E, Haas S. Surfactant irritation: in vitro corneosurfametry and in vivo bioengineering. Skin Res Technol. 2001;7(1):49-55.

22 Gfatter R, Hackl P, Braun F. Effects of soap and detergents on skin surface pH; stratum corneum hydration and fat content in infants. Dermatology. 1997;195(3):358-62.

23 Korting H, Braun-Falco O. The effect of detergents on skin pH and its consequences. Clin Dermatol. 1996;14(1):23-7.

24 Schmid M, Korting H. The concept of the acid mantle of the skin: its relevance for the choice of skin cleansers. Dermatology. 1995;191(4):276-80.

25 Lakshmi C, Srinivas C, Anand C, Mathew A. Irritancy ranking of 31 cleansers in the Indian market in a 24-h patch test. Int J Cosmet Sci. 2008;30(4):277-83.

26 Baranda L, González-Amaro R, Torres-Alvarez B, Alvarez C, Ramírez V. Correlation between pH and irritant effect of cleansers marketed for dry skin. Int J Dermatol. 2002;41(8):494-9.

27 Kurokawa I, Danby F, Ju Q, Wang X, Xiang L, Xia L, Chen W, Nagy I, Picardo M, Suh D, et al. New developments in our understanding of acne pathogenesis and treatment. Exp Dermatol. 2009;18(10):821-32.

28 Toyoda M, Nakamura M, Morohashi M. Neuropeptides and sebaceous glands. Eur J Dermatol. 2002;12(5):422-7.

29 Toyoda M, Morohashi M. New aspects in acne inflammation. Dermatology. 2003;206(1):17-23.

30 Engel R, Gutmann M, Hartisch C, Kolodziej H, Nahrstedt A. Study on the composition of the volatile fraction of Hamamelis virginiana. Planta Med. 1998;64(3):251-8.

31 Kornhauser A, Coelho S, Hearing V. Applications of hydroxy acids: classification; mechanisms; and photoactivity. Clin Cosmet Investig Dermatol. 2010;20(3):135-142.

32 Babilas P, Knie U, Abels C. Cosmetic and dermatologic use of alpha hydroxy acids. J Dtsch Dermatol Ges. 2012;10(7):488-91.

33 Bowe W, Shalita A. Effective Over-the-Counter Acne Treatments. Semin Cutan Med Surg. 2008;27(3):170-176.

34 Strauss J, Krowchuk D, Leyden J, Lucky A, Shalita A, Siegfried E, Thiboutot D, Van-Voorhees A, Beutner K, Sieck C, et al. Guidelines of care for acne vulgaris management. J Am Acad Dermatol. 2007;56(4):651-63.

35 Fartasch M, Teal J, Menon G. Mode of action of glycolic acid on human stratum corneum: ultrastructural and functional evaluation of the epidermal barrier. Arch Dermatol Res. 1997;289(7):404-9.

36 Kootiratrakarn T, Kampirapap K, Chunhasewee C. Epidermal permeability barrier in the treatment of keratosis pilaris. Dermatol Res Pract. 2015;2015:205012.

37 Flament F, Bazin R, Laquieze S, Rubert V, Simonpietri E, Piot B. Effect of the sun on visible clinical signs of aging in Caucasian skin. Clin Cosmet Investig Dermatol. 2013;6:221-232.

38 McKnight A, Momoh A, Bullocks J. Variations of Structural Components: Specific Intercultural Differences in Facial Morphology; Skin Type; and Structures. Semin Plast Surg. 2009;23(3):163-167.

39 Shadfar S, Perkins S. Anatomy and physiology of the aging neck. Facial Plast Surg Clin North Am. 2014;22(2):161-70.

40 Sykes J. Rejuvenation of the aging neck. Facial Plast Surg. 2001;17(2):99-107.

41 Yano K, Kadoya K, Kajiya K, Hong Y, Detmar M. Ultraviolet B irradiation of human skin induces an angiogenic switch that is mediated by upregulation of vascular endothelial growth factor and by downregulation of thrombospondin-1. Br J Dermatol. 2005;152(1):115-21.

42 Varani J, Dame M, Rittie L, Fligiel S, Kang S, Fisher G, Voorhees J. Decreased collagen

production in chronologically aged skin: roles of age-dependent alteration in fibroblast function and defective mechanical stimulation. Am J Pathol. 2006;168(6):1861-8.

43 D'Orazio J, Jarrett S, Amaro-Ortiz A, Scott T. UV Radiation and the Skin. Int J Mol Sci. 2013;14(6):12222-12248.

44 Fisher G, Datta S, Talwar H, Wang Z, Varani J, Kang S, Voorhees J. Molecular basis of sun-induced premature skin ageing and retinoid antagonism. Nature. 1996;379(6563):335-9.

45 Cole C, Appa Y, Ou-Yang H. A broad-spectrum high-SPF photostable sunscreen with a high UVA-PF can protect against cellular damage at high UV exposure doses. Photodermatol Photoimmunol Photomed. 2014;30(4):212-9.

46 Liu W, Wang X, Lai W, Yan T, Wu Y, Wan M, Yi J, MS. M. Sunburn protection as a function of sunscreen application thickness differs between high and low SPFs. Photodermatol Photoimmunol Photomed. 2012;28(3):120-6.

47 Diffey B. When should sunscreen be reapplied? J Am Acad Dermatol. 2001;45(6):882-5.

48 U.S. Food and Drug Administration. Labeling and effectiveness testing; sunscreen drug products for over-the-counter human use (final rule). [Internet]. 2011 [cited 2015]. Available from: http://www.gpo.gov/fdsys/pkg/FR-2011-06-17/pdf/2011-14766.pdf.

49 Almutawa F, Vandal R, Wang S, Lim H. Current status of photoprotection by window glass; automobile glass; window films; and sunglasses. Photodermatol Photoimmunol Photomed. 2003;29(2):65-72.

50 U.S. Food and Drug Administration. FDA Sunscreen Monograph Re: "Tentative Final Monograph for OTC Sunscreen. [Internet]. 2011 [cited 2015]. Available from: http://www. fda.gov/ohrms/dockets/dailys/00/Sep00/090600/c000573_10_Attachment_F.pdf.

51 Latha M, Martis J, Shobha V, Sham-Shinde R, Bangera S, Krishnankutty B, Bellary S, Varughese S, Rao P, Naveen-Kumar B. Sunscreening agents: a review. J Clin Aesthet Dermatol. 2013;6(1):16-26.

52 Jou P, Feldman R, Tomecki K. UV protection and sunscreens: what to tell patients. Cleve Clin J Med. 2012;79(6):427-36.

53 Bhate K, Williams H. Epidemiology of acne vulgaris. Br J Dermatol. 2013;168(3):474-485.

54 Plewig G, Wolff H. Sebaceous filaments. Arch Dermatol Res. 1976;255(1):9-21.

55 Thornton M. Estrogens and aging skin. Dermatoendocrinol. 2103;5(2):264-70.

56 Suh D, Kwon H. What's new in the physiopathology of acne? Br J Dermatol. 2015;172(S1):13-19.

57 Ale I, Maibach H. Irritant contact dermatitis. Rev Environ Health. 2014;29(3):195-206.

58 Goodman G. Cleansing and moisturizing in acne patients. Am J Clin Dermatol. 2009;10(S1):1-6.

59 Melnik B. Evidence for acne-promoting effects of milk and other insulinotropic dairy products. Nestle Nutr Workshop Ser Pediatr Program. 2011;67:131-45.

60 Adebamowo C, Spiegelman D, Berkey C, Danby F, Rockett H, Colditz G, Willett W, Holmes M. Milk consumption and acne in teenaged boys. J Am Acad Dermatol. 2008;58(5):787-93.

61 Adebamowo C, Spiegelman D, Danby F, Frazier A, Willett W, Holmes M. High school dietary dairy intake and teenage acne. J Am Acad Dermatol. 2005;58(5):207-14.

62 Reynolds R, Lee S, Choi J, Atkinson F, Stockmann K, Petocz P, Brand-Miller J. Effect of the glycemic index of carbohydrates on Acne vulgaris. Nutrients. 2010;2(10):60-72.

63 Spencer E, Ferdowsian H, Barnard N. Diet and acne: a review of the evidence. Int J Dermatol. 2009;48(4):339-47.

64 Cunliffe W, Holland D, Jeremy A. Comedone formation: etiology; clinical presentation; and treatment. Clin Dermatol. 2004;22(5):367-74.

65 Kligman A, Kwong T. An improved rabbit ear model for assessing comedogenic substances.

Br J Dermatol. 1979;100(6):699-702.

66 Kligman A, Mills OJ. Acne cosmetica. Arch Dermatol. 1972;6(6):843-50.

67 Salminen A, Kaarniranta K, Kauppinen A. Inflammaging: disturbed interplay between autophagy and inflammasomes. Aging. 2012;4(3):166-75.

68 Simonart T. Newer approaches to the treatment of acne vulgaris. Am J Clin Dermatol. 2012;13(6):357-64.

69 Pannu J, McCarthy A, Martin A, Hamouda T, Ciotti S, Ma L, Sutcliffe J, Baker JJ. In vitro antibacterial activity of NB-003 against Propionibacterium acnes. Antimicrob Agents Chemother. 2011;55(9):4211-7.

70 Cosmetic Ingredient Review Expert Panel. Safety assessment of Salicylic Acid; Butyloctyl Salicylate; Calcium Salicylate; C12-15 Alkyl Salicylate; Capryloyl Salicylic Acid; Hexyldodecyl Salicylate; Isocetyl Salicylate; Isodecyl Salicylate; Magnesium Salicylate; MEA-Salicylate. Int J Toxicol. 2003;22(S1):1-108.

71 Sagransky M, Yentzer B, Feldman S. Benzoyl peroxide: a review of its current use in the treatment of acne vulgaris. Expert Opin Pharmacother. 2009;10(15):2555-62.

72 Bowe W. Antibiotic Resistance and Acne: Where We Stand and What the Future Holds. J Drugs Dermatol. 2014;13(6):S66-S70.

73 Del Rosso J, Kircik L, Gallagher C. Comparative efficacy and tolerability of dapsone 5% gel in adult versus adolescent females with acne vulgaris. J Clin Aesthet Dermatol. 2015;8(1):31-7.

74 Thielitz A, Gollnick H. Topical retinoids in acne vulgaris: update on efficacy and safety. Am J Clin Dermatol. 2008;9(6):369-81.

75 Del Rosso J, Pillai R, Moore R. Absence of Degradation of Tretinoin When Benzoyl Peroxide is Combined with an Optimized Formulation of Tretinoin Gel (0.05%). J Clin Aesthet Dermatol. 2010;3(10):26-28.

76 Sieber M, Hegel J. Azelaic acid: Properties and mode of action. Skin Pharmacol Physiol. 2014;27(S1):9-17.

77 Dreno B, Thiboutot D, Gollnick H, Bettoli V, Kang S, Leyden J, Shalita A, Torres V. Antibiotic stewardship in dermatology: limiting antibiotic use in acne. Eur J Dermatol. 2014;24(3):330-4.

78 Brynhildsen J. Combined hormonal contraceptives: prescribing patterns; compliance; and benefits versus risks. Ther Adv Drug Saf. 2014;5(5):201-13.

79 Gehring W. Nicotinic acid/niacinamide and the skin. J Cosmet Dermatol. 2004;3(2):88-93.

80 Grange P, Raingeaud J, Calvez V, Dupin N. Nicotinamide inhibits Propionibacterium acnes-induced IL-8 production in keratinocytes through the NF-κB and MAPK pathways. J Dermatol Sci. 2009;56(2):6-112.

81 Baquerizo N, Yim E, Keri J. Probiotics and prebiotics in dermatology. J Dermatol Sci. 2014;71(4):814-821.

82 Desbois A, Lawlor K. Antibacterial Activity of Long-Chain Polyunsaturated Fatty Acids against Propionibacterium acnes and Staphylococcus aureus. Mar Drugs. 2013;11(11):4544-57.

83 Nakatsuji T, Kao M, Fang J, Zouboulis C, Zhang L, Gallo R, Huang C. Antimicrobial property of lauric acid against Propionibacterium acnes: its therapeutic potential for inflammatory acne vulgaris. J Invest Dermatol. 2009;129(10):2480-8.

84 Burris J, Rietkerk W, Woolf K. Relationships of self-reported dietary factors and perceived acne severity in a cohort of New York young adults. J Acad Nutr Diet. 2014;114(3):384-92.

85 Rao J. Treatment of Acne Scarring. Facial Plast Surg Clin North Am. 2011;19(2):275-291.

86 Goodman G. Treatment of acne scarring. Int J Dermatol. 2011;50(10):1179-94.

87 Franceschi C, Capri M, Monti D, Giunta S, Olivieri F, Sevini F, Panourgia M, Invidia L, Celani L, Scurti M, et al. Inflammaging and anti-inflammaging: a systemic perspective on

aging and longevity emerged from studies in humans. Mech Ageing Dev. 2007;128(1):92-5.

88 Davis E, Callender V. Postinflammatory Hyperpigmentation. J Clin Aesthet Dermatol. 2010;3(7):20-3.

89 Sandoval S, Cox J, Koshy J, Hatef D, Hollier L. Facial Fat Compartments: A Guide to Filler Placement. Semin Plast Surg. 2009;23(4):283-287.

90 Sherratt M. Tissue elasticity and the ageing elastic fibre. Age (Dordr). 2009;31(4):305-325.

91 Wehr R, Krochmal L. Considerations in selection a moisturizer. Cutis. 1987;39(6):512-5.

92 Thomas J, Dixon T, Bhattacharyya T. Effects of Topicals on the Aging Skin Process. Facial Plast Surg Clin North Am. 2013;21(1):55-60.

93 Papakonstantinou E, Roth M, Karakiulakis G. Hyaluronic acid: A key molecule in skin aging. Dermatoendocrinol. 2012;4(3):253-258.

94 Oe M, Mitsugi K, Odanaka W, Yoshida H, Matsuoka R, Seino S, Kanemitsu T, Masuda Y. Dietary hyaluronic acid migrates into the skin of rats. ScientificWorldJournal. 2014;2014(378024).

95 Mukherjee S, Date A, Patravale V, Korting H, Roeder A, Weindl G. Retinoids in the treatment of skin aging: an overview of clinical efficacy and safety. Clin Interv Aging. 2006;1(4):327-348.

96 Kang S, Duell E, Fisher G, Datta S, Wang Z, Reddy A, Tavakkol A, Yi J, Griffiths C, Elder J, et al. Application of retinol to human skin in vivo induces epidermal hyperplasia and cellular retinoid binding proteins characteristic of retinoic acid but without measurable retinoic acid levels or irritation. J Invest Dermatol. 1995;5(4):549-56.

97 Tucker-Samaras S, Zedayko T, Cole C, Miller D, Wallo W, Leyden J. A stabilized 0.1% retinol facial moisturizer improves the appearance of photodamaged skin in an eight-week; double-blind; vehicle-controlled study. J Drugs Dermatol. 2009;8(10):932-6.

98 Varani J. Vitamin A antagonizes decreased cell growth and elevated collagen-degrading matrix metalloproteinases and stimulates collagen accumulation in naturally aged human skin. J Invest Dermatol. 2000;114(3):480-6.

99 Kockaert M, Neumann M. Systemic and topical drugs for aging skin. J Drugs Dermatol. 2003;2(4):435-41.

100 Gianeti M, Gaspar L, Camargo FJ, Campos P. Benefits of Combinations of Vitamin A; C and E Derivatives in the Stability of Cosmetic Formulations. Molecules. 2012;17(2):2219-2230.

101 Carlotti M. Photodegradation of retinol and anti-aging effectiveness of two commercial emulsions. J Cosmet Sci. 2006;57(4):261-77.

102 Törmä H, Vahlquist A. Vitamin A esterification in human epidermis: a relation to keratinocyte differentiation. J Invest Dermatol. 1990;94(1):132-8.

103 Campos P, Ricci G, Semprini M, Lopes R. Histopathological; morphometric; and stereologic studies of dermocosmetic skin formulations containing vitamin A and/or glycolic acid. J Cosmet Sci. 1999;50(3):159-170.

104 Yoshimura K, Momosawa A, Aiba E, Sato K, Matsumoto D, Mitoma Y, Harii K, Aoyama T, Iga T. Clinical trial of bleaching treatment with % all-trans retinol gel. Dermatol Surg. 2003;29(2):155-60.

105 Gaspar L, Campos P. Photostability and efficacy studies of topical formulations containing UV-filters combination and vitamins A; C and E. Int J Pharm. 2007;342(1-2):181-9.

106 Gaspar L, Campos P. A HPLC method to evaluate the influence of photostabilizers on cosmetic formulations containing UV-filters and vitamins A and E. Talanta. 2010;82(4):1490-4.

107 Carlotti M, Rossatto V, Gallarate M, Trotta M, Debernardi F. Vitamin A palmitate photostability and stability over time. J Cosmet Sci. 2004;55(3):233-52.

108 Telang P. Vitamin C in dermatology. Indian Dermatol Online J. 2013;4(2):143-146.

109 Darr D, Combs S, Dunston S, Manning T, Pinnell S. Topical Vitamin-C Protects Porcine Skin From Ultraviolet Radiation-Induced Damage. Br J Dermatol. 1992;127(3):247-253.

110 Nusgens B, Humbert P, Rougier A, Colige A, Haftek M, Lambert C, Richard A, Creidi P, Lapière C. Topically applied vitamin C enhances the mRNA level of collagens I and III; their processing enzymes and tissue inhibitor of matrix metalloproteinase 1 in the human dermis. J Invest Dermatol. 2001;116(6):853-9.

111 Klock J, Ikeno H, Ohmori K, Nishikawa T, Vollhardt J, Schehlmann V. Sodium ascorbyl phosphate shows in vitro and in vivo efficacy in the prevention and treatment of acne vulgaris. Int J Cosmet Sci. 2005;27(3):171-6.

112 Fitzpatrick R, Rostan E. Double-Blind; Half-Face Study Comparing Topical Vitamin C and Vehicle for Rejuvenation of Photodamage. Dermatol Surg. 2002;28(3):231-6.

113 Abdulmajed K, Heard C. Topical delivery of retinyl ascorbate co-drug: 1. Synthesis; penetration into and permeation across human skin. Int J Pharm. 2004;280(1-2):113-24.

114 Perricone N. The use of topical ascorbyl palmitate and alpha lipoic acid for aging skin. Drug Cosmet Industr. 1998;162(2):20-24.

115 Murracy J, Burch J, Streilein R, Iannacchione M, Hall R, Pinnell S. A topical antioxidant solution containing vitamins C and E stabilized by ferulic acid provides protection for human skin against damage caused by ultraviolet irradiation. J Am Acad Dermatol. 2008;59(3):418-25.

116 Xu T, Chen J, Li Y, Wu Y, Luo Y, Gao X, Chen H. Split-face study of topical 23.8% L-ascorbic acid serum in treating photo-aged skin. J Am Acad Dermatol. 2008;11(1):51-6.

117 Campos P, Gonçalves G, Gaspar L. In vitro antioxidant activity and in vivo efficacy of topical formulations containing vitamin C and its derivatives studied by non-invasive methods. Skin Res Technol. 2008;14(3):376-80.

118 Sauermann K, Jaspers S, Koop U, Wenck H. Topically applied vitamin C increases the density of dermal papillae in aged human skin. BMC Dermatol. 2004;4(1):13.

119 Brandner J, Zorn-Kruppa M, Yoshida T, Moll I, Beck L, De-Benedetto A. Epidermal tight junctions in health and disease. Tissue Barriers. 2015;3(1-2):e974451.

120 Harris E, Rayton J, Balthrop J, DiSilvestro R, Garcia-de-Quevedo M. Copper and the synthesis of elastin and collagen. Ciba Found Symp. 1980;79:163-82.

121 Huang P, Huang Y, Su M, Yang T, Huang J, Jiang C. In vitro observations on the influence of copper peptide aids for the LED photoirradiation of fibroblast collagen synthesis. Photomed Laser Surg. 2007;25(3):183-90.

122 Ferguson L, Laing W. Chronic inflammation, mutation and human disease. Mutat Res. 2010;690(1-2):1-2.

123 Ramasamy R, Vannucci S, Yan S, Herold K, Yan S, Schmidt A. Advanced glycation end products and RAGE: a common thread in aging, diabetes, neurodegeneration, and inflammation. Glycobiology. 2005;15(7):16R-28R.

124 Basu A, Devaraj S, Jialal I. Dietary factors that promote or retard inflammation. Arterioscler Thromb Vasc Biol. 2006;26(5):995-1001.

125 Wu X, Schauss A. Mitigation of inflammation with foods. J Agric Food Chem. 2012;60(27):6703-17.

126 Danby F. Nutrition and aging skin: sugar and glycation. Clin Dermatol. 2010;28(4):409-11.

127 Jiao L, Kramer JR, Chen L, Rugge M, Parente P, Verstovsek G, El-Serag H. Dietary consumption of meat; fat; animal products and advanced glycation end-products and the risk of Barrett's oesophagus. Aliment Pharmacol Ther. 2013;38(7):817-24.

128 Semba R, Nicklett E, Ferrucci L. Does accumulation of advanced glycation end products

contribute to the aging phenotype?. J Gerontol A Biol Sci Med Sci. 2010;65(9):963-75.

[129] Shaheen B, Gonzalez M. Acne sans P. acnes. J Eur Acad Dermatol Venereol. 2013;27(1):1-10.

[130] Seo Y, Li Z, Choi D, Sohn K, Kim H, Lee Y, Kim C, Lee Y, Shi G, Lee J, et al. Regional difference in sebum production by androgen susceptibility in human facial skin. Exp Dermatol. 2014;23(1):70-2.

[131] Smith K, Thiboutot D. Thematic review series: skin lipids.Sebaceous gland lipids: friend or foe? J Lipid Res. 2008;49(2):271-81.

[132] Picardo M, Ottaviani M, Camera E, Mastrofrancesco A. Sebaceous gland lipids. Dermatoendocrinol. 2009;1(2):68-71.

[133] Grice E, Segre J. The skin microbiome. Nat Rev Microbiol. 2011;9(4):244-253.

[134] Rossi A, Perez M. Treatment of Hyperpigmentation. Facial Plast Surg Clin North Am. 2011;19(2):313-324.

[135] Warner R, Stone K, Boissy Y. Hydration disrupts human stratum corneum ultrastructure. J Invest Dermatol. 2003;120(2):275-84.

[136] Madison K. Barrier Function of the Skin: "La Raison d'Être" of the Epidermis. J Invest Dermatol. 2003;121(2):231-41.

[137] Vestergaard C, Hvid M, Johansen C, Kemp K, Deleuran B, Deleuran M. Inflammation-induced alterations in the skin barrier function: implications in atopic dermatitis. Chem Immunol Allergy. 96:77-80. 2012;96:77-80.

[138] Matthaus B, Özcan M, Al-Juhaimi F. Fatty acid composition and tocopherol profiles of safflower (Carthamus tinctorius L.) seed oils. Nat Prod Res. 2015;29(2):193-6.

[139] Kejlová K, Jírová D, Bendová H, Gajdoš P, Kolářová H. Phototoxicity of essential oils intended for cosmetic use. Toxicol In Vitro. 2010;24(8):2084-9.

[140] Wa C, Maibach H. Mapping the human face: biophysical properties. Skin Res Technol. 2010;16(1):38-54.

[141] Jansen T. Clinical presentations and classification of rosacea. Ann Dermatol Venereol. 138 Suppl 3.S192-200. 2011;138(S3):192-200.

[142] Reinholz M, Ruzicka T, Schauber J. Cathelicidin LL-37: An Antimicrobial Peptide with a Role in Inflammatory Skin Disease. Ann Dermatol. 24(2): 126-135. 2012;24(2):126-135.

[143] Two A, Del-Rosso J. Kallikrein 5-Mediated Inflammation in Rosacea. J Clin Aesthet Dermatol. 2014;7(1):20-25.

[144] Jarmuda S, O'Reilly N, Zaba R, Jakubowicz O, Szkaradkiewicz A, Kavanagh K. Potential role of Demodex mites and bacteria in the induction of rosacea. J Med Microbiol. 2012;61(Pt 11):1504-10.

[145] Forton F, Seys B. Density of Demodex folliculorum in rosacea: a case-control study using standardized skin-surface biopsy. Br J Dermatol. 1993;128(6):650-9.

[146] Del Rosso J. Advances in Understanding and Managing Rosacea: Part 2. J Clin Aesthet Dermatol. 2012;5(3):26-36.

[147] Crawford G, Pelle M, James W. Rosacea: I. Etiology; pathogenesis; and subtype classification. J Am Acad Dermatol. 2004;51(3):327-41.

[148] Tschiggerl C, Bucar F. Volatile fraction of lavender and bitter fennel infusion extracts. Nat Prod Commun. 2010;5(9):1431-6.

[149] Levin J, Miller R. A Guide to the Ingredients and Potential Benefits of Over-the-Counter Cleansers and Moisturizers for Rosacea Patients. J Clin Aesthet Dermatol. 2011;4(8):31-49.

[150] Torok H. Rosacea skin care. Cutis. 2000;66(4):14-6.

[151] Salzer S, Kresse S, Hirai Y, Koglin S, Reinholz M, Ruzicka T, Schauber J. Cathelicidin peptide LL-37 increases UVB-triggered inflammasome activation: possible implications for rosacea. J Dermatol Sci. 2014;76(3):173-9.

152 Culp B, Scheinfeld N. Rosacea: A Review. P T. 2009;34(1):38-45.

153 Cohen A, Tiemstra J. Diagnosis and treatment of rosacea. J Am Board Fam Pract. 2002;15(3):214-7.

154 Weinkle A, Doktor V, Emer J. Update on the management of rosacea. Clin Cosmet Investig Dermatol. 8:159-77. 2015;8:159-77.

155 Levin J, Miller R. A Guide to the Ingredients and Potential Benefits of Over-the-Counter Cleansers and Moisturizers for Rosacea Patients. J Clin Aesthet Dermatol. 2011;4(8):31-49.

156 Park H, Del Rosso J. Use of Oral Isotretinoin in the Management of Rosacea. J Clin Aesthet Dermatol. 2011;4(9):54-61.

157 Lim H, Lee S, Won Y, Lee J. The efficacy of intense pulsed light for treating erythematotelangiectatic rosacea is related to severity and age. Ann Dermatol. 2014;26(4):491-5.

158 Liu J, Liu J, Ren Y, Li B, Lu S. Comparative efficacy of intense pulsed light for different erythema associated with rosacea. J Cosmet Laser Ther. 2014;16(6):324-7.

159 Brenner M, Hearing V. The Protective Role of Melanin Against UV Damage in Human Skin. Photochem Photobiol. 2008;84(3):539-549.

160 Brenner M, Hearing V. Modifying skin pigmentation - approaches through intrinsic biochemistry and exogenous agents. Drug Discov Today Dis Mech. 2008;5(2):e189-e199.

161 Seité S, Colige A, Piquemal-Vivenot P, Montastier C, Fourtanier A, Lapière C, Nusgens B. A full-UV spectrum absorbing daily use cream protects human skin against biological changes occurring in photoaging. Photodermatol Photoimmunol Photomed. 2000;16(4):147-55.

162 Ionescu M, Gougerot A. Sun protection and sunscreen labeling--an update. Acta Dermatovenerol Croat. 2007;15(2):92-5.

163 Han A, Chien A, Kang S. Photoaging. Dermatol Clin. 2014;32(3):291-9.

164 Hande IA, Miot L, Miot H. Melasma: a clinical and epidemiological review. An Bras Dermatol. 2014;89(5):771-82.

165 Elmets C, Athar M. Milestones in photocarcinogenesis. J Invest Dermatol. 2013;133(E1):E13-7.

166 Arora P, Sarkar R, Garg V, Arya L. Lasers for treatment of melasma and post-inflammatory hyperpigmentation. J Cutan Aesthet Surg. 2012;5(2):93-103.

167 Desai S. Hyperpigmentation therapy: a review. J Clin Aesthet Dermatol. 2014;7(8):13-7.

168 Rychlinska I, Nowak S. Quantitative Determination of Arbutin and Hydroquinone in Different Plant Materials by HPLC. Not Bot Horti Agrobo. 2012;40(2):109-113.

169 Breathnach A. Melanin hyperpigmentation of skin: melasma; topical treatment with azelaic acid; and other therapies. Cutis. 1996;57(1):36-45.

170 Pérez-Bernal A, Muñoz-Pérez M, Camacho F. Management of facial hyperpigmentation. Am J Clin Dermatol. 2000;1(5):261-8.

171 Lajis A, Hamid M, Ariff A. Depigmenting effect of Kojic acid esters in hyperpigmented B16F1 melanoma cells. J Biomed Biotechnol. 2012;2012:952452.

172 Farris P. Topical vitamin C: a useful agent for treating photoaging and other dermatologic conditions. Dermatol Surg. 2005;31(7 Pt. 2):814-7; Discussion 818.

173 Sehgal V, Verma P, Srivastava G, Aggarwal A, Verma S. Melasma: treatment strategy. J Cosmet Laser Ther. 2011;13(6):265-79.

174 Guerrero D. Dermocosmetic management of hyperpigmentations. Ann Dermatol Venereol. 2012;139(S4):S166-9.

175 Berk D, Bayliss S. Milia: a review and classification. J Am Acad Dermatol. 2008;59(6):1050-63.

176 Kim J, Park H, Lee W, Kang J. Sebaceous hyperplasia effectively improved by the pin-hole technique with squeezing. Ann Dermatol. 2013;25(2):257-8.

177 Zampeli V, Makrantonaki E, Tzellos T, Zouboulis C. New pharmaceutical concepts for sebaceous gland diseases: implementing today's pre-clinical data into tomorrow's daily clinical practice. Curr Pharm Biotechnol. 2012;13(10):1898-913.

178 Simmons B, Griffith R, Falto-Aizpurua L, Bray F, Nouri K. Light and laser therapies for the treatment of sebaceous gland hyperplasia a review of the literature. J Eur Acad Dermatol Venereol. [Internet]. 2015 March [cited 2015 July]. Available from: http://www.ncbi.nlm.nih.gov/pubmed/25731611.

179 Eisen D, Michael D. Sebaceous lesions and their associated syndromes: part l. J Am Acad Dermatol. 2009;61(4):549-60.

180 Schmidt N, Gans E. Tretinoin: A Review of Its Anti-inflammatory Properties in the Treatment of Acne. J Clin Aesthet Dermatol. 2011;4(11):22-29.

181 Draelos Z, Matsubara A, Smiles K. The effect of 2% niacinamide on facial sebum production. J Cosmet Laser Ther. 2006;8(2):96-101.

182 Bissett D, Oblong J, Berge C. Niacinamide: A B vitamin that improves aging facial skin appearance. Dermatol Surg. 2005;31(7 Pt. 2):860-5; Discussion 865.

183 Thomas M, Khopkar U. Keratosis Pilaris Revisited: Is It More Than Just a Follicular Keratosis?. Int J Trichology. 2012;4(4):255-258.

184 Gruber R, Sugarman J, Crumrine D, Hupe M, Mauro T, Mauldin E, Thyssen J, Brandner J, Hennies H, Schmuth M, et al. Sebaceous gland; hair shaft; and epidermal barrier abnormalities in keratosis pilaris with and without filaggrin deficiency. Am J Pathol. 2015;185(4):1012-21.

185 Hwang S, Schwartz R. Keratosis pilaris: a common follicular hyperkeratosis. Cutis. 2008;82(3):177-80.

186 Ibrahim O, Khan M, Bolotin D, Dubina M, Nodzenski M, Disphanurat W, Kakar R, Yoo S, Whiting D, West D, et al. Treatment of keratosis pilaris with 810-nm diode laser: a randomized clinical trial. JAMA Dermatol. 2015;151(2):187-91.

187 Saelim P, Pongprutthipan M, Pootongkam S, Jariyasethavong V, Asawanonda P. Long-pulsed 1064-nm Nd:YAG laser significantly improves keratosis pilaris: a randomized; evaluator-blind study. J Dermatolog Treat. 2013;24(4):318-22.

188 Rodríguez-Lojo R, Pozo J, Barja J, Piñeyro F, L. PV. Keratosis pilaris atrophicans: treatment with intense pulsed light in four patients. J Cosmet Laser Ther. 2010;12(4):188-90.

189 Alcántara G, Boixeda P, Truchuelo D, Fleta A. Keratosis pilaris rubra and keratosis pilaris atrophicans faciei treated with pulsed dye laser: report of 10 cases. J Eur Acad Dermatol Venereol. 2011;25(6):710-4.

190 Peate l. Eczema: causes; symptoms and treatment in the community. Br J Community Nurs. 2011;16(7):324;326-31.

191 Abuabara K, Margolis D. Do children really outgrow their eczema; or is there more than one eczema?. J Allergy Clin Immunol. 2013;132(5):1139-40.

192 Mao W, Mao J, Zhang J, Wang L, Cao D, Qu Y. Atopic eczema: a disease modulated by gene and environment. Front Biosci (Landmark Ed). 2014;19:707-17.

193 Brown S, McLean W. Eczema genetics: current state of knowledge and future goals. J Invest Dermatol. 2009;129(3):543-52.

194 Nosbaum A, Vocanson M, Rozieres A, Hennino A, Nicolas J. Allergic and irritant contact dermatitis. Eur J Dermatol. 19(4):325-32. 2009;19(4):325-32.

195 Williams J, Eichenfield L, Burke B, Barnes-Eley M, Friedlander S. Prevalence of scalp scaling in prepubertal children. Pediatrics. 2005;115(1):e1-6.

196 Wannanukul S, Chiabunkana J. Comparative study of 2% ketoconazole cream and 1% hydrocortisone cream in the treatment of infantile seborrheic dermatitis. J Med Assoc Thai. 2004;87(S2):S68-71.

197 Bukvić M, Kralj M, Basta-Juzbašić A, LakošJukić I. Seborrheic dermatitis: an update. Acta Dermatovenerol Croat. 2012;20(2):98-104.

198 Bonamonte D, Foti C, Vestita M, Ranieri L, G. A. Nummular eczema and contact allergy: a retrospective study. Dermatitis. 2012;23(4):153-7.

199 Cheong W. Gentle cleansing and moisturizing for patients with atopic dermatitis and sensitive skin. Am J Clin Dermatol. 2009;10(S1):13-7.

200 Sivaranjani N, Rao S, Rajeev G. Role of reactive oxygen species and antioxidants in atopic dermatitis. J Clin Diagn Res. 2013;7(12):2683-5.

201 Williams C, Wilkinson S, McShane P, Lewis J, Pennington D, Pierce S, Fernandez C. A double-blind; randomized study to assess the effectiveness of different moisturizers in preventing dermatitis induced by hand washing to simulate healthcare use. Br J Dermatol. 2010;162(5):1088-92.

202 Chong M, Fonacier L. Treatment of Eczema: Corticosteroids and Beyond. Clin Rev Allergy Immunol. [Internet]. 2015 Apr [cited 2015 July]. Available from: http://www.ncbi.nlm.nih.gov/pubmed/25869743.

203 Watson W, Sandeep K. Atopic dermatitis. Allergy Asthma Clin Immunol. 2011;7(S1):S4.

204 Zöller N, Kippenberger S, Thaçi D, Mewes K, Spiegel M, Sättler A, Schultz M, Bereiter-Hahn J, Kaufmann R, A. B. Evaluation of beneficial and adverse effects of glucocorticoids on a newly developed full-thickness skin model. Toxicol In Vitro. 2008;22(3):747-59.

205 Nguyen T, Zuniga R. Skin conditions: new drugs for managing skin disorders. FP Essent. 2013;407:11-6.

206 Ando T, Matsumoto K, Namiranian S, Yamashita H, Glatthorn H, Kimura M, Dolan B, Lee J, Galli S, Kawakami Y, et al. Mast cells are required for full expression of allergen/SEB-induced skin inflammation. J Invest Dermatol. 2013;133(12):2695-705.

207 U.S. Food and Drug Administration. Public Health Advisory for Elidel and Protopic (3/10/2005). [Internet]. 2005 [cited 2015 July]. Available from: http://www.fda.gov/drugs/drugsafety/postmarketdrugsafetyinformationforpatientsandproviders/ucm153956.htm.

208 Dogra S, Mahajan R. Phototherapy for atopic dermatitis. Indian J Dermatol Venereol Leprol. 2015;81(1):10-5.

209 Adişen E, Karaca F, Oztaş M, Gürer M. Efficacy of local psoralen ultraviolet A treatments in psoriasis; vitiligo and eczema. Clin Exp Dermatol. 2008;33(3):344-5.

210 Archier E, Devaux S, Castela E, Gallini A, Aubin F, LeMaître M, Aractingi S, Bachelez H, Cribier B, Joly P, et al. Carcinogenic risks of psoralen UV-A therapy and narrowband UV-B therapy in chronic plaque psoriasis: a systematic literature review. J Eur Acad Dermatol Venereol. 2012;26(3):22-31.

211 Williams H. Evening primrose oil for atopic dermatitis. BMJ. 2003;327(7428):1358-1359.

212 Greenhawt M. The role of food allergy in atopic dermatitis. Allergy Asthma Proc. 2010;31(5):392-7.

213 Hong E, Smith S, Fischer G. Evaluation of the atrophogenic potential of topical corticosteroids in pediatric dermatology patients. Pediatr Dermatol. 2011;28(4):393-6.

214 Charman C, Morris A, Williams H. Topical corticosteroid phobia in patients with atopic eczema. Br J Dermatol. 2000;142(5):931-6.

215 Chung V, Kelley L, Marra D, Jiang S. Onion extract gel versus petrolatum emollient on new surgical scars: prospective double-blinded study. Dermatol Surg. 2006;32(2):193-7.

216 Harcharik S, Emer J. Steroid-sparing properties of emollients in dermatology. Skin Therapy Lett. 2014;19(1):5-10.

217 Soleymani T, Hung T, Soung J. The role of vitamin D in psoriasis: a review. Int J Dermatol. 2015;54(4):383-92.

[218] Cather J, Crowley J. Use of biologic agents in combination with other therapies for the treatment of psoriasis. Am J Clin Dermatol. 2014;15(6):467-78.

[219] Jacobi A, Mayer A, Augustin M. Keratolytics and emollients and their role in the therapy of psoriasis: a systematic review. Dermatol Ther (Heidelb). 2015;5(1):1-18.

[220] Roelofzen J, Aben K, Van de Kerkhof P, PG VdV, LA. K. Dermatological exposure to coal tar and bladder cancer risk: a case-control study. Urol Oncol. 2015;33(1):e19-22.

[221] Situm M, Bulat V, Majcen K, Dzapo A, Jezovita J. Benefits of controlled ultraviolet radiation in the treatment of dermatological diseases. Coll Antropol. 2014;38(4):1249-53.

[222] Takeshita J, Wang S, Shin D, Callis Duffin K, Krueger G, Kalb R, Weisman J, Sperber B, Stierstorfer M, Brod B, et al. Comparative effectiveness of less commonly used systemic monotherapies and common combination therapies for moderate to severe psoriasis in the clinical setting. J Am Acad Dermatol. 2014;71(6):1167-75.

[223] Chan C, Van Voorhees A, Lebwohl M, Korman N, Young M, Bebo BJ, Kalb R, Hsu S. Treatment of severe scalp psoriasis: from the Medical Board of the National Psoriasis Foundation. J Am Acad Dermatol. 2009;60(6):962-71.

[224] U.S. Food and Drug Administration. Unintentional Injection of Soft Tissue Filler into Blood Vessels in the Face: FDA Safety Communication. [Internet]. 2015 [cited 2015 July]. Available from: http://www.fda.gov/MedicalDevices/Safety/AlertsandNotices/ucm448255.htm?source=govdelivery&utm_medium=email&utm_source=govdelivery.

[225] Trindade A, Carruthers J, Cox S, Goldman M, Wheeler S, Gallagher C. Patient satisfaction and safety with aesthetic onabotulinumtoxinA after at least 5 years: a retrospective cross-sectional analysis of 4;402 glabellar treatments. Dermatol Surg. 2015;41(S1):S19-28.

[226] Brin M, Boodhoo T, Pogoda J, James L, Demos G, Terashima Y, Gu J, Eadie N, Bowen B. Safety and tolerability of onabotulinumtoxinA in the treatment of facial lines: a meta-analysis of individual patient data from global clinical registration studies in 1678 participants. J Am Acad Dermatol. 2009;61(6):e1-11.

[227] Kollewe K, Mohammadi B, Köhler S, Pickenbrock H, Dengler R, Dressler D. Blepharospasm: long-term treatment with either Botox; Xeomin or Dysport. J Neural Transm. 2015;122(3):427-31.

[228] Wollina U, Goldman A. Dermal fillers: facts and controversies. Clin Dermatol. 2013;31(6):731-6.

[229] Lipozenčić J, Mokos Z. Will nonablative rejuvenation replace ablative lasers? Facts and controversies. Clin Dermatol. 2013;31(6):718-24.

[230] Beasley K, Dai J, Brown P, Lenz B, Hivnor C. Ablative fractional versus nonablative fractional lasers-where are we and how do we compare differing products?. Curr Dermatol Rep. 2013;2:135–143. 2013;2(2):135-143.

[231] Kauvar A. Fractional nonablative laser resurfacing: is there a skin tightening effect?. Dermatol Surg. 2014;41(S12):S157-63.

[232] Miller L, Mishra V, Alsaad S, Winstanley D, Blalock T, Tingey C, Qiu J, Romine S, Ross E. Clinical evaluation of a non-ablative 1940 nm fractional laser. J Drugs Dermatol. 2014;13(11):1324-9.

[233] Preissig J, Hamilton K, Markus R. Current Laser Resurfacing Technologies: A Review that Delves Beneath the Surface. Semin Plast Surg. 2012;26(3):109-116.

[234] El-Domyati M, El-Ammawi T, Moawad O, Medhat W, Mahoney M, Uitto J. Intense pulsed light photorejuvenation: a histological and immunohistochemical evaluation. J Drugs Dermatol. 2011;10(11):1246-52.

[235] Wu D, Friedmann D, Fabi S, Goldman M, Fitzpatrick R. Comparison of intense pulsed light with 1;927-nm fractionated thulium fiber laser for the rejuvenation of the chest. Dermatol Surg. 2014;40(2):129-33.

236 Babilas P, Schreml S, Szeimies R, Landthaler M. Intense pulsed light (IPL): a review. Lasers Surg Med. 2010;42(2):93-104.

237 Brazil J, Owens P. Long-term clinical results of IPL photorejuvenation. J Cosmet Laser Ther. 2003;5(3-4):168-74.

238 Goldberg D. Current Trends in Intense Pulsed Light. J Clin Aesthet Dermatol. 2012;5(6):45-53.

239 Stampar M. The Pelleve procedure: an effective method for facial wrinkle reduction and skin tightening. Facial Plast Surg Clin North Am. 2011;19(2):335-45.

240 Polder K, Bruce S. Radiofrequency: Thermage. Facial Plast Surg Clin North Am. 2011;19(2):347-59.

241 Belenky I, Margulis A, Elman M, Bar-Yosef U, Paun S. Exploring channeling optimized radiofrequency energy: a review of radiofrequency history and applications in esthetic fields. Adv Ther. 2012;29(3):249-66.

242 Oni G, Hoxworth R, Teotia S, Brown S, Kenkel J. Evaluation of a microfocused ultrasound system for improving skin laxity and tightening in the lower face. Aesthet Surg J. 2014;34(7):1099-110.

243 Fabi S. Noninvasive skin tightening: focus on new ultrasound techniques. Clin Cosmet Investig Dermatol. 2015;5(8):47-52.

244 Hitchcock T, Dobke M. Review of the safety profile for microfocused ultrasound with visualization. J Cosmet Dermatol. 2014;13(4):329-35.

245 Dogra S, Yadav S, Sarangal R. Microneedling for acne scars in Asian skin type: an effective low cost treatment modality. J Cosmet Dermatol. 2014;13(3):180-7.

246 Liebl H, Kloth L. Skin cell proliferation stimulated by microneedles. J Am Coll Clin Wound Spec. 2012;4(1):2-6.

247 Chawla S. Split Face Comparative Study of Microneedling with PRP Versus Microneedling with Vitamin C in Treating Atrophic Post Acne Scars. J Cutan Aesthet Surg. 2014;7(4):209-212.

248 Lodish H, Berk A, Zipursky SMP, Baltimore D, Darnell J. Molecular Cell Biology. New York: W. H. Freeman; 2000. p. Section 22.3.

249 Cahill E, O'Cearbhaill E. Toward Biofunctional Microneedles for Stimulus Responsive Drug Delivery. Bioconjug Chem. [Internet]. 2015 Jun [cited 2015 Jul]. Available from: http://pubs.acs.org/doi/abs/10.1021/acs.bioconjchem.5b00211.

250 Al-Qallaf B, Das D. Optimizing microneedle arrays to increase skin permeability for transdermal drug delivery. Ann N Y Acad Sci. 2009;1161:83-94.

251 Narayan R. Transdermal delivery of insulin via microneedles. J Biomed Nanotechnol. 2014;10(9):2244-60.

252 Zhang H, Zhai Y, Yang X, Zhai G. Breaking the skin barrier: achievements and future directions. Curr Pharm Des. 2015;21(20):2713-24.

253 Seo K, Kim D, Lee S, Yoon M, Lee H. Skin rejuvenation by microneedle fractional radiofrequency and a human stem cell conditioned medium in Asian skin: a randomized controlled investigator blinded split-face study. J Cosmet Laser Ther. 2013;15(1):25-33.

254 Ma Y, Liu Y, Wang Q, Ren J, Xiang L. Prospective study of topical 5-aminolevulinic acid photodynamic therapy for the treatment of severe adolescent acne in Chinese patients. J Dermatol. 2015;42(5):504-7.

255 Ash C, Harrison A, Drew S, Whittall R. A randomized controlled study for the treatment of acne vulgaris using high-intensity 414 nm solid state diode arrays. J Cosmet Laser Ther. 2015;20:1-7.

256 Dai T, Gupta A, Murray C, Vrahas M, Tegos G, Hamblin M. Blue light for infectious diseases: Propionibacterium acnes; Helicobacter pylori; and beyond? Drug Resist Updat.

2012;15(4):223-36.

[257] Liu L, Fan X, An Y, Zhang J, Wang C, Yang R. Randomized trial of three phototherapy methods for the treatment of acne vulgaris in Chinese patients. Photodermatol Photoimmunol Photomed. 2014;30(5):246-53.

[258] YR JY, Kim S, Sohn K, Lee Y, Seo Y, Lee Y, Whang K, Kim C, Lee J, Im M. Regulation of lipid production by light-emitting diodes in human sebocytes. Arch Dermatol Res. 2015;307(3):265-73.

[259] Mamalis A, Garcha M, Jagdeo J. Light emitting diode-generated blue light modulates fibrosis characteristics: fibroblast proliferation; migration speed; and reactive oxygen species generation. Lasers Surg Med. 2015;47(2):210-5.

[260] Das S, Reynolds R. Recent advances in acne pathogenesis: implications for therapy. Am J Clin Dermatol. 2014;15(6):479-88.

[261] Wunsch A, Matuschka K. A controlled trial to determine the efficacy of red and near-infrared light treatment in patient satisfaction; reduction of fine lines; wrinkles; skin roughness; and intradermal collagen density increase. Photomed Laser Surg. 2014;32(2):93-100.

[262] Sadick N. A study to determine the efficacy of a novel handheld light-emitting diode device in the treatment of photoaged skin. J Cosmet Dermatol. 2008;7(4):263-7.

[263] Russell B, Kellett N, Reilly L. A study to determine the efficacy of combination LED light therapy (633 nm and 830 nm) in facial skin rejuvenation. J Cosmet Laser Ther. 2005;7(3-4):196-200.

[264] de Vasconcelos Catão M, Nonaka C, de Albuquerque Jr R, Bento P, de Oliveira Costa R. Effects of red laser; infrared; photodynamic therapy; and green LED on the healing process of third-degree burns: clinical and histological study in rats. Lasers Med Sci. 2015;30(1):421-8.

[265] Dungel P, Hartinger J, Chaudary S, Slezak P, Hofmann A, Hausner T, Strassl M, Wintner E, Redl H, Mittermayr R. Low level light therapy by LED of different wavelength induces angiogenesis and improves ischemic wound healing. Lasers Surg Med. 2014;46(10):773-80.

[266] Niu T, Tian Y, Ren Q, Wei L, Li X, Cai Q. Red light interferes in UVA-induced photoaging of human skin fibroblast cells. Photochem Photobiol. 2014;90(6):1349-58.

[267] Keller E. Home-use devices in aesthetic dermatology. Semin Cutan Med Surg. 2014;33(4):198-204.

[268] Seité S, Bredoux C, Compan D, Zucchi H, Lombard D, Medaisko C, Fourtanier A. Histological evaluation of a topically applied retinol-vitamin C combination. Skin Pharmacol Physiol. 2005;18(2):81-7.

[269] Bernardini F, Cetinkaya A, Devoto M, Zambelli A. Calcium hydroxyl-apatite (Radiesse) for the correction of periorbital hollows; dark circles; and lower eyelid bags. Ophthal Plast Reconstr Surg. 2014;30(1):34-9.

[270] Paolo F, Nefer F, Paola P, Nicolò S. Periorbital area rejuvenation using carbon dioxide therapy. J Cosmet Dermatol. 2012;11(3):223-8.

[271] Vavouli C. Chemical peeling with trichloroacetic acid and lactic acid for infraorbital dark circles. J Cosmet Dermatol. 2013;12(3):204-9.

[272] Xu T, Yang Z, Li Y, Chen J, Guo S, Wu Y, Liu W, Gao X, He C, Geng L, et al. Treatment of infraorbital dark circles using a low-fluence Q-switched 1;064-nm laser. Dermatol Surg. 2011;37(6):797-803.

[273] Darcy S, Miller T, Goldberg R, Villablanca J, Demer J, Rudkin G. Magnetic resonance imaging characterization of orbital changes with age and associated contributions to lower eyelid prominence. Plastic and reconstructive surgery. 2008;122(3):921-9.

[274] Murphy L, White I, Rastogi S. Is hypoallergenic a credible term?. Clin Exp Dermatol. 2004;29(3):325-7.

275 Wolf R, Wolf D, Tüzün B, Tüzün Y. Cosmetics and contact dermatitis. Dermatol Therapy. 2001;14:181–7. 2001;14(3):181-7.

276 Kwak S, Brief E, Langlais D, Kitson N, Lafleur M, Thewalt J. Ethanol perturbs lipid organization in models of stratum corneum membranes: An investigation combining differential scanning calorimetry; infrared and (2)H NMR spectroscopy. Biochim Biophys Acta. 2012;1818(5):1410-9.

277 Kownatzki E. Hand hygiene and skin health. J Hosp Infect. 2003;55(4):239-45.

278 Makrantonaki E, Ganceviciene R, Zouboulis C. An update on the role of the sebaceous gland in the pathogenesis of acne. Dermatoendocrinol. 2011;3(1):41-49.

279 Roy A, Sahu R, Matlam M, Deshmukh V, Dwivedi J, Jha A. In vitro techniques to assess the proficiency of skincare cosmetic formulations. Pharmacogn Rev. 2013;7(14):97-106.

280 Darvin M, Sterry W, Lademann J. Resonance Raman spectroscopy as an effective tool for the determination of antioxidative stability of cosmetic formulations. J Biophotonics. 2010;3(1-2):82-8.

281 Seité S, Fourtanier A, Moyal D, Young A. Photodamage to human skin by suberythemal exposure to solar ultraviolet radiation can be attenuated by sunscreens: a review. Br J Dermatol. 2010;163(5):903-14.

282 Hacker E, Boyce Z, Kimlin M, Wockner L, Pollak T, Vaartjes S, Hayward N, Whiteman D. The effect of MC1R variants and sunscreen on the response of human melanocytes in vivo to ultraviolet radiation and implications for melanoma. Pigment Cell Melanoma Res. 2013;26(6):835-44.

283 Robinson J, Bigby M. Prevention of Melanoma With Regular Sunscreen Use. JAMA. 2011;306(3):302-303.

284 Siegel R, Naishadham D, Jemal A. Cancer statistics; 2013. CA Cancer J Clin. 2013;63(1):11-30.

285 Antille C, Tran C, Sorg O, Carraux P, Didierjean L, Saurat J. Vitamin A exerts a photoprotective action in skin by absorbing ultraviolet B radiation. J Invest Dermatol. 2003;1212(5):1163-7.

286 McKenna D, Murphy G. Skin cancer chemoprophylaxis in renal transplant recipients: 5 years of experience using low-dose acitretin. Br J Dermatol. 1999;140(4):656-660.

287 Benavides F, Oberyszyn T, VanBuskirk A, Reeve V, Kusewitt D. The hairless mouse in skin research. J Dermatol Sci. 2009;53(1):10-8.

288 Morison W, Wang S. Sunscreens: Safe and Effective? Web. 13 Oct. 2014. [Internet]. 2014 [cited 2015 July]. Available from: http://www.skincancer.org/prevention/sun-protection/sunscreen/sunscreens-safe-and-effective.

289 Burnett M, Wang S. Current sunscreen controversies: a critical review. Photodermatol Photoimmunol Photomed. 2011;27(2):58-67.

290 Calafat A, Wong L, Ye X, Reidy J, Needham L. Concentrations of the Sunscreen Agent Benzophenone-3 in Residents of the United States: National Health and Nutrition Examination Survey 2003–2004. Environ Health Perspect. 2008;116(7):893-897.

291 Janjua N, Mogensen B, Andersson A, Petersen J, Henriksen M, Skakkebaek N, Wulf H. Systemic absorption of the sunscreens benzophenone-3; octyl-methoxycinnamate; and 3-(4-methyl-benzylidene) camphor after whole-body topical application and reproductive hormone levels in humans. J Invest Dermatol. 2004;123(1):57-61.

292 Janjua N, Kongshoj B, Andersson A, Wulf H. Sunscreens in human plasma and urine after repeated whole-body topical application. J Eur Acad Dermatol Venereol. 2008;22(4):456-61.

293 American Academy of Dermatology. Is sunscreen safe? [Internet]. 2014 [cited 2015 July]. Available from: https://www.aad.org/spot-skin-cancer/learn-about-skin-cancer/prevent-skin-cancer/is-sunscreen-safe.

294 Morison W, Wang S. Sunscreens Are Safe. [Internet]. 2010 [cited 2015 July]. Available from:

https://people.creighton.edu/~tri88836/TheSkinCancerJournal/Sunscreens-Safe%20 and%20Effective.pdf.

295 European Commission Directorate General for Health and Consumers. Opinion on Benzophenone-3. [Internet]. 2008 [cited 2015 July]. Available from: http://ec.europa.eu/ health/ph_risk/committees/04_sccp/docs/sccp_o_159.pdf.

296 Hayden C, Cross S, Anderson C, Saunders N, Roberts M. Sunscreen penetration of human skin and related keratinocyte toxicity after topical application. Skin Pharmacol Physiol. 2005;18(4):170-4.

297 European Commission Directorate General for Health and Consumers. Cosmetic Ingredient Glossary; Substance: 2-Ethylhexyl 4-methoxycinnamate / Octinoxate. [Internet]. 2009 [cited 2015 July]. Available from: http://ec.europa.eu/consumers/cosmetics/cosing/ index.cfm?fuseaction=search.details_v2&id=28816.

298 Nohynek G, Lademann J, Ribaud C, Roberts M. Grey goo on the skin? Nanotechnology; cosmetic and sunscreen safety. Crit Rev Toxicol. 2007;37(3):251-77.

299 Krasnikov I, Popov A, Seteikin A, Myllylä R. Influence of titanium dioxide nanoparticles on skin surface temperature at sunlight irradiation. Biomed Opt Express. 2011;2(12):3278-3283.

300 Environmental Protection Agency. Nanomaterial Case Studies: Nanoscale Titanium Dioxide. [Internet]. 2010 [cited 2015 July]. Available from: http://cfpub.epa.gov/ncea/cfm/ recorddisplay.cfm?deid=210206.

301 Mancebo S, Wang S. Skin cancer: role of ultraviolet radiation in carcinogenesis. Rev Environ Health. 2014;29(3):265-73.

302 Jou P, Tomecki K. Sunscreens in the United States: current status and future outlook. Adv Exp Med Biol. 2014;810:464-84.

303 Norval M, Wulf H. Does chronic sunscreen use reduce vitamin D production to insufficient levels?. Br J Dermatol. 2009;161(4):732-6.

304 Diehl J, Chiu M. Effects of ambient sunlight and photoprotection on vitamin D status. Dermatol Ther. 2010;23(1):48-60.

305 Webb A, Engelsen O. Ultraviolet exposure scenarios: risks of erythema from recommendations on cutaneous vitamin D synthesis. Adv Exp Med Biol. 2014;810:406-22.

306 Terushkin V, Bender A, Psaty F, Engelsen O, Wang S, Halpern A. Estimated equivalency of vitamin D production from natural sun exposure versus oral vitamin D supplementation across seasons at two US latitudes. J Am Acad Dermatol. 2010;62(6):92.

307 Kaur P, Mishra S, Mithal A. Vitamin D toxicity resulting from overzealous correction of vitamin D deficiency. Clin Endocrinol (Oxf). [Internet]. 2015 Jun [cited 2015 July]. Available from: http://www.ncbi.nlm.nih.gov/pubmed/26053339.

308 McKenna M, Murray B, O'Keane M, Kilbane M. Rising trend in vitamin D status from 1993 to 2013: dual concerns for the future. Endocr Connect. 2015 ;4(3):163-71.

309 Autier P. Cutaneous malignant melanoma: facts about sunbeds and sunscreen. Expert Rev Anticancer Ther. 2005;5(5):821-33.

310 Darbre P, Aljarrah A, Miller W, NG C, MJ S, GS. P. Concentrations of parabens in human breast tumours. J Appl Toxicol. 2004;24(1):5-13.

311 Darbre P, Aljarrah A, Miller W, Coldham N, Sauer M, Pope G. Reply to Alan M. Jeffrey and Gary M. Williams. J Appl Toxicol. 2004;24(4):304-305.

312 Golden R, Gandy J, Vollmer G. A review of the endocrine activity of parabens and implications for potential risks to human health. Crit Rev Toxicol. 2005;35(5):435-58.

313 U.S. Food and Drug Administration. Parabens. [Internet]. 2007 [cited 2015 July]. Available from: http://www.fda.gov/cosmetics/productsingredients/ingredients/ucm128042.htm.

314 Scientific Committee on Consumer Safety. Opinion on Parabens. [Internet]. 2011 [cited 2015 July]. Available from: http://ec.europa.eu/health/scientific_committees/consumer_safety/docs/sccs_o_041.pdf.

315 Japan Ministry of Health, Labour and Welfare. Standards for Cosmetics: Ministry of Health and Welfare Notification No.331 of 2000. [Internet]. 2001 [cited 2015 July]. Available from: http://www.mhlw.go.jp/file/06-Seisakujouhou-11120000-Iyakushokuhinkyoku/0000032704.pdf.

316 Canada. H. Safety of Cosmetic Ingredients; Parabens. [Internet]. 2015 [cited 2015 July]. Available from: http://www.hc-sc.gc.ca/cps-spc/cosmet-person/labelling-etiquetage/ingredients-eng.php#a4.7.

317 American Cancer Society. Antiperspirants and Breast Cancer Risk. [Internet]. 2014 [cited 2015 July]. Available from: http://www.cancer.org/cancer/cancercauses/othercarcinogens/athome/antiperspirants-and-breast-cancer-risk.

318 Council) TPCPC(. Paraben Information. [Internet]. 2015 [cited 2015 July]. Available from: http://www.cosmeticsinfo.org/paraben-information.

319 Kang Y, Parker C, Smith A, Waldron K. Characterization and distribution of phenolics in carrot cell walls. J Agric Food Chem. 2008;56(18):8558-64.

320 Gao L, Mazza G. Characterization; Quantitation; and Distribution of Anthocyanins and Colorless Phenolics in Sweet Cherries. J. Agric. Food Chem. 1995;43(2):343-346.

321 Huang W, Zhang H, Liu W, Li C. Survey of antioxidant capacity and phenolic composition of blueberry; blackberry; and strawberry in Nanjing. J Zhejiang Univ Sci B. 2012;13(2):94-102.

322 Sellappan S, Akoh C, Krewer G. Phenolic compounds and antioxidant capacity of Georgia-grown blueberries and blackberries. J Agric Food Chem. 2002;50(8):2432-8.

323 Kim E, Ro H, Kim S, Kim H, Chung I. Analysis of phenolic compounds and isoflavones in soybean seeds (Glycine max (L.) Merill) and sprouts grown under different conditions. J Agric Food Chem. 2012;60(23):6045-55.

324 Giacomel C, Dartora G, Dienfethaeler H, Haas S. Investigation on the use of expired make-up and microbiological contamination of mascaras. Int J Cosmet Sci. 2013;35(4):375-80.

325 Avram M. Cellulite: a review of its physiology and treatment. J Cosmet Laser Ther. 2004;6(4):181-5.

326 Luebberding S, Krueger N, Sadick N. Cellulite: An Evidence-Based Review. Am J Clin Dermatol. [Internet]. 2015 May [cited 2015 July]. Available from: http://www.ncbi.nlm.nih.gov/pubmed/25940753.

327 Turati F, Pelucchi C, Marzatico F, Ferraroni M, Decarli A, Gallus S, La Vecchia C, Galeone C. Efficacy of cosmetic products in cellulite reduction: systematic review and meta-analysis. J Eur Acad Dermatol Venereol. 2014;28(1):1-15.

328 De La Casa Almeida M, Suarez Serrano C, Medrano Sánchez E, Diaz Mohedo E, Chamorro Moriana G, Rebollo Salas M. The efficacy of capacitive radio-frequency diathermy in reducing buttock and posterior thigh cellulite measured through the cellulite severity scale. J Cosmet Laser Ther. 2014;16(5):214-24.

329 Mlosek R, Dębowska R, Lewandowski M, Malinowska S, Nowicki A, Eris I. Imaging of the skin and subcutaneous tissue using classical and high-frequency ultrasonographies in anti-cellulite therapy. Skin Res Technol. 2011;17(4):461-8.

330 Rossi A, Katz B. A modern approach to the treatment of cellulite. Dermatol Clin. 2014;32(1):51-6.

331 Schauss A, Wu X, Prior R, Ou B, Huang D, Owens J, Agarwal A, Jensen G, Hart A, Shanbrom E. Antioxidant capacity and other bioactivities of the freeze-dried Amazonian palm berry, Euterpe oleraceae mart. (acai). J Agric Food Chem. 2006;54(22):8604-10.

332 Muzzarelli R. Human enzymatic activities related to the therapeutic administration of

chitin derivatives. Cell Mol Life Sci. 1997;53(2):131-40.

[333] Ueno H, Murakami M, Okumura M, Kadosawa T, Uede T, Fujinaga T. Chitosan accelerates the production of osteopontin from polymorphonuclear leukocytes. Biomaterials. 2001;22(12):1667-73.

[334] Mammone T, Gan D, Fthenakis C, Marenus K. The effect of N-acetyl-glucosamine on stratum corneum desquamation and water content in human skin. J Cosmet Sci. 2009;60(4):423-8.

[335] Millikin C, Robinson M, Reichling T, Hurley G. Topical N-acetyl glucosamine and niacinamide affect pigmentation-relevant gene expression in in vitro genomics experimentation. J Am Acad Dermatol. 2007;56(2):AB169.

[336] Kimball A, Kaczvinsky J, Li J, Robinson L, Matts P, Berge C, Miyamoto K, Bissett D. Reduction in the appearance of facial hyperpigmentation after use of moisturizers with a combination of topical niacinamide and N-acetyl glucosamine: results of a randomized; double-blind; vehicle-controlled trial. Br J Dermatol. 2010;162(2):435-41.

[337] Bissett D, Farmer T, McPhail S, Reichling T, Tiesman J, Juhlin K, Hurley G, Robinson M. Genomic expression changes induced by topical N-acetyl glucosamine in skin equivalent cultures in vitro. J Cosmet Dermatol. 2007;6(4):232-8.

[338] Bissett D. Glucosamine: an ingredient with skin and other benefits. J Cosmet Dermatol. 2006 Dec;5(4):309-15. 2006;5(4):309-15.

[339] Trindade de Almeida A, Carruthers J, Cox S, Goldman M, Wheeler S, Gallagher C. Patient satisfaction and safety with aesthetic onabotulinumtoxinA after at least 5 years: a retrospective cross-sectional analysis of 4;402 glabellar treatments. Dermatol Surg. 2015;41(S1):S19-28.

[340] Blanes-Mira C, Clemente J, Jodas G, Gil A, Fernández-Ballester G, Ponsati B, Gutierrez L, Pérez-Payá E, Ferrer-Montiel A. A synthetic hexapeptide (Argireline) with antiwrinkle activity. Int J Cosmet Sci. 2002;24(5):303-10.

[341] Wilson C. Adenosine receptors and asthma in humans. Br J Pharmacol. 2008;155(4):475-486.

[342] Georgiou J, Skarratt K, Fuller S, Martin C, Christopherson R, Wiley J, Sluyter R. Human Epidermal and Monocyte-Derived Langerhans Cells Express Functional P2X7 Receptors. J Invest Dermatol. 2005;125(3):482-90.

[343] Holzer A, Granstein R. Role of Extracellular Adenosine Triphosphate in Human Skin. J Cutan Med Surg. 2004;8(2):90-6.

[344] Kaidbey K, Sutherland B, Bennett P, Wamer W, Barton C, Dennis D, Kornhauser A. Topical glycolic acid enhances photodamage by ultraviolet light. Photodermatol Photoimmunol Photomed. 2003;19(1):21-7.

[345] Okuda M, Donahue D, Kaufman L, Avalos J, Simion F, Story D, Sakaguchi H, Fautz R, Fuchs A. Negligible penetration of incidental amounts of alpha-hydroxy acid from rinse-off personal care products in human skin using an in vitro static diffusion cell model. Toxicol In Vitro. 2011;25(8):2041-7.

[346] Neuman M, Haber J, Malkiewicz I, Cameron R, Katz G, Shear N. Ethanol signals for apoptosis in cultured skin cells. Alcohol. 2002;26(3):179-90.

[347] Neilan B. The molecular evolution and DNA profiling of toxic cyanobacteria. Curr Issues Mol Biol. 2002;4(1):1-11.

[348] Shih M, Cherng J. Potential protective effect of fresh grown unicellular green algae component (resilient factor) against PMA- and UVB-induced MMP1 expression in skin fibroblasts. Eur J Dermatol. 2008;18(3):303-7.

[349] Rupérez P, Ahrazem O, Leal J. Potential Antioxidant Capacity of Sulfated Polysaccharides from the Edible Marine Brown Seaweed Fucus vesiculosus. J Agric Food Chem. 2002;50(4):840-5.

350 Surjushe A, Vasani R, Saple D. Aloe vera: a short review. Indian J Dermatol. 2008;53(4):163-6.

351 Reynolds T, Dweck A. Aloe vera leaf gel: a review update. J Ethnopharmacol. 1999;68(1-3):3-37.

352 Lee K, Weintraub S, Yu B. Isolation and identification of a phenolic antioxidant from Aloe barbadensis. Free Radic Biol Med. 2000;28(2):261-5.

353 DalBelo S, Gaspar L, Maia Campos P. Moisturizing effect of cosmetic formulations containing Aloe vera extract in different concentrations assessed by skin bioengineering techniques. Skin Res Technol. 2006;12(4):241-6.

354 del Nogal Sánchez M, Pérez-Pavón J, Moreno Cordero B. Determination of suspected allergens in cosmetic products by headspace-programmed temperature vaporization-fast gas chromatography-quadrupole mass spectrometry. Anal Bioanal Chem. 2010;397(6):2579-91.

355 Sgorbini B, Ruosi M, Cordero C, Liberto E, Rubiolo P, Bicchi C. Quantitative determination of some volatile suspected allergens in cosmetic creams spread on skin by direct contact sorptive tape extraction–gas chromatography–mass spectrometry. J Chromatogr A. 2010;1217(16):2599-605.

356 An S, Lee A, Lee C, Kim D, Hahm J, Kim K, Moon K, Won Y, Ro Y, Eun H. Fragrance contact dermatitis in Korea: a joint study. Contact Dermatitis. 2005;53(6):320-3.

357 Beitner H. Randomized; placebo-controlled; double blind study on the clinical efficacy of a cream containing 5% alpha-lipoic acid related to photoageing of facial skin. Br J Dermatol. 2003;149(4):841-9.

358 Podda M, Grundmann-Kollmann M. Low molecular weight antioxidants and their role in skin ageing. Clin Exp Dermatol. 2001;26(7):578-82.

359 Wada T, Wakami H, Konishi T, Matsugo S. The Degradation and Regeneration of α-Lipoic Acid under the Irradiation of UV Light in the Existence of Homocysteine. J Clin Biochem Nutr. 2009;44(3):218–222.

360 Robinson V, Bergfeld W, Belsito D, Hill R, Klaassen C, Marks JJ, Shank R, Slaga T, Snyder P, Andersen A. Final report of the amended safety assessment of sodium laureth sulfate and related salts of sulfated ethoxylated alcohols. Int J Toxicol. 2010;29(4S):151S-61S.

361 Wei A, Shibamoto T. Antioxidant activities and volatile constituents of various essential oils. J Agric Food Chem. 2007;55(5):1737-42.

362 Ford C, Maibach H. Anti-Irritants: Myth or Reality?. Exog Dermatol. 2004;3:154–160.

363 Kim B, Lee Y, Kang K. The mechanism of retinol-induced irritation and its application to anti-irritant development. Toxicol Lett. 2003;146(1):65-73.

364 Hori I, Nihei K, Kubo I. Structural criteria for depigmenting mechanism of arbutin. Phytother Res. 2004;18(6):475-9.

365 Sugimoto K, Nishimura T, Nomura K, Sugimoto K, T. K. Inhibitory effects of alpha-arbutin on melanin synthesis in cultured human melanoma cells and a three-dimensional human skin model. Biol Pharm Bull. 2004;27(4):510-4.

366 Drissi A, Girona J, Cherki M, Godàs G, Derouiche A, El Messal M, Saile R, Kettani A, Solà R, Masana L, et al. Evidence of hypolipemiant and antioxidant properties of argan oil derived from the argan tree (Argania spinosa). Clin Nutr. 2004;23(5):1159-66.

367 Monfalouti H. Therapeutic potential of argan oil: a review. J Pharm Pharmacol. 2010;62(12):1669-75.

368 Dobrev H. Clinical and instrumental study of the efficacy of a new sebum control cream. J Cosmet Dermatol. 2007;6(2):113-8.

369 Charrouf Z, Guillaume D. Ethnoeconomical; ethnomedical; and phytochemical study of Argania spinosa (L.) Skeels. J Ethnopharmacol. 1999;67(1):7-14.

370 Witte M, Barbul A, Schick M, Vogt N, Becker H. Upregulation of arginase expression in wound-derived fibroblasts. J Surg Res. 2002;105(1):35-42.

[371] Angele M, Nitsch S, Hatz R, Angele P, Hernandez-Richter T, Wichmann M, Chaudry I, Schildberg F. L-arginine: a unique amino acid for improving depressed wound immune function following hemorrhage. Eur Surg Res. 2002 ;34(1-2):53-60.

[372] Seeley B, Denton A, Ahn M, Maas C. Effect of homeopathic Arnica montana on bruising in face-lifts: results of a randomized; double-blind; placebo-controlled clinical trial. Arch Facial Plast Surg. 2006;8(1):54-9.

[373] Hofmann U, Priem M, Bartzsch C, Winckler T, Feller K. A sensitive sensor cell line for the detection of oxidative stress responses in cultured human keratinocytes. Sensors (Basel). 2014;14(7):11293-307.

[374] Hausen B. A 6-year experience with compositae mix. Am J Contact Dermat. 1996;7(2):94-9.

[375] Stamford N. Stability; transdermal penetration; and cutaneous effects of ascorbic acid and its derivatives. J Cosmet Dermatol. 2012;11(4):310-7.

[376] Gallarate M, Carlotti M, Trotta M, Bovo S. On the stability of ascorbic acid in emulsified systems for topical and cosmetic use. Int J Pharm. 1999;188(2):233-41.

[377] Tsai F, Wang Y, Chen C, Hsieh C, Cheng Z, Wu Y. Evaluation of the antioxidative capability of commonly used antioxidants in dermocosmetics by in vivo detection of protein carbonylation in human stratum corneum. J Photochem Photobiol B. 2012;112:7-15.

[378] Hakozaki T, Takiwaki H, Miyamoto K. Ultrasound enhanced skin-lightening effect of vitamin C and niacinamide. Skin Res Technol. 2006;12(2):105-13.

[379] Carlotti M, Ugazio E, Gastaldi L, Sapino S, Vione D, Fenoglio I, Fubini B. Specific effects of single antioxidants in the lipid peroxidation caused by nano-titania used in sunscreen lotions. J Photochem Photobiol B. 2009;96(2):130-5.

[380] Kleinová M, Hewitt M, Brezová V, Madden J, Cronin M, Valko M. Antioxidant properties of carotenoids: QSAR prediction of their redox potentials. Gen Physiol Biophys. 2007;26(2):97-103.

[381] Niwano T, Terazawa S, Nakajima H, Wakabayashi Y, Imokawa G. Astaxanthin and withaferin A block paracrine cytokine interactions between UVB-exposed human keratinocytes and human melanocytes via the attenuation of endothelin-1 secretion and its downstream intracellular signaling. Cytokine. 2015;72(2):184-97.

[382] Amber K, Bloom R, Staropoli P, Dhiman S, Hu S. Assessing the Current Market of Sunscreen: A Cross-Sectional Study of Sunscreen Availability in Three Metropolitan Counties in the United States. Journal of Skin Cancer. 2014;2014:285357.

[383] Jansen R, Osterwalder U, Wang S, Burnett M, Lim H. Photoprotection: part II. Sunscreen: development, efficacy, and controversies. J Am Acad Dermatol. 2013;69(6):867.e1-14.

[384] Jutley G, Rajaratnam R, Halpern J, Salim A, Emmett C. Systematic review of randomized controlled trials on interventions for melasma: an abridged Cochrane Review. J Am Acad Dematol. 2014;7(2):369-73.

[385] Fleischer Jr A. Inflammation in rosacea and acne: Implications for patient care. J Drugs Dermatol. 2011;10(6):614-20.

[386] Kircik L. Efficacy and safety of azelaic acid (AzA) gel 15% in the treatment of post-inflammatory hyperpigmentation and acne: a 16-week, baseline-controlled study. J Drugs Dermatol. 2011;10(6):586-90.

[387] Koytchev R, Alken R, Dundarov S. Balm mint extract (Lo-701) for topical treatment of recurring herpes labialis. Phytomedicine. 1999;6(4):225-30.

[388] Duh P, Yen G, Yen W, Chang L. Antioxidant Effects of Water Extracts from Barley (Hordeum vulgare L.) Prepared under Different Roasting Temperatures. J. Agric. Food Chem. 2001;49(3):1455-1463.

[389] Iguchi T, Kawata A, Watanabe T, Mazumder T, Tanabe S. Fermented barley extract suppresses the development of atopic dermatitis-like skin lesions in NC/Nga mice, probably

by inhibiting inflammatory cytokines. Biosci Biotechnol Biochem. 2009;73(3):489-93.

390 Dykesa G, Amarowiczb R, Pegga R. Enhancement of nisin antibacterial activity by a bearberry (Arctostaphylos uva-ursi) leaf extract. Food Microbiol. 2003;20(2):211-216.

391 Haddad A, Matos L, Brunstein F, Ferreira L, Silva A, Costa Jr D. A clinical, prospective, randomized, double-blind trial comparing skin whitening complex with hydroquinone vs. placebo in the treatment of melasma. Int J Dermatol. 2003;42(2):153-6.

392 Parejo I, Viladomat F, Bastida J, Codina C. A single extraction step in the quantitative analysis of arbutin in bearberry (Arctostaphylos uva-ursi) leaves by high-performance liquid chromatography. Phytochem Anal. 2001;12(5):336-9.

393 Matsuda H, Higashino M, Nakai Y, Iinuma M, Kubo M, Lang F. Studies of cuticle drugs from natural sources. IV. Inhibitory effects of some Arctostaphylos plants on melanin biosynthesis. Biol Pharm Bull. 1996;19(1):153-6.

394 Epstein H. Anatomy of a Skin Cleanser. Skinmed. 2005;4(3):183-185.

395 Schnuch A, Mildau G, Kratz E, Uter W. Risk of sensitization to preservatives estimated on the basis of patch test data and exposure, according to a sample of 3541 leave-on products. Contact Dermatitis. 2011;65(3):167-74.

396 Nair B. Final report on the safety assessment of Benzyl Alcohol, Benzoic Acid, and Sodium Benzoate. Int J Toxicol. 2001;20(S3):23-50.

397 Kaddu S, Ker lH, Wolf P. Accidental bullous phototoxic reactions to bergamot aromatherapy oil. J Am Acad Dermatol. 2001;45(3):458-61.

398 Yasui Y, Hirone T. Action spectrum for bergamot-oil phototoxicity measured by sunburn cell counting. J Dermatol. 1994;21(5):319-22.

399 Kurtz E, Wallo W. Colloidal oatmeal: history, chemistry and clinical properties. J Drugs Dermatol. 2007;6(2):167-70.

400 Tsiapali E, Whaley S, Kalbfleisch J, Ensley H, Browder I, Williams D. Glucans exhibit weak antioxidant activity, but stimulate macrophage free radical activity. Free Radic Biol Med. 2001;30(4):393-402.

401 Maurya A, Singh M, Dubey V, Srivastava S, Luqman S, Bawankule D. α-(-)-bisabolol reduces pro-inflammatory cytokine production and ameliorates skin inflammation. Curr Pharm Biotechnol. 2014;15(2):173-81.

402 Miyazawa M, Okuno Y, Fukuyama M, Nakamura S, Kosaka H. Antimutagenic activity of polymethoxyflavonoids from Citrus aurantium. J Agric Food Chem. 1999;47(12):5239-44.

403 Nardelli A, D'Hooghe E, Drieghe J, Dooms M, Goossens A. Allergic contact dermatitis from fragrance components in specific topical pharmaceutical products in Belgium. Contact Dermatitis. 2009;60(6):303-13.

404 Pereira D, Faria J, Gaspar L, Valentão P, de Pinho P, Andrade P. Boerhaavia diffusa: metabolite profiling of a medicinal plant from Nyctaginaceae. Food Chem Toxicol. 2009;47(8):2142-9.

405 Ferreres F, Sousa C, Justin M, Valentão P, Andrade P, Llorach R, Rodrigues A, Seabra R, Leitão A. Characterisation of the phenolic profile of Boerhaavia diffusa L. by HPLC-PAD-MS/MS as a tool for quality control. Phytochem Anal. 2005;16(6):451-8.

406 Asadi-Samani M, Bahmani M, Rafieian-Kopaei M. The chemical composition, botanical characteristic and biological activities of Borago officinalis: a review. Asian Pac J Trop Med. 2014;7S1:S22-8.

407 Cosmetic Ingredient Review Expert Panel. Final Report of the Cosmetic Ingredient Review Expert Panel: Amended Safety Assessment of Cocos Nucifera (Coconut) Oil, Coconut Acid, Hydrogenated Coconut Acid, Hydrogenated Coconut Oil, and its Derivatives. [Internet]. 2008 [cited 2015 July]. Available from: http://www.cir-safety.org/sites/default/files/115_buff3e_suppl.pdf.

[408] Yazar K, Johnsson S, Lind M, Boman A, Lidén C. Preservatives and fragrances in selected consumer-available cosmetics and detergents. Contact Dermatitis. 2011;64(5):265-72.

[409] Kerzendorfer C, O'Driscoll M. UVB and caffeine: inhibiting the DNA damage response to protect against the adverse effects of UVB. J Invest Dermatol. 2009;129(7):161-3.

[410] Conney A, Kramata P, Lou Y, Lu Y. Effect of caffeine on UVB-induced carcinogenesis, apoptosis, and the elimination of UVB-induced patches of p53 mutant epidermal cells in SKH-1 mice. Photochem Photobiol. 2008;84(2):330-8.

[411] Lu Y, Lou Y, Liao J, Xie J, Peng Q, Yang C, Conney A. Administration of green tea or caffeine enhances the disappearance of UVB-induced patches of mutant p53 positive epidermal cells in SKH-1 mice. Carcinogenesis. 2005;26(8):1465-72.

[412] Yazheng L, Kitts D. Activation of antioxidant response element (ARE)-dependent genes by roasted coffee extracts. Food Funct. 2012;3(9):950-4.

[413] Ribeiro J, Sebastião A, de Mendonca A. Adenosine receptors in the nervous system: pathophysiological implications. Prog Neurobiol. 2002;68(6):377-92.

[414] Velasco M, Tano C, Machado-Santelli G, Consiglieri V, Kaneko T, Baby R. Effects of caffeine and siloxanetriol alginate caffeine, as anticellulite agents, on fatty tissue: histological evaluation. J Cosmet Dermatol. 2008;7(1):23-9.

[415] Herman A, Herman A. Caffeine's mechanisms of action and its cosmetic use. Skin Pharmacol Physiol. 2013;26(1):8-14.

[416] Shimoda H, Seki E, Michio A. Inhibitory effect of green coffee bean extract on fat accumulation and body weight gain in mice. BMC Complement Altern Med. 2006;6(9):17.

[417] Kobayashi-Hattori K, Mogi A, Matsumoto Y, Takita T. Effect of caffeine on the body fat and lipid metabolism of rats fed on a high-fat diet. Biosci Biotechnol Biochem. 2005;69(11):2219-23.

[418] Reider N, Komericki P, Hausen B, Fritsch P, Aberer W. The seamy side of natural medicines: contact sensitization to arnica (Arnica montana L.) and marigold (Calendula officinalis L.). Contact Dermatitis. 2001;45(5):269-72.

[419] Chen W, Vermaak I, Viljoen A. Camphor—A Fumigant during the Black Death and a Coveted Fragrant Wood in Ancient Egypt and Babylon—A Review. Molecules. 2013;18(5):5334-5454.

[420] Ernst E. Adverse effects of herbal drugs in dermatology. Br J Dermatol. 2000;143(5):923-929.

[421] Lloyd S, Modlin R. Toll-like receptors in the skin. Semin Immunopathol. 2007.;29(1):15-26.

[422] Kim M, Kim Y, Eun H, Cho K, Chung J. All-Trans Retinoic Acid Antagonizes UV-Induced VEGF Production and Angiogenesis via the Inhibition of ERK Activation in Human Skin Keratinocytes. J Invest Dermatol. 2006;126(12):2697-2706.

[423] Li J, Zhang Y, Kirsner R. Angiogenesis in wound repair: angiogenic growth factors and the extracellular matrix. Microsc Res Tech. 2003;60(1):107-14.

[424] He Z, Ong C, Halper J, Bateman A. Progranulin is a mediator of the wound response. Nat Med. 2003;9(2):225-9.

[425] Quan T, He T, Kang S, Voorhees J, Fisher G. Connective tissue growth factor: expression in human skin in vivo and inhibition by ultraviolet irradiation. J Invest Dermatol. 2002;118(3):402-8.

[426] Denning M. Epidermal keratinocytes: regulation of multiple cell phenotypes by multiple protein kinase C isoforms. Int J Biochem Cell Biol. 2004;36(7):1141-6.

[427] Boudjelal M, Voorhees J, Fisher G. Retinoid signaling is attenuated by proteasome-mediated degradation of retinoid receptors in human keratinocyte HaCaT cells. Exp Cell Res. 2002;274(1):130-7.

[428] de Gruijl F. Photocarcinogenesis: UVA vs. UVB Radiation. Skin Pharmacol Appl Skin

Physiol. 2002;15:316–320.

[429] Kwon Y, Kim C, Youm J, Gwak H, Park B, Lee S, Jeon S, Kim B, Seo Y, Park J, et al. Novel synthetic ceramide derivatives increase intracellular calcium levels and promote epidermal keratinocyte differentiation. J Lipid Res. 2007;48(9):1936-43.

[430] Vielhaber G, Pfeiffer S, Brade L, Lindner B, Goldmann T, Vollmer E, Hintze U, Wittern K, Wepf R. Localization of ceramide and glucosylceramide in human epidermis by immunogold electron microscopy. J Invest Deratol. 2001;117(5):1126-36.

[431] Schwarz T. Biological effects of UV radiation on keratinocytes and Langerhans cells. Exp Dermatol. 2005;14(10):788-9.

[432] Choi M, Maibach H. Role of ceramides in barrier function of healthy and diseased skin. Am J Clin Dematol. 2005;6(4):215-23.

[433] Proksch E, Fölster-Holst R, Jensen J. Skin barrier function, epidermal proliferation and differentiation in eczema. J Dermatol Sci. 2006;43(3):159-69.

[434] Geilen C, Barz S, Bektas M. Sphingolipid Signaling in Epidermal Homeostasis. Skin Pharmacol Appl Skin Physiol. 2001;14:261-271.

[435] Meckfessel M, Brandt S. The structure, function, and importance of ceramides in skin and their use as therapeutic agents in skin-care products. J Am Acad Dermatol. 2014;71(1):177-84.

[436] Mojumdar E, Kariman Z, van Kerckhove L, Gooris G, Bouwstra J. The role of ceramide chain length distribution on the barrier properties of the skin lipid membranes. Biochim Biophys Acta. 2014;1838(10):2473-2483.

[437] Srivastava J, Shankar E, Gupta S. Chamomile: A herbal medicine of the past with bright future. Mol Med Report. 2010;3(6):895-901.

[438] Thornfeldt C. Cosmeceuticals containing herbs: fact, fiction, and future. Dermatol Surg. 2005;31(7 Pt. 2):873-80.

[439] McKay D, Blumberg J. A review of the bioactivity and potential health benefits of chamomile tea (Matricaria recutita L.). Phytother Res. 2006;20(7):519-30.

[440] Norlén L, Gil I, Simonsen A, Descouts P. Human stratum corneum lipid organization as observed by atomic force microscopy on Langmuir-Blodgett films. J Struct Biol. 2007;158(3):386-400.

[441] Meding B. Skin symptoms among workers in a spice factory. Contact Dermatitis. 1993;29(4):202-5.

[442] We A, Shibamoto T. Antioxidant activities of essential oil mixtures toward skin lipid squalene oxidized by UV irradiation. Cutan Ocul Toxicol. 2007;26(3):227-33.

[443] Fiume M, Heldreth B, Bergfeld W, Belsito D, Hill R, Klaassen C, Liebler D, Marks Jr J, Shank R, Slaga T, et al. Safety assessment of diethanolamides as used in cosmetics. Int J Toxicol. 2013;32(3S):26S-58S.

[444] Gasser P, Lati E, Peno-Mazzarino L, Bouzoud D, Allegaert L, Bernaert H. Cocoa polyphenols and their influence on parameters involved in ex vivo skin restructuring. Int J Cosmet Sci. 2008;30(5):339-45.

[445] Buchanan K, Fletcher H, Reid M. Prevention of striae gravidarum with cocoa butter cream. Int J Gynaecol Obstet. 2010;108(1):65-8.

[446] Osman H, Usta I, Rubeiz N, Abu-Rustum R, Charara I, Nassar A. Cocoa butter lotion for prevention of striae gravidarum: a double-blind, randomised and placebo-controlled trial. BJOG. 2008;115(9):1138-42.

[447] Evangelista M, Abad-Casintahan F, Lopez-Villafuerte L. The effect of topical virgin coconut oil on SCORAD index, transepidermal water loss, and skin capacitance in mild to moderate pediatric atopic dermatitis: a randomized, double-blind, clinical trial. Int J Dermatol. 2014;53(1):100-8.

[448] Verallo-Rowell V, Dillague K, Syah-Tjundawan B. Novel antibacterial and emollient effects of coconut and virgin olive oils in adult atopic dermatitis. Dermatitis. 2008;19(6):308-15.

[449] Yang D, Pornpattananangkul D, Nakatsuji T, Chan M, Carson D, Huang C, Zhang L. The antimicrobial activity of liposomal lauric acids against Propionibacterium acnes. Biomaterials. 2009;30(30):6035-40.

[450] Kaur C, Swarnlata S. In vitro sun protection factor determination of herbal oils used in cosmetics. Pharmacognosy Res. 2010;2(1):22-25.

[451] Fu PXQ, Lin G, MW. C. Genotoxic Pyrrolizidine Alkaloids — Mechanisms Leading to DNA Adduct Formation and Tumorigenicity. Int. J. Mol. Sci. 2002;3:948-964.

[452] Johnson B, Bolton J, van Breeman R. Screening Botanical Extracts for Quinoid Metabolites. Chem. Res. Toxicol. 2001;14(11):1546-1551.

[453] Pickart L, Vasquez-Soltero J, Margolina A. The Human Tripeptide GHK-Cu in Prevention of Oxidative Stress and Degenerative Conditions of Aging: Implications for Cognitive Health. Oxid Med Cell Longev. 2012 324832.

[454] Zuang V, Rona C, Archer G, Berardesca E. Detection of Skin Irritation Potential of Cosmetics by Non-Invasive Measurements. Skin Pharmacol Appl Skin Physiol. 2000.;13:358-371.

[455] Yosipovitch G, Szolar C, Hui X, Maibach H. Effect of topically applied menthol on thermal, pain and itch sensations and biophysical properties of the skin. Arch Dermatol Res. 1996;288(5-6):245-8.

[456] Perkins M, Osterhues M, Farage M, Robinson M. A noninvasive method to assess skin irritation and compromised skin conditions using simple tape adsorption of molecular markers of inflammation. Skin Res Technol. 2001;7(4):224-37.

[457] Kai H, Baba M, Okuyama T. Inhibitory effect of Cucumis sativus on melanin production in melanoma B16 cells by downregulation of tyrosinase expression. Planta Med. 2008;74(15):1785-8.

[458] Villaseñor I, Simon M, Villanueva A. Comparative potencies of nutraceuticals in chemically induced skin tumor prevention. Nutr Cancer. 2002;44(1):66-71.

[459] Kumar D, Kumar S, Singh J, Narender R, Vashistha B, Singh N. Free Radical Scavenging and Analgesic Activities of Cucumis sativus L. Fruit Extract. J Young Pharm. 2010;2(4):365-8.

[460] Ibrahim T, El-Hefnawy H, El-Hela A. Antioxidant potential and phenolic acid content of certain cucurbitaceous plants cultivated in Egypt. Nat Prod Res. 2010;24(16):1537-45.

[461] Ismail H, Chan K, Mariod A, Ismail M. Phenolic content and antioxidant activity of cantaloupe (Cucumis melo) methanolic extracts. Food Chem. 2010;119:643-647.

[462] Vouldoukis I, Lacan D, Kamate C, Coste P, Calenda A, Mazier D, Conti M, Dugas B. Antioxidant and anti-inflammatory properties of a Cucumis melo LC. extract rich in superoxide dismutase activity. J Ethnopharmacol. 2004;94(1):67-75.

[463] Goel A, Kunnumakkara A, Aggarwal B. Curcumin as "Curecumin": from kitchen to clinic. Biochem Pharmacol. 2008;75(4):787-809.

[464] Menon V, Sudheer A. Antioxidant and Anti-Inflammatory Properties of Curcumin. Springer US; 2007. p. 105-125.

[465] International Journal of Toxicology. Final Report on the Safety Assessment of Diazolidinyl Urea. Int J Toxicol. 1990;9(2):229-245.

[466] Rastogi S. Analytical control of preservative labelling on skin creams. Contact Dermatitis. 2000;43(6):339-43.

[467] National Toxicology Program. NTP Toxicology and Carcinogenesis Studies of Diethanolamine (CAS No. 111-42-2) in F344/N Rats and B6C3F1 Mice (Dermal Studies). Natl Toxicol Program Tech Rep Ser. 1999;478:1-212.

468 U.S. Food and Drug Administration. Diethanolamine. [Internet]. 2006 [cited 2015 July]. Available from: http://www.fda.gov/cosmetics/productsingredients/ingredients/ucm109655.htm.

469 Brain K, Walters K, Green D, Brain S, Loretz L, Sharma R, Dressler W. Percutaneous penetration of diethanolamine through human skin in vitro: application from cosmetic vehicles. Food Chem Toxicol. 2005;43(5):681-90.

470 Fu J, Dusza S, Halpern A. Sunless tanning. J Am Acad Dermatol. 2004;50(5):706-13.

471 Teixeira V, Cabral R, Gonçalo M. Exuberant connubial allergic contact dermatitis from diphenhydramine. Cutan Ocul Toxicol. 2014;33(1):82-4.

472 Shaughnessy C, Malajian D, Belsito D. Cutaneous delayed-type hypersensitivity in patients with atopic dermatitis: reactivity to topical preservatives. J Am Acad Dermatol. 2014;70(1):102-7.

473 Chow E, Avolio A, Lee A, Nixon R. Frequency of positive patch test reactions to preservatives: The Australian experience. Australas J Dermatol. 2013;54(1):31-5.

474 The Personal Care Products Council (the Council). DMDM Hydantoin. [Internet]. 2015 [cited 2015 July]. Available from: http://www.cosmeticsinfo.org/ingredient/dmdm-hydantoin.

475 Rai R, Shanmuga S, Srinivas C. Update on Photoprotection. Indian J Dermatol. 2012;57(5):335-342.

476 Young D. Classification of enzymes and current status of enzyme nomenclature and units. Ann Clin Lab Sci. 93-8;7(2):1977.

477 Cai Y, Chou K. Predicting enzyme subclass by functional domain composition and pseudo amino acid composition. J Proteome Res. 2005;4(3):967-71.

478 Lods L, Dres C, Johnson C, Scholz D, Brooks G. The future of enzymes in cosmetics. Int J Cosmet Sci. 2000;22(2):85-94.

479 Garone Jr M, Howard J, Fabrikant J. A Review of Common Tanning Methods. J Clin Aesthet Dermatol. 2015;8(2):43-47.

480 Higgins C, Palmer A, Nixon R. Eucalyptus oil: contact allergy and safety. Contact Dermatitis. 2015;72(5):344-6.

481 Nielsen J. Natural oils affect the human skin integrity and the percutaneous penetration of benzoic acid dose-dependently. Basic Clin Pharmacol Toxicol. 2006;98(6):575-81.

482 Turić P, Lipozencić J, Milavec-Puretić V, Kulisić S. Contact allergy caused by fragrance mix and Myroxylon pereirae (balsam of Peru)--a retrospective study. Coll Antropol. 2011;35(1):83-7.

483 Takeyoshi M, Noda S, Yamazaki S, Kakishima H, Yamasaki K, Kimber I. Assessment of the skin sensitization potency of eugenol and its dimers using a non-radioisotopic modification of the local lymph node assay. J Appl Toxicol. 2004;24(1):77-81.

484 Svedman C, Engfeldt M, Api A, Politano V, Belsito D, Gruvberger B, Bruze M. Does the new standard for eugenol designed to protect against contact sensitization protect those sensitized from elicitation of the reaction? Dermatitis. 2012;23(1):32-8.

485 Prashar A, Locke I, Evans C. Cytotoxicity of clove (Syzygium aromaticum) oil and its major components to human skin cells. Cell Prolif. 2006;39(4):241-8.

486 Akiyama H, Oono T, Huh W, Yamasaki O, Ogawa S, Katsuyama M, Ichikawa H, Iwatsuki K. Actions of farnesol and xylitol against Staphylococcus aureus. Chemotherapy. 2002;48(3):122-8.

487 Chaudhary S, Alam M, Siddiqui M, Athar M. Chemopreventive effect of farnesol on DMBA/TPA-induced skin tumorigenesis: involvement of inflammation, Ras-ERK pathway and apoptosis. Life Sci. 2009;85(5-6):196-205.

[488] Machida K, Tanaka T, Fujita K, Taniguchi M. Farnesol-induced generation of reactive oxygen species via indirect inhibition of the mitochondrial electron transport chain in the yeast Saccharomyces cerevisiae. J Bacteriol. 1998;180(17):4460-5.

[489] U.S. Food and Drug Administration. Color Additive Status List. [Internet]. 2015 [cited 2015 July]. Available from: http://www.fda.gov/ForIndustry/ColorAdditives/ ColorAdditiveInventories/ucm106626.htm.

[490] Zhang L, Al-Suwayeh S, Hsieh P, Fang J. A comparison of skin delivery of ferulic acid and its derivatives: evaluation of their efficacy and safety. Int J Pharm. 2010;399(1-2):44-51.

[491] Monti D, Tampucci S, Chetoni P, Burgalassi S, Saino V, Centini M, Anselmi C. Permeation and Distribution of Ferulic Acid and Its α-Cyclodextrin Complex from Different Formulations in Hairless Rat Skin. AAPS PharmSciTech. 2011;12(2):514-520.

[492] Ichihashi M, Funasaka Y, Ohashi A, Chacraborty A, Ahmed N, Ueda M, Osawa T. The inhibitory effect of DL-alpha-tocopheryl ferulate in lecithin on melanogenesis. Anticancer Res. 1999;19(5A):3796-74.

[493] Rodriguez K, Wong H, Oddos T, Southall M, Frei B, Kaur S. A purified feverfew extract protects from oxidative damage by inducing DNA repair in skin cells via a PI3-kinase-dependent Nrf2/ARE pathway. J Dermatol Sci. 2013;72(3):304-10.

[494] Martin K, Sur R, Liebel F, Tierney N, Lyte P, Garay M, Oddos T, Anthonavage M, Shapiro S, Southall M. Parthenolide-depleted Feverfew (Tanacetum parthenium) protects skin from UV irradiation and external aggression. Arch Dermatol Res. 2008;300(2):69-80.

[495] Pareek A, Suthar M, Rathore G, Bansal V. Feverfew (Tanacetum parthenium L.): A systematic review. Pharmacogn Rev. 2011;5(9):103-110.

[496] Dearman R, Betts C, Farr C, McLaughlin J, Berdasco N, Wiench K, Kimber I. Comparative analysis of skin sensitization potency of acrylates (methyl acrylate, ethyl acrylate, butyl acrylate, and ethylhexyl acrylate) using the local lymph node assay. Contact Dermatitis. 2007;57(4):242-7.

[497] Dinkloh A, Worm M, Geier J, Schnuch A, Wollenberg A. Contact sensitization in patients with suspected cosmetic intolerance: results of the IVDK 2006-2011. J Eur Acad Dermatol Venereol. 2015;29(6):1071-81.

[498] Huang Z, Hung C, Lin Y, Fang J. In vitro and in vivo evaluation of topical delivery and potential dermal use of soy isoflavones genistein and daidzein. Int J Pharm. 2008;364(1):36-44.

[499] Wang Y, Wu W, Chen H, Fang H. Genistein protects against UVB-induced senescence-like characteristics in human dermal fibroblast by p66Shc down-regulation. J Dermatol Sci. 2010;58(1):19-27.

[500] Emmerson E, Campbell L, Ashcroft G, Hardman M. The phytoestrogen genistein promotes wound healing by multiple independent mechanisms. Mol Cell Endocrinol. 2010;321(1):184-93.

[501] Larsen W, Nakayama H, Fischer T, Elsner P, Frosch P, Burrows D, Jordan W, Shaw S, Wilkinson J, Marks Jr J, et al. Fragrance contact dermatitis: a worldwide multicenter investigation (Part II). Contact Dermatitis. 2001;44(6):244-6.

[502] Dorman H, Deans S. Antimicrobial agents from plants: antibacterial activity of plant volatile oils. J Appl Microbiol. 2000;88(2):308-16.

[503] Radulović N, Stojković M, Mitić S, Randjelović P, Ilić I, Stojanović N, Stojanović-Radić Z. Exploitation of the antioxidant potential of Geranium macrorrhizum (Geraniaceae): hepatoprotective and antimicrobial activities. Nat Prod Commun. 2012;7(12):1609-14.

[504] Murakami A, Takahashi D, Kinoshita T, Koshimizu K, Kim H, Yoshihiro A, Nakamura Y, Jiwajinda S, Terao J, Ohigashi H. Zerumbone, a Southeast Asian ginger sesquiterpene, markedly suppresses free radical generation, proinflammatory protein production, and cancer cell proliferation accompanied by apoptosis: the alpha,beta-unsaturated carbonyl

group is a prerequisite. Carcinogenesis. 2002;23(5):795-802.

505 Surh Y. Anti-tumor promoting potential of selected spice ingredients with antioxidative and anti-inflammatory activities: a short review. Food Chem Toxicol. 2002;40(8):1097-7.

506 Minghetti P, Sosa S, Cilurzo F, Casiraghi A, Alberti E, Tubaro A, Loggia R, Montanari L. Evaluation of the topical anti-inflammatory activity of ginger dry extracts from solutions and plasters. Planta Med. 2007;73(15):1525-30.

507 Boelsma E, Lamers R, Hendriks H, van Nesselrooij J, Roza L. Evidence of the regulatory effect of Ginkgo biloba extract on skin blood flow and study of its effects on urinary metabolites in healthy humans. Planta Med. 2004;70(11):1052-7.

508 Di Mambro V, Fonseca M. Assays of physical stability and antioxidant activity of a topical formulation added with different plant extracts. J Pharm Biomed Anal. 2005;37(2):287-95.

509 Eli R, Fasciano J. An adjunctive preventive treatment for cancer: ultraviolet light and ginkgo biloba, together with other antioxidants, are a safe and powerful, but largely ignored, treatment option for the prevention of cancer. Med Hypotheses. 2006;66(6):1152-6.

510 Chuarienthong P, Lourith N, Leelapornpisid P. Clinical efficacy comparison of anti-wrinkle cosmetics containing herbal flavonoids. Int J Cosmet Sci. 2010;32(2):99-106.

511 Dal Belo S, Gaspar L, Maia Campos P. Photoprotective effects of topical formulations containing a combination of Ginkgo biloba and green tea extracts. Phytother Res. 2011;25(12):1854-60.

512 Elmets C, Singh D, Tubesing K, Matsui M, Katiyar S, Mukhtar H. Cutaneous photoprotection from ultraviolet injury by green tea polyphenols. J Am Acad Dermatol. 2001;44(3):425-32.

513 Thompson T, Grace T. Gluten in cosmetics: is there a reason for concern? J Acad Nutr Diet. 2012;112(23):1316-23.

514 Kraft J, Lynde C. Moisturizers: what they are and a practical approach to product selection. Skin Therapy Lett. 2005;10(5):1-8.

515 Lorencini M, Brohem C, Dieamant G, Zanchin N, Maibach H. Active ingredients against human epidermal aging. Ageing Res Rev. 2014;15:100-15.

516 Short R, Chan J, Choi J, Egbert B, Rehmus W, Kimball A. Effects of moisturization on epidermal homeostasis and differentiation. Clin Exp Dermatol. 2007;32(1):88-90.

517 Roure R, Lanctin M, Nollent V, Bertin C. Methods to Assess the Protective Efficacy of Emollients against Climatic and Chemical Aggressors. Dermatol Res Pract. 2012;2012:864734.

518 Fowler Jr J. Efficacy of a skin-protective foam in the treatment of chronic hand dermatitis. Am J Contact Dermat. 2000;11(3):165-9.

519 Garner L. Contact dermatitis to metals. Dermatol Ther. 2004;17(4):321-7.

520 Forte G, Petrucci F, Bocca B. Metal allergens of growing significance: epidemiology, immunotoxicology, strategies for testing and prevention. Inflamm Allergy Drug Targets. 2008;7(3):146-62.

521 Ehrlich A, Belsito D. Allergic contact dermatitis to gold. Cutis. 2000;65(5):323-6.

522 Vazirnia A, Jacob S. Review ACDS' Allergen of the Year 2000-2015. The Dermatologist. 2014;22(11).

523 Paciotti G, Myer L, Weinreich D, Goia D, Pavel N, McLaughlin R, Tamarkin L. Colloidal gold: a novel nanoparticle vector for tumor directed drug delivery. Drug Deliv. 2004;11(3):169-83.

524 Shi J, Yu J, Pohorly J, Kakuda Y. Polyphenolics in grape seeds-biochemistry and functionality. J Med Food. 2003;6(4):291-9.

525 Leifert W, Abeywardena M. Cardioprotective actions of grape polyphenols. Nutr Res.

2008;28(11):729-37.

[526] Khanna S, Venojarvi M, Roy S, Sharma N, Trikha P, Bagchi D, Bagchi M, Sen C. Dermal wound healing properties of redox-active grape seed proanthocyanidins. Free Radic Biol Med. 2002;33(8):1089-96.

[527] Hemmati A, Aghel N, Rashidi I, Gholampur-Aghdami A. Topical grape (Vitis vinifera) seed extract promotes repair of full thickness wound in rabbit. Int Wound J. 2011;8(5):514-20.

[528] Yuan X, Liu W, Hao J, Gu W, Zhao Y. Topical grape seed proanthocyandin extract reduces sunburn cells and mutant p53 positive epidermal cell formation, and prevents depletion of Langerhans cells in an acute sunburn model. Photomed Laser Surg. 2012;30(1):20-5.

[529] Kaur M, Agarwal C, Agarwal R. Anticancer and cancer chemopreventive potential of grape seed extract and other grape-based products. J Nutr. 2009;139(9):1806S-12S.

[530] Ibuki Y, Toyooka T. Evaluation of chemical phototoxicity, focusing on phosphorylated histone H2AX. J Radiat Res. 2015;56(2):220-228.

[531] Hata T, Sakaguchi I, Mori M, Ikeda N, Kato Y, Minamino M, Watabe K. Induction of apoptosis by Citrus paradisi essential oil in human leukemic (HL-60) cells. In Vivo. 2003;17(6):553-9.

[532] Njoroge S, Koaze H, Karanja P, Sawamura M. Volatile constituents of redblush grapefruit (Citrus paradisi) and pummelo (Citrus grandis) peel essential oils from Kenya. J Agric Food Chem. 2005;53(25):9790-4.

[533] Dugrand A, Olry A, Duval T, Hehn A, Froelicher Y, Bourgaud F. Coumarin and furanocoumarin quantitation in citrus peel via ultraperformance liquid chromatography coupled with mass spectrometry (UPLC-MS). J Agric Food Chem. 2013;61(45):10677-84.

[534] von Woedtke T, Schlüter B, Pflegel P, Lindequist U, Jülich W. Aspects of the antimicrobial efficacy of grapefruit seed extract and its relation to preservative substances contained. Pharmazie. 1999;54(6):452-6.

[535] Cvetnić Z, Vladimir-Knezević S. Antimicrobial activity of grapefruit seed and pulp ethanolic extract. Acta Pharm. 2004;54(3):243-50.

[536] Takeoka G, Dao L, Wong R, Lundin R, Mahoney N. Identification of benzethonium chloride in commercial grapefruit seed extracts. J Agric Food Chem. 2001;49(7):3316-20.

[537] Heinrich U, Moore C, De Spirt S, Tronnier H, Stahl W. Green tea polyphenols provide photoprotection, increase microcirculation, and modulate skin properties of women. J Nutr. 2011;141(6):1202-8.

[538] Katiyar S, Bergamo B, Vyalil P, Elmets C. Green tea polyphenols: DNA photodamage and photoimmunology. J Photochem Photobiol B. 2001;65(2-3):109-14.

[539] Oyetakin White P, Tribout H, Baron E. Protective mechanisms of green tea polyphenols in skin. Oxid Med Cell Longev. 2012;2012:560682.

[540] Katiyar S. Skin photoprotection by green tea: antioxidant and immunomodulatory effects. Curr Drug Targets Immune Endocr Metabol Disord. 2003;3(3):234-42.

[541] Katiyar S, Perez A, Mukhtar H. Green tea polyphenol treatment to human skin prevents formation of ultraviolet light B-induced pyrimidine dimers in DNA. Clin Cancer Res. 2000;6(10):3864-9.

[542] Katiyar S, Afaq F, Perez A, Mukhtar H. Green tea polyphenol (-)-epigallocatechin-3-gallate treatment of human skin inhibits ultraviolet radiation-induced oxidative stress. Carcinogenesis. 2001;22(2):287-94.

[543] Buckley D. Fragrance ingredient labelling in products on sale in the U.K. Br J Dermatol. 2007;157(2):295-300.

[544] Krautheim A, Uter W, Frosch P, Schnuch A, Geier J. Patch testing with fragrance mix II: results of the IVDK 2005-2008. Contact Dermatitis. 2010;63(5):262-9.

545 Burlando B, Cornara L. Honey in dermatology and skin care: a review. J Cosmet Dermatol. 2013;12(4):306-13.

546 Lu J, Carter D, Turnbull L, Rosendale D, Hedderley D, Stephens J, Gannabathula S, Steinhorn G, Schlothauer R, Whitchurch C, et al. The effect of New Zealand kanuka, manuka and clover honeys on bacterial growth dynamics and cellular morphology varies according to the species. PLoS One. 2013;8(2):e55898.

547 Oelschlaegel S, Gruner M, Wang P, Boettcher A, Koelling-Speer I, Speer K. Classification and characterization of manuka honeys based on phenolic compounds and methylglyoxal. J Agric Food Chem. 2012;60(29):7229-37.

548 Rahmasari K, Matsunaga A, Haruyama T, Kobayashi N. Anti-influenza viral effects of honey in vitro: potent high activity of manuka honey. Arch Med Res. 2014;45(5):359-65.

549 Ernst E, Pittler M, Stevinson C. Complementary/Alternative Medicine in Dermatology. Am J Clin Dermatol. 2002;3(5):341-8.

550 Koch R. Comparative study of Venostasin and Pycnogenol in chronic venous insufficiency. Koch R1. 2002;16(S1):S1-5.

551 Gründemann C, Lengen K, Sauer B, Garcia-Käufer M, Zehl M, Huber R. Equisetum arvense (common horsetail) modulates the function of inflammatory immunocompetent cells. BMC Complement Altern Med. 2014;14:283.

552 Schlesinger T, Rowland P. Efficacy and safety of a low-molecular weight hyaluronic Acid topical gel in the treatment of facial seborrheic dermatitis. J Clin Aesthet Dermatol. 2012;5(10):20-3.

553 Pavicic T, Gauglitz G, Lersch P, Schwach-Abdellaoui K, Malle B, Korting H, Farwick M. Efficacy of cream-based novel formulations of hyaluronic acid of different molecular weights in anti-wrinkle treatment. J Drugs Dermatol. 2011;10(9):990-1000.

554 Yoshimura K, Tsukamoto K, Okazaki M, Virador V, Lei T, Suzuki Y, Uchida G, Kitano Y, Harii K. Effects of all-trans retinoic acid on melanogenesis in pigmented skin equivalents and monolayer culture of melanocytes. J Dermatol Sci. 2001;27(S1):S68-75.

555 Grimes P, Kelly A, Torok H, Willis I. Community-based trial of a triple-combination agent for the treatment of facial melasma. Cutis. 2006;77(3):177-84.

556 Fabi S, Goldman M. Comparative Study of Hydroquinone-Free and Hydroquinone-Based Hyperpigmentation Regimens in Treating Facial Hyperpigmentation and Photoaging. J Drugs Dermatol. 2013;12(3):S32-7.

557 Wester R, Melendres J, Hui X, Cox R, Serranzana S, Zhai H, Quan D, Maibach H. Human in vivo and in vitro hydroquinone topical bioavailability, metabolism, and disposition. J Toxicol Environ Health A. 1998;54(4):301-17.

558 Draelos Z. Skin lightening preparations and the hydroquinone controversy. Dermatol Ther. 2007;20(5):308-13.

559 Tse T. Hydroquinone for skin lightening: safety profile, duration of use and when should we stop? J Dermatolog Treat. 2010;21(5):272-5.

560 DeCaprio A. The toxicology of hydroquinone--relevance to occupational and environmental exposure. Crit Rev Toxicol. 1999;29(3):283-330.

561 McGregor D. Hydroquinone: an evaluation of the human risks from its carcinogenic and mutagenic properties. Crit Rev Toxicol. 2007;37(10):887-914.

562 Levitt J. The safety of hydroquinone: a dermatologist's response to the 2006 Federal Register. J Am Acad Dermatol. 2007;57(5):854-72.

563 Steinberg D. Preservatives for Cosmetics. Carol Stream: Allured Pub Corp; 2006. p. 51-52.

564 Fulton Jr J, Pay S, Fulton 3rd J. Comedogenicity of current therapeutic products, cosmetics, and ingredients in the rabbit ear. J Am Acad Dermatol. 1984;10(1):96-105.

565 Draelos Z, DiNardo J. A re-evaluation of the comedogenicity concept. J Am Acad Dermatol. 2006;54(3):507-12.

566 Paulsen E, Christensen L, Andersen K. Dermatitis from common ivy (Hedera helix L. subsp. helix) in Europe: past, present, and future. Contact Dermatitis. 2010;62(4):201-9.

567 Mahillon V, Saussez S, Michel O. High incidence of sensitization to ornamental plants in allergic rhinitis. Allergy. 2006;61(9):1138-40.

568 Paibon W, Yimnoi C, Tembab N, Boonlue W, Jampachaisri K, Nuengchamnong N, Waranuch N, Ingkaninan K. Comparison and evaluation of volatile oils from three different extraction methods for some Thai fragrant flowers. Int J Cosmet Sci. 2011;33(2):150-6.

569 Laresen W. How to test for fragrance allergy. Cutis. 2006;65(1):39-41.

570 Jain S, Agrawal S. Fungistatic activity of some perfumes against otomycotic pathogens. Mycoses. 2002;45(3-4):88-90.

571 Meyer J, Marshall B, Gacula Jr M, Rheins L. Evaluation of additive effects of hydrolyzed jojoba (Simmondsia chinensis) esters and glycerol: a preliminary study. J Cosmet Dermatol. 2008;7(4):268-74.

572 Patzelt A, Lademann J, Richter H, Darvin M, Schanzer S, Thiede G, Sterry W, Vergou T, Hauser M. In vivo investigations on the penetration of various oils and their influence on the skin barrier. Skin Res Technol. 2012;18(3):364-9.

573 Ranzato E, Martinotti S, Burlando B. Wound healing properties of jojoba liquid wax: an in vitro study. J Ethnopharmacol. 2011;134(2):443-9.

574 Pazyar N, Yaghoobi R, Ghassemi M, Kazerouni A, Rafeie E, Jamshydian N. Jojoba in dermatology: a succinct review. G Ital Dermatol Venereol. 2013;148(6):687-91.

575 Moreno L, Bello R, Beltrán B, Calatayud S, Primo-Yúfera E, Esplugues J. Pharmacological screening of different Juniperus oxycedrus L. extracts. Pharmacol Toxicol. 1998;82(2):108-12.

576 International Journal of Toxicology. Final report on the safety assessment of Juniperus communis Extract, Juniperus oxycedrus Extract, Juniperus oxycedrus Tar, Juniperus phoenicea extract, and Juniperus virginiana Extract. Int J Toxicol. 2001;20(S2):41-56.

577 Lee S, Choi S, Kim H, Hwang J, Lee B, Gao J, Kim S. Mulberroside F isolated from the leaves of Morus alba inhibits melanin biosynthesis. Biol Pharm Bull. 2002;25(8):1045-8.

578 Sarkar R, Arora P, Garg K. Cosmeceuticals for Hyperpigmentation: What is Available? J Cutan Aesthet Surg. 2013;6(1):4-11.

579 Gonçalez M, Marcussi DCG, Corrêa M, Chorilli M. Structural characterization and in vitro antioxidant activity of kojic dipalmitate loaded w/o/w multiple emulsions intended for skin disorders. Biomed Res Int. 2015;2015:304591.

580 Brown A, Koett J, Johnson D, Semaskvich N, Holck P, Lally D, Cruz L, Young R, Higa B, Lo S. Effectiveness of kukui nut oil as a topical treatment for psoriasis. Int J Dermatol. 2005;44(8):684-7.

581 Afaq F, Mukhtar H. Botanical antioxidants in the prevention of photocarcinogenesis and photoaging. Exp Dermatol. 2006;15(9):678-84.

582 Deng S, May B, Zhang A, Lu C, Xue C. Plant extracts for the topical management of psoriasis: a systematic review and meta-analysis. Br J Dermatol. 2013;169(4):769-82.

583 Pinnell S, Yang H, Omar M, Monteiro-Riviere N, DeBuys H, Walker L, Wang Y, Levine M. Topical L-ascorbic acid: percutaneous absorption studies. Dermatol Surg. 2001;27(2):137-42.

584 European Commission Directorate General for Health and Consumers. Cosmetic Ingredient Glossary; Substance: Ascorbic Acid. [Internet]. 2015 [cited 2015 July]. Available from: http://ec.europa.eu/consumers/cosmetics/cosing/index.cfm?fuseaction=search.details&id=74328.

585 Naidu K. Vitamin C in human health and disease is still a mystery ? An overview. Nutr J.

2003;2(7).

586 Loden M. Role of topical emollients and moisturizers in the treatment of dry skin barrier disorders. Am J Clin Dermatol. 2003;4(11):771-88.

587 Wakelin S, Smith H, White I, Rycroft R, McFadden J. A retrospective analysis of contact allergy to lanolin. Br J Dermatol. 2001;145(1):28-31.

588 Suzuki M, Nigawara T, Yumoto M, Kimura M, Shirai H, Hanabusa K. L-lysine based gemini organogelators: their organogelation properties and thermally stable organogels. Org Biomol Chem. 2003;1(22):4125-34.

589 Prashar A, Locke I, Evans C. Cytotoxicity of lavender oil and its major components to human skin cells. Cell Prolif. 2004;37(3):221-9.

590 Jager W, Buchbauer G, Jirovetz L, Fritzer M. Percutaneous absorption of lavender oil from a massage oil. J Cosmet Sci. 1992;43(1):49-57.

591 Hagvall L, Sköld M, Bråred-Christensson J, Börje A, Karlberg A. Lavender oil lacks natural protection against autoxidation, forming strong contact allergens on air exposure. Contact Dermatitis. 2008;59(3):143-50.

592 Fiume Z. Final report on the safety assessment of Lecithin and Hydrogenated Lecithin. Int J Toxicol. 2001;20(S1):21-45.

593 Matura M, Goossens A, Bordalo O, Garcia-Bravo B, Magnusson K, Wrangsjö K, Karlberg A. Oxidized citrus oil (R-limonene): a frequent skin sensitizer in Europe. J Am Acad Dermatol. 2002;47(5):709-14.

594 Naganuma M, Hirose S, Nakayama Y, Nakajima K, Someya T. A study of the phototoxicity of lemon oil. Arch Dermatol Res. 1985;278(1):31-6.

595 Oyedele A, Gbolade A, Sosan M, Adewoyin F, Soyelu O, Orafidiya O. Formulation of an effective mosquito-repellent topical product from lemongrass oil. Phytomedicine. 2002;9(3):259-62.

596 Rahnama M, Mehrabani D, Japoni S, Edjtehadi M, Saberi M. The healing effect of licorice (Glycyrrhiza glabra) on Helicobacter pylori infected peptic ulcers. J Res Med Sci. 2013;18(6):532-533.

597 Ebanks J, Wickett R, Boissy R. Mechanisms Regulating Skin Pigmentation: The Rise and Fall of Complexion Coloration. Int J Mol Sci. 2009;10(9):4066-4087.

598 Nam C, Kim S, Sim Y, Chang I. Anti-Acne Effects of Oriental Herb Extracts: A Novel Screening Method to Select Anti-Acne Agents. Skin Pharmacol Appl Skin Physiol. 2003;16:84-90.

599 Simmler C, Pauli G, Chen S. Phytochemistry and biological properties of glabridin. Fitoterapia. 2013;90:160-84.

600 Veratti E, Rossi T, Giudice S, Benassi L, Bertazzoni G, Morini D, Azzoni P, Bruni E, Giannetti A, Magnoni C. 18beta-glycyrrhetinic acid and glabridin prevent oxidative DNA fragmentation in UVB-irradiated human keratinocyte cultures. Anticancer Res. 2011;31(6):2209-15.

601 Placzek M, Frömel W, Eberlein B, Gilbertz K, Przybilla B. Evaluation of phototoxic properties of fragrances. Acta Derm Venereol. 2007;87(4):312-6.

602 Nigg H, Nordby H, Beier R, Dillman A, Macias C, Hansen R. Phototoxic coumarins in limes. Food Chem Toxicol. 1993;31(5):331-5.

603 Kim Y, Kim M, Chung B, Bang du Y, Lim S, Choi S, Lim D, Cho M, Yoon K, Kim H, et al. Safety evaluation and risk assessment of d-Limonene. J Toxicol Environ Health B Crit Rev. 2013;16(1):17-38.

604 Chandrashekar N, Hiremath S. In vivo immunomodulatory, cumulative skin irritation, sensitization and effect of d-limonene on permeation of 6-mercaptopurine through transdermal drug delivery. Biol Pharm Bull. 2008;31(4):656-61.

[605] Christensson J, Hellsén S, Börje A, Karlberg A. Limonene hydroperoxide analogues show specific patch test reactions. Contact Dermatitis. 2014;70(5):291-9.

[606] Ando H, Ryu A, Hashimoto A, Oka M, Ichihashi M. Linoleic acid and alpha-linolenic acid lightens ultraviolet-induced hyperpigmentation of the skin. Arch Dermatol Res. 1998;290(7):375-81.

[607] Letawe C, Boone M, Piérard G. Digital image analysis of the effect of topically applied linoleic acid on acne microcomedones. Clin Exp Dermatol. 1998;23(2):56-8.

[608] Valdman-Grinshpoun Y, Ben-Amitai D, Zvulunov A. Barrier-Restoring Therapies in Atopic Dermatitis: Current Approaches and Future Perspectives. Dermatol Res Pract. 2012;2012:923134.

[609] McCusker M, Grant-Kels J. Healing fats of the skin: the structural and immunologic roles of the omega-6 and omega-3 fatty acids. Clin Dermatol. 2010;28(4):440-51.

[610] Cardoso C, Souza M, Ferro E, Favoreto Jr S, Pena J. Influence of topical administration of n-3 and n-6 essential and n-9 nonessential fatty acids on the healing of cutaneous wounds. Wound Repair Regen. 2004;12(2):235-43.

[611] Segall A, Moyano M. Stability of vitamin C derivatives in topical formulations containing lipoic acid, vitamins A and E. Int J Cosmet Sci. 2008;30(6):453-8.

[612] Pandel R, Poljšak B, Godic A, Dahmane R. Skin Photoaging and the Role of Antioxidants in Its Prevention. ISRN Dermatol. 2013;2013:930164.

[613] Shaikh Z, Mashood A. Treatment of refractory melasma with combination of topical 5% magnesium ascorbyl phosphate and fluorescent pulsed light in Asian patients. Int J Dermatol. 2014;53(1):93-9.

[614] Parvez S, Kang M, Chung H, Cho C, Hong M, Shin M, H. B. Survey and mechanism of skin depigmenting and lightening agents. Phytother Res. 2006;20(11):921-34.

[615] Ash M. Handbook of Cosmetic and Personal Care Additives. Synapse Information Resources, Inc.; 2002.

[616] Solís-Fuentes J, Durán-de-Bazúa M. Mango seed uses: thermal behaviour of mango seed almond fat and its mixtures with cocoa butter. Bioresour Technol. 2004;92(1):71-8.

[617] Dhara R, Bhattacharyya D, Ghosh M. Analysis of sterol and other components present in unsaponifiable matters of mahua, sal and mango kernel oil. J Oleo Sci. 2010;59(4):169-76.

[618] Green B. The sensory effects of l-menthol on human skin. Somatosens Mot Res. 1992;9(3):235-44.

[619] Franken L, de Groot A, Laheij-de Boer A. Allergic contact dermatitis caused by menthoxypropanediol in a lip cosmetic. Contact Dermatitis. 2013;69(6):377-8.

[620] Reinhard E, Waeber R, Niederer M, Maurer T, Maly P, Scherer S. Preservation of products with MCI/MI in Switzerland. Contact Dermatitis. 2001;45(5):257-64.

[621] Krasteva M, Kehren J, Ducluzeau M, Sayag M, Dupuis M, Kanitakis J, Nicolas J. Contact dermatitis II. Clinical aspects and diagnosis. Eur J Dermatol. 1999;9(2):144-160.

[622] Travassos A, Claes L, Boey L, Drieghe J, Goossens A. Non-fragrance allergens in specific cosmetic products. Contact Dermatitis. 2011;65(5):276-285.

[623] Scherrer M, Rocha V. Increasing trend of sensitization to Methylchloroisothiazolinone/methylisothiazolinone (MCI/MI). An Bras Dermatol. 2014;89(3):527.

[624] Flower C, Meredith E. Preserving with Methylisothiazolinone. Cosm & Toil. 2014;129(2):24.

[625] Geier J, Lessmann H, Schnuch A, Uter W. Recent increase in allergic reactions to methylchloroisothiazolinone/methylisothiazolinone: is methylisothiazolinone the culprit?. Contact Dermatitis. 2012;67(6):334-41.

[626] Gaspar L, Campos M. Evaluation of the photostability of different UV filter combinations in a sunscreen. Int. J. Pharm. 2006;307(2):123-328.

627 Chatelain E, Gabard B. Photostabilization of butyl methoxydibenzoylmethane (Avobenzone) and ethylhexyl methoxycinnamate by bis-ethylhexyloxyphenol methoxyphenyl triazine (Tinosorb S); a new UV broadband filter. Photochem Photobiol. 2001;72(3):401-6.

628 Rawlings A, Lombard K. A review on the extensive skin benefits of mineral oil. Int J Cosmet Sci. 2012;34(6):511-8.

629 Agero A, Verallo-Rowell V. A randomized double-blind controlled trial comparing extra virgin coconut oil with mineral oil as a moisturizer for mild to moderate xerosis. Dermatitis. 2004;15(3):109-16.

630 Sahlin A, Edlund F, Loden M. A double-blind and controlled study on the influence of the vehicle on the skin susceptibility from lactic acid. Int J Cosmetic Sci. 2007;29(5):385-90.

631 Wang I, Lin I, Hu F, Hou Y. A comparison of the effect of carbomer-; cellulose-; and mineral-oil based artificial tear formulations. Eur J Ophthalmol. 2007;17(2):151-159.

632 Brigido S. The use of an acellular dermal regenerative tissue matrix in the treatment of lower extremity wounds: a prospective 16-week pilot study. Int Wound J. 2006;3(3):181-87.

633 Hoggarth A, Waring M, Alexander J, Greenwood A, Callaghan T. A Controlled Three-Part Trial to Investigate the Barrier Function and Skin Hydration Properties of Six Skin Protectants. Ostomy Wound Manage. 2005;51(12):30-42.

634 Wang S, Liu X, Zhang J, Zang Y. An efficient preparation of mulberroside a from the branch bark of mulberry and its effect on the inhibition of tyosinase activity. PLoS One. 2014;9(10):e109396.

635 Park K, Kim J, Hwang D, Yoo Y, Lim Y. Inhibitory effect of mulberroside A and its derivatives on melanogenesis induced by ultraviolet B radiation. Food Chem Toxicol. 2011;49(12):3038-45.

636 Lewis C. Clearing Up Cosmetic Confusion. FDA Consumer Magazine. 1998;32(3):6-11.

637 Ao Y, Satoh K, Shibano K, Kawahito Y, Shioda S. Singlet Oxygen Scavenging Activity and Cytotoxicity of Essential Oils from Rutacae. J Clin Biochem Nutr. 2008;43(1):6-12.

638 Ammar A, Bouajila J, Mathieu F, Romdhane M, Zagrouba F. Chemical composition and in vitro antimicrobial and antioxidant activities of Citrus Aurantium l. flowers essential oil (Neroli oil). Pak J Biol Sci. 2012;15(21):1034-40.

639 Feng B, Ma L, Fang Y, Mei Y, Wei S. Protective effect of oat bran extracts on human dermal fibroblast injury induced by hydrogen peroxide. J Zhejiang Univ Sci B. 2013;14(2):97-105.

640 Vie K, Cours-Darne S, Vienne M, Boyer F, Dupuy P. Modulating effects of oatmeal extracts in the sodium lauryl sulfate skin irritancy model. Skin Pharmacol Appl Skin Physiol. 2002;15(2):120-24.

641 Montenegro L, Puglisi G. Evaluation of sunscreen safety by in vitro skin permeation studies: effects of vehicle composition. Pharmazie. 2013;68(1):34-40.

642 U.S. Food and Drug Administration. CFR - Code of Federal Regulations Title 21--FOOD AND DRUGS. [Internet]. 2014 [cited 2015 July]. Available from: www.accessdata.fda.gov/scripts/cdrh/cfdocs/cfCFR/CFRSearch.cfm?fr=352.50.

643 Bissonnette R. Update on sunscreens. Skin Therapy Lett. 2008;13(6):5-7.

644 deGroot A, Roberts D. Contact and photocontact allergy to octocrylene: a review. Contact Dermatitis. 2014;70(4):193-204.

645 Jimenez-Diaz J, Molina-Molina J, Zafra-Gomez A, Ballesteros O, Navalon A, Real M, Saenz J, Fernandez M, Olea N. Simultaneous determination of the UV-filters benzyl salicylate; phenyl salicylate; octyl salicylate; homosalate; 3-(4-methylbenzylidene) camphor and 3-benzylidene camphor in human placental tissue by LC-MS/MS. J Chromatogr B Analyt Technol Biomed Life Sci. 2013;936:80-7.

646 Zarrouk W, Carrasco-Pancorbo A, Zarrouk M, Segura-Carretero A, Fernandez-Gutierrez

A. A. Multi-component analysis (sterols; tocopherols; and triterpenic dialcohols) of the unsaponifiable fraction of vegetable oils by liquid chromatography-atmospheric pressure chemical ionization-ion trap mass spectrometry. Talanta. 2008;80(2):924-34.

[647] Raederstorff D. Antioxidant activity of olive polyphenols in humans: a review. Int J Vitam Nutr Res. 2009;79(3):152-65.

[648] Covas M, Nyyssonen K, Poulsen H, Kaikkonen J, Zunft H, Kiesewetter H, Gaddi A, de la Torre R, Mursu J, Baumler H, et al. The effect of polyphenols in olive oil on heart disease risk factors: a randomized trial. Ann Intern Med. 2006;145(5):331-41.

[649] Danby S, Al Enezi T, Sultan A, Lavender T, Chittock J, Brown K, Cork M. Effect of Olive and Sunflower Seed Oil on the Adult Skin Barrier: Implications for Neonatal Skin Care. Pediatr Dermatol. 2013;30(1):42-50.

[650] Kranke B, Komericki P, Aberer W. Olive oil – contact sensitizer or irritant?. Contact Dermatitis. 1997;36(1):5-10.

[651] Lautenschlager H. Essential fatty acids – cosmetic from inside and outside. Dermaviduals. 2003;4:54-56.

[652] Garidel P, Folting B, Schaller I, Kerth A. The microstructure of the stratum corneum lipid barrier: Mid-infrared spectroscopic studies of hydrated ceramide:palmitic acid:cholesterol model systems. Biophys Chem. 2010;150(1-3):144-156.

[653] Robinson L, Fitzgerald N, Doughty D, Dawes N, Berge C, Bissett D. Topical palmitoyl pentapeptide provides improvement in photoaged human facial skin. Int J Cosmet Sci. 2005;27(3):155-60.

[654] Mondon P, Hillion M, Peschard O, Andre N, Marchand T, Doridot E, Feuilloley M, Pionneau C, Chardonnet S. Evaluation of dermal extracellular matrix and epidermal-dermal junction modifications using matrix-assisted laser desorption/ionization mass spectrometric imaging; in vivo reflectance confocal microscopy; echography; [and other factors]. J Cosmet Dermatol. 2015;14(2):152-60.

[655] Trookman N, Rizer R, Ford R, Ho E, Gotz V. Immediate and Long-term Clinical Benefits of a Topical Treatment for Facial Lines and Wrinkles. J Clin Aesthet Dermatol. 2009;2(3):38-43.

[656] Ki S, Yokozawa T, Kim H, Park J. Study on the Nitric Oxide Scavenging Effects of Ginseng and Its Compounds. J Agric Food Chem. 2006;54(7):2558-2562.

[657] Panwar M, Kumar M, Samarth R, Kumar A. Evaluation of chemopreventive action and antimutagenic effect of the standardized Panax ginseng extract; EFLA400; in Swiss albino mice. Phytother Res. 2005;19(1):65-71.

[658] Camargo F, Gaspar L, Campos P. Skin moisturizing effects of panthenol-based formulations. J Cosmet Sci. 2011;62(4):361-70.

[659] Stremnitzer C, Manzano-Szalai K, Willensdorfer A, Starkl P, Pieper M, König P, Mildner M, Tschachler E, Reichart U, Jensen-Jarolim E. Papain Degrades Tight Junction Proteins of Human Keratinocytes In Vitro and Sensitizes C57BL/6 Mice via the Skin Independent of its Enzymatic Activity or TLR4 Activation. J Invest Dermatol. 2015;135(7):1790-800.

[660] Murthy M, Murthy B, Bhave S. Comparison of safety and efficacy of papaya dressing with hydrogen peroxide solution on wound bed preparation in patients with wound gape. Indian J Pharmacol. 2012;44(6):784-7.

[661] International Journal of Toxicology. Final report on the safety assessment of Triethylene Glycol and PEG-4. Int J Toxicol. 2006;25(s2):121-38.

[662] Fruijtier-Pölloth C. Safety assessment on polyethylene glycols (PEGs) and their derivatives as used in cosmetic products. Toxicology. 2005;214(1-2):1-38.

[663] Işcan G, Kirimer N, Kürkcüoğlu M, Başer K, Demirci F. Antimicrobial screening of Mentha piperita essential oils. J Agric Food Chem. 2002;50(14):3973-6.

[664] Posadzki P, Alotaibi A, Ernst E. Adverse effects of aromatherapy: a systematic review of case

reports and case series. Int J Risk Saf Med. 2012;24(3):147-61.

665 Herro E, Jacob S. Mentha piperita (Peppermint). Dermatitis. 2010;21(6):327-29.

666 Robbins P, Oliver S, Sheu S, Goodnough J, Wender P, Khavari P. Peptide delivery to tissues via reversibly linked protein transduction sequences. Biotechniques. 2002;33(1):190-2; 194.

667 Huq A, Jamal J, Stanslas J. Ethnobotanical, Phytochemical, Pharmacological, and Toxicological Aspects of Persicaria hydropiper (L.) Delarbre. Evid Based Complement Alternat Med. 2014;2014:782830.

668 Kim Y, Kim K, Han C, Yang H, Park S, Ko K, Lee S, Kim K, Lee N, Kim J, et al. Inhibitory effects of natural plants of Jeju Island on elastase and MMP-1 expression. J Cosmet Sci. 2007;58(1):19-33.

669 Khatun A, Imam M, Rana M. Antinociceptive effect of methanol extract of leaves of Persicaria hydropiper in mice. BMC Complement Altern Med. 2015;15:63.

670 Chan L, Cheah E, Saw C, Weng W, Heng P. Antimicrobial and antioxidant activities of Cortex Magnoliae Officinalis and some other medicinal plants commonly used in South-East Asia. Chin Med. 2008;28(3):15.

671 Lodén M, Bárány E. Skin-identical lipids versus petrolatum in the treatment of tape-stripped and detergent-perturbed human skin. Acta Derm Venereol. 2000;80(6):412-5.

672 Ghadially R, Halkier-Sorensen L, Elias P. Effects of petrolatum on stratum corneum structure and function. J Am Acad Dermatol. 1992;26(3 Pt 2):387-96.

673 Krowka J, Loretz L, Brzuska K, Almeida J, Diehl M, Gonsior S, Johnson A, Sellam S, Bade S, Champ S. Phenoxyethanol as a Safe and Important Preservative in Personal Care. Cosm & Toil. 2014;129(5):24-27.

674 Dreher F, Draelos Z, Gold M, Goldman M, Fabi S, Puissegur M. Efficacy of hydroquinone-free skin-lightening cream for photoaging. J Cosmet Dermatol. 2013;12(1):12-17.

675 Gold M, Biron J. Efficacy of a novel hydroquinone-free skin-brightening cream in patients with melasma. J Cosmet Dermatol. 2011;10(3):189-96.

676 Han N, Kim H, Jeong H. The β-sitosterol attenuates atopic dermatitis-like skin lesions through down-regulation of TSLP. Exp Biol Med (Maywood). 2014;239(4):454-64.

677 Grether-Beck S, Muhlberg K, Brenden H, Krutmann J. Topische Applikation von Vitaminen; Phytosterolen und Ceramiden. Der Hautarzt. 2008;59(7):557-562.

678 Puglia C, Bonina F. In vivo spectrophotometric evaluation of skin barrier recovery after topical application of soybean phytosterols. J Cosmet Sci. 2008;59(3):217-24.

679 Pavan R, Jain S, Shraddha, Kumar A. Properties and Therapeutic Application of Bromelain: A Review. Biotechnol Res Int. 2012;2012:976203.

680 Taussig S, Batkin S. Bromelain, the enzyme complex of pineapple (Ananas comosus) and its clinical application. An update. J Ethnopharmacol. 1988;22(2):191-203.

681 Eriksen M, Mason S, Wilson S, Box C, Zellers A, Edwards W, Farley H, Amato S. Microplastic pollution in the surface waters of the Laurentian Great Lakes. Mar Pollut Bull. 2013;77(1-2):177-82.

682 Browne M, Niven S, Galloway T, Rowland S, Thompson R. Microplastic moves pollutants and additives to worms; reducing functions linked to health and biodiversity. Curr Biol. 2013;23(23):2388-92.

683 Johnson & Johnson Consumer Companies, Inc. Our Safety & Care Commitment: Microbeads. [Internet]. 2015 [cited 2015 July]. Available from: http://www.safetyandcarecommitment.com/ingredient-info/other/microbeads.

684 Unilever. Micro-plastics. [Internet]. 2015 [cited 2015 July]. Available from: http://www.unilever.com/sustainable-living/what-matters-to-you/micro-plastics.html.

685 The Personal Care Products Council (the Council). Methyl Methacrylate/Glycol

Dimethacrylate Crosspolymer. [Internet]. 2015 [cited 2015 July]. Available from: http://www.cosmeticsinfo.org/ingredient/methyl-methacrylateglycol-dimethacrylate-crosspolymer.

[686] Fowler Jr J, Woolery-Lloyd H, Waldorf H, Saini R. Innovations in natural ingredients and their use in skin care. J Drugs Dermatol. 2010;9(S6):S72-81.

[687] Baumann L, Woolery-Lloyd H, Friedman A. "Natural" ingredients in cosmetic dermatology. J Drugs Dermatol. 2009;8(S6):S5-9.

[688] Noda Y, Kaneyuki T, Mori A, Packer L. Antioxidant activities of pomegranate fruit extract and its anthocyanidins: delphinidin; cyanidin; and pelargonidin. J Agric Food Chem. 2002;50(1):166-71.

[689] Steinberg D. Preservatives for Cosmetics. Carol Stream: Allured Publishing Corp; 2012. p. 36-38.

[690] Lundov M, Moesby L, Zachariae C, Johansen J. Contamination versus preservation of cosmetics: a review on legislation; usage; infections; and contact allergy. Contact Dermatitis. 2009;60(2):70-8.

[691] Fowles J, Banton M, Pottenger L. A toxicological review of the propylene glycols. Crit Rev Toxicol. 2013;43(4):363-90.

[692] Agency for Toxic Substances and Disease Registry. Public Health Statement: Ethylene Glycol and Propylene Glycol. [Internet]. 1997 [cited 2015 July]. Available from: http://www.atsdr.cdc.gov/toxprofiles/tp96-c1-b.pdf.

[693] Becker L, Bergfeld W, Belsito D, Klaassen C, Hill R, Leibler D, Marks Jr J, Shank R, Slaga T, Snyder P, et al. Final report of the amended safety assessment of Quaternium-15 as used in cosmetics. Int J Toxicol. 2010;29(S3):98S-114S.

[694] Bose S, Du Y, Takhistov P, Michniak-Kohn B. Formulation optimization and topical delivery of quercetin from solid lipid based nanosystems. Int J Pharm. 2013;441(1-2):56-66.

[695] Scalia S, Franceschinis E, Bertelli D, Iannuccelli V. Comparative Evaluation of the Effect of Permeation Enhancers, Lipid Nanoparticles and Colloidal Silica on in vivo Human Skin Penetration of Quercetin. Skin Pharmacol Physiol. 2013;26(2):57-67.

[696] Lin C, Leu Y, Al-Suwayeh S, Ku M, Hwang T, Fang J. Anti-inflammatory activity and percutaneous absorption of quercetin and its polymethoxylated compound and glycosides: the relationships to chemical structures. Eur J Pharm Sci. 2012;47(5):857-64.

[697] Cho J, Cho S, Lee S, Lee K. Onion extract and quercetin induce matrix metalloproteinase-1 in vitro and in vivo. Int J Mol Med. 2010;25(3):347-52.

[698] Phan T, Lim I, Chan S, Tan E, Lee S, Longaker M. Suppression of transforming growth factor beta/smad signaling in keloid-derived fibroblasts by quercetin: implications for the treatment of excessive scars. J Trauma. 2004;57(5):1032-7.

[699] Soeur J, Eilstein J, Léreaux G, Jones C, Marrot L. Skin resistance to oxidative stress induced by resveratrol: from Nrf2 activation to GSH biosynthesis. Free Radic Biol Med. 2015;78:213-23.

[700] Aggarwal B, Bhardwaj A, Aggarwal R, Seeram N, Shishodia S, Takada Y. Role of resveratrol in prevention and therapy of cancer: preclinical and clinical studies. Anticancer Res. 2004;24(5A):2783-840.

[701] de la Lastra C, Villegas I. Resveratrol as an anti-inflammatory and anti-aging agent: mechanisms and clinical implications. Mol Nutr Food Res. 2005;49(5):405-30.

[702] Bhat K, Kosmeder 2nd J, Pezzuto J. Biological effects of resveratrol. Antioxid Redox Signal. 2001;3(6):1041-64.

[703] Duell E, Kang S, Voorhees J. Unoccluded retinol penetrates human skin in vivo more effectively than unoccluded retinyl palmitate or retinoic acid. J Invest Dermatol. 1997;109(3):301-5.

[704] Kim B, Kim J, Kim H, Lee J, Choi K, Lee S. Co-treatment with retinyl retinoate and a PPARα

agonist reduces retinoid dermatitis. Int J Dermatol. 2012;51(6):733-41.

[705] Kim H, Koh J, Baek J, Seo Y, Kim B, Kim J, Lee J, Ryoo H, Jung H. Retinyl retinoate; a novel hybrid vitamin derivative; improves photoaged skin: a double-blind; randomized-controlled trial. Skin Res Technol. 2011;17(3):380-5.

[706] Kim J, Kim B, Kim H, Kim H, Lee J, Kim H, Choi K, Lee S. Retinyl retinoate induces hyaluronan production and less irritation than other retinoids. J Dermatol. 2010;37(5):448-54.

[707] Boskabady M, Shafei M, Saberi Z, Amini S. Pharmacological Effects of Rosa Damascena. Iran J Basic Med Sci. 2011;14(4):295-307.

[708] Halvorsen B, Holte K, Myhrstad M, Barikmo I, Hvattum E, Remberg S, Wold A, Haffner K, Baugerød H, Andersen L, et al. A systematic screening of total antioxidants in dietary plants. J Nutr. 2002;132(3):461-71.

[709] Hornero-Méndez D, Mínguez-Mosquera M. Carotenoid pigments in Rosa mosqueta hips; an alternative carotenoid source for foods. J Agric Food Chem. 2000;48(3):825-8.

[710] Kähkönen M, Hopia A, Vuorela H, Rauha J, Pihlaja K, Kujala T, Heinonen M. Antioxidant activity of plant extracts containing phenolic compounds. J Agric Food Chem. 1999;47(10):3954-62.

[711] Tabassum N, Hamdani M. Plants used to treat skin diseases. Pharmacogn Rev. 2014;8(15):52-60.

[712] Sienkiewicz M, Łysakowska M, Pastuszka M, Bienias W, Kowalczyk E. The potential of use basil and rosemary essential oils as effective antibacterial agents. Molecules. 2013;18(8):9334-51.

[713] Sayorwan W, Ruangrungsi N, Piriyapunyporn T, Hongratanaworakit T, Kotchabhakdi N, Siripornpanich V. Effects of inhaled rosemary oil on subjective feelings and activities of the nervous system. Sci Pharm. 2013;81(2):531-42.

[714] Sœur J, Marrot L, Perez P, Iraqui I, Kienda G, Dardalhon M, Meunier JR AD, Huang M. Selective cytotoxicity of Aniba rosaeodora essential oil towards epidermoid cancer cells through induction of apoptosis. Mutat Res. 2011;718(1-2):24-32.

[715] d'Acampora Z, Lo Presti M, Barata L, Dugo P, Dugo G, Mondello L. Evaluation of leaf-derived extracts as an environmentally sustainable source of essential oils by using gas chromatography-mass spectrometry and enantioselective gas chromatography-olfactometry. Anal Chem. 2006;78(3):883-90.

[716] Hartmann A. The influence of various factors on the human resident skin flora. Semin Dermatol. 1990;9(4):305-8.

[717] Dwivedi C, Zhang Y. Sandalwood oil prevent skin tumour development in CD1 mice. Eur J Cancer Prev. 1999;8(5):449-55.

[718] Gupta A, Kumar R, Pal K, Banerjee P, Sawhney R. A preclinical study of the effects of seabuckthorn (Hippophae rhamnoides L.) leaf extract on cutaneous wound healing in albino rats. Int J Low Extrem Wounds. 2005;4(2):88-92.

[719] Vijayaraghavan R, Gautam A, Kumar O, Pant S, Sharma M, Singh S, Kumar H, Singh A, Nivsarkar M, Kaushik M, et al. Protective effect of ethanolic and water extracts of sea buckthorn (Hippophae rhamnoides L.) against the toxic effects of mustard gas. Indian J Exp Biol. 2006;44(10):821-31.

[720] Hwang I, Kim J, Choi S, Lee H, Lee Y, Jang M, Son H, Lee H, Oh C, Kim B, et al. UV radiation-induced skin aging in hairless mice is effectively prevented by oral intake of sea buckthorn (Hippophae rhamnoides L.) fruit blend for 6 weeks through MMP suppression and increase of SOD activity. Int J Mol Med. 2012;30(2):392-400.

[721] Maranz S, Wiesman Z, Garti N. Phenolic constituents of shea (Vitellaria paradoxa) kernels. J Agric Food Chem. 2003;51(21):6268-73.

[722] Klopp R, Niemer W, Fraenkel M, von der Weth A. Effect of four treatment variants on the

functional and cosmetic state of mature scars. J Wound Care. 2000;9(7):319-24.

[723] Schlossman M. The Chemistry and Manufacture of Cosmetics. Carol Stream: Allured Publishing Corp; 2002. p. 833-839.

[724] Draelos Z, Callender V, Young C, Dhawan S. The effect of vehicle formulation on acne medication tolerability. Cutis. 2008;82(4):281-4.

[725] Fabbrocini G, Annunziata M, D'Arco V, De Vita V, Lodi G, Mauriello M, Pastore F, Monfrecola G. Acne Scars: Pathogenesis; Classification and Treatment. Dermatol Res Pract. 2010;2010:893080.

[726] Ruamrak C, Lourith N, Natakankitkul S. Comparison of clinical efficacies of sodium ascorbyl phosphate; retinol and their combination in acne treatment. Int J Cosmet Sci. 2009;31(1):41-6.

[727] Seidenari S, Pepe P, Di Nardo A. Sodium hydroxide-induced irritant dermatitis as assessed by computerized elaboration of 20 MHz B-scan images and by TEWL measurement: a method for investigating skin barrier function. Acta Derm Venereol. 1995;75(2):97-101.

[728] Charbonnier V, Morrison Jr B, Paye M, Maibach H. Subclinical; non-erythematous irritation with an open assay model (washing): sodium lauryl sulfate (SLS) versus sodium laureth sulfate (SLES). Food Chem Toxicol. 2001;39(3):279-86.

[729] Löffler H, Pirker C, Aramaki J, Frosch P, Happle R, I. E. Evaluation of skin susceptibility to irritancy by routine patch testing with sodium lauryl sulfate. Eur J Dermatol. 2001;11(5):416-9.

[730] Löffler H, Freyschmidt-Paul P, Effendy I, Maibach H. Pitfalls of irritant patch testing using different test chamber sizes. Am J Contact Dermat. 2001;12(1):28-32.

[731] Dastychová E, Necas M, Pěncíková K, Cerný P. Contact sensitization to pharmaceutic aids in dermatologic cosmetic and external use preparations. Ceska Slov Farm. 2004;53(3):151-6.

[732] Stallings ALM. Practical Uses of Botanicals in Skin Care. J Clin Aesthet Dermatol. 2009;2(1):36-40.

[733] Schmid D, Zülli F. Topically-Applied Soy Isoflavones Increase Skin Thickness. Cosm & Toil. 2002 45-50.

[734] Miyazaki K, Hanamizu T, Sone T, Chiba K, Kinoshita T, Yoshikawa S. Topical application of Bifidobacterium-fermented soy milk extract containing genistein and daidzein improves rheological and physiological properties of skin. J Cosmet Sci. 2004;55(5):473-9.

[735] Südel K, Venzke K, Mielke H, Breitenbach U, C M, Jaspers S, Koop U, Sauermann K, Knussman-Hartig E, Moll I, et al. Novel aspects of intrinsic and extrinsic aging of human skin: beneficial effects of soy extract. Photochem Photobiol. 2005;81(3):581-7.

[736] Park N, Park J, Kang Y, Bae J, Lee H, Yeom M, Cho J, Na Y. Soybean extract showed modulation of retinoic acid-related gene expression of skin and photo-protective effects in keratinocytes. Int J Cosmet Sci. 2013;35(2.):136-42.

[737] Chiang H, Wu W, Fang H, Chen B, Kao T, Chen Y, Hung C. UVB-Protective Effects of Isoflavone Extracts from Soybean Cake in Human Keratinocytes. Int J Mol Sci. 2007;8(7):651-661.

[738] Toxicology. IJo. Final report of the amended safety assessment of PEG-5; -10; -16; -25; -30; and -40 soy sterol. Int J Toxicol. 2004;23(S2):23-47.

[739] Passi S, De Pità O, Puddu P, Littarru G. Lipophilic antioxidants in human sebum and aging. Free Radic Res. 2002;36(4):471-7.

[740] Owen R, Giacosa A, Hull W, Haubner R, Würtele G, Spiegelhalder B, Bartsch H. Olive-oil consumption and health: the possible role of antioxidants. Lancet Oncol. 2000;1:107-12.

[741] Boiy A, Roelandts R, van den Oord J, de Witte P. Photosensitizing activity of hypericin and hypericin acetate after topical application on normal mouse skin. Br J Dermatol. 2008;158(2):360-9.

[742] Zheng W, Wang S. Antioxidant activity and phenolic compounds in selected herbs. J Agric Food Chem. 2001;49(11):5165-70.

[743] Saddiqe Z, Naeem I, Maimoona A. A review of the antibacterial activity of Hypericum perforatum L. J Ethnopharmacol. 2010;131(3):511-21.

[744] Haake H, Marten S, Seipel W, Eisfeld W. Hair breakage--how to measure and counteract. J Cosmet Sci. 2009;60(2):143-51.

[745] Bergfeld W, Belsito D, Marks Jr J, Andersen F. Safety of ingredients used in cosmetics. J Am Acad Dermatol. 2005;52(1):125-32.

[746] Turkoglu M, Sakr A. Evaulation of irritation potential of surfactant mixtures. Int J Cosmet Sci. 1999;21(6):371-82.

[747] Sander C, Chang H, Salzmann S, Müller C, Ekanayake-Mudiyanselage S, Elsner P, Thiele J. Photoaging is associated with protein oxidation in human skin in vivo. J Invest Dermatol. 2002;118(4):618-25.

[748] Afaq F, Mukhtar H. Effects of solar radiation on cutaneous detoxification pathways. J Photochem Photobiol B. 2001;63(1-3):61-9.

[749] Vorauer-Uhl K, Fürnschlief E, Wagner A, Ferko B, Katinger H. Topically applied liposome encapsulated superoxide dismutase reduces postburn wound size and edema formation. Eur J Pharm Sci. 2001;14(1):63-7.

[750] Wild P. Lung cancer risk and talc not containing asbestiform fibres: a review of the epidemiological evidence. Occup Environ Med. 2006;63:4-9.

[751] Mills P, Riordan D, Cress R, Young H. Perineal talc exposure and epithelial ovarian cancer risk in the Central Valley of California. Int J Cancer. 2004;112(3):458-64.

[752] Huncharek M, Geschwind J, Kupelnick B. Perineal application of cosmetic talc and risk of invasive epithelial ovarian cancer: a meta-analysis of 11;933 subjects from sixteen observational studies. Anticancer Res. 2003;23(2C):1955-60.

[753] Wehner A. Cosmetic Talc Should Not Be Listed as a Carcinogen; Comments on NTP's Deliberations to List Talc as a Carcinogen. Regul Toxicol Pharm. 2002;36(1):40-50.

[754] Iqbal M, Kim K, Ahn J. Monoterpenes released from fruit; plant; and vegetable systems. Sensors (Basel). 2014;14(10):18286-301.

[755] Pazyar N, Yaghoobi R, Bagherani N, Kazerouni A. A review of applications of tea tree oil in dermatology. Int J Dermatol. 2013;52(7):784-90.

[756] Cox S, Mann C, Markham J, Bell H, Gustafson J, Warmington J, Wyllie S. The mode of antimicrobial action of the essential oil of Melaleuca alternifolia (tea tree oil). J Appl Microbiol. 2000;88(1):170-5.

[757] Carson C, Ashton L, Dry L, Smith D, Riley T. Melaleuca alternifolia (tea tree) oil gel (6%) for the treatment of recurrent herpes labialis. J Antimicrob Chemother. 2001;48(3):450-1.

[758] Raman A, Weir U, Bloomfield S. Antimicrobial effects of tea-tree oil and its major components on Staphylococcus aureus; Staph. epidermidis and Propionibacterium acnes. Lett Appl Microbiol. 1995;21(4):242-5.

[759] Bassett I, Pannowitz D, Barnetson R. A comparative study of tea-tree oil versus benzoylperoxide in the treatment of acne. Med J Aust. 1990;153(8):455-8.

[760] D'Arrigo M, Ginestra G, Mandalari G, Furneri P, Bisignano G. Synergism and postantibiotic effect of tobramycin and Melaleuca alternifolia (tea tree) oil against Staphylococcus aureus and Escherichia coli. Phytomedicine. 2010;17(5):317-22.

[761] Zug K, Warshaw E, Fowler Jr J, Maibach H, Belsito D, Pratt M, Sasseville D, Storrs F, Taylor J, Mathias C, et al. Patch-test results of the North American Contact Dermatitis Group 2005-2006. Dermatitis. 2009;20(3):149-60.

[762] Miura K, Kikuzaki H, Nakatani N. Antioxidant activity of chemical components from sage

(Salvia officinalis L.) and thyme (Thymus vulgaris L.) measured by the oil stability index method. J Agric Food Chem. 2002;50(7):1845-51.

[763] Shimelis N, Asticcioli S, Baraldo M, Tirillini B, Lulekal E, Murgia V. Researching accessible and affordable treatment for common dermatological problems in developing countries. An Ethiopian experience. Int J Dermatol. 2012;51(7):790-5.

[764] Sienkiewicz M, Łysakowska M, Denys P, Kowalczyk E. The antimicrobial activity of thyme essential oil against multidrug resistant clinical bacterial strains. Microb Drug Resist. 2012;18(2):137-48.

[765] Strobel C, Torrano A, Herrmann R, Malissek M, Bräuchle C, Reller A, Treuel L, Hilger I. Effects of the physicochemical properties of titanium dioxide nanoparticles; commonly used as sun protection agents; on microvascular endothelial cells. J Nanopart Re. 2014;16:2130.

[766] Fiume M, Heldreth B, Bergfeld W, Belsito D, Hill R, Klaassen C, Liebler D, Marks Jr J, Shank R, Slaga T, et al. Safety assessment of triethanolamine and triethanolamine-containing ingredients as used in cosmetics. Int J Toxicol. 2013;32(S3):59S-83S.

[767] Wohlrab J, Siemes C, Marsch W. The influence of L-arginine on the regulation of epidermal arginase. Skin Pharmacol Appl Skin Physiol. 2002;15(1):44-54.

[768] Sinha A, Verma SSU. Development and validation of an RP-HPLC method for quantitative determination of vanillin and related phenolic compounds in Vanilla planifolia. J Sep Sci. 2007;30:15-20.

[769] Stone W, LeClair I, Ponder T, Baggs G, Reis B. Infants discriminate between natural and synthetic vitamin E. Am J Clin Nutr. 2003;77(4):899-906.

[770] Baumann L, Spencer J. The effects of topical vitamin E on the cosmetic appearance of scars. Dermatol Surg. 1999;25(4):311-5.

[771] Khoosal D, Goldman R. Vitamin E for treating children's scars. Does it help reduce scarring?. Can Fam Physician. 2006;52:855-6.

[772] Miettinen H, Johansson G, Gobom S, Swanbeck G. Studies on constituents of moisturizers: water-binding properties of urea and NaCl in aqueous solutions. Skin Pharmacol Appl Skin Physiol. 1999;12(6):344-51.

[773] Martin K. Direct measurement of moisture in skin by NIR spectroscopy. J Cosmet Sci. 1993;44(5):249-62.

[774] Tsai T, Maibach H. How irritant is water? An overview. Contact Dermatitis. 1999;41(6):311-4.

[775] Tsuruta D, Green K, Getsios S, Jones J. The barrier function of skin: how to keep a tight lid on water loss. Trends Cell Biol. 2002;12(8):355-7.

[776] Chamlin S, Kao J, Frieden I, Sheu M, Fowler A, Fluhr J, Williams M, Elias P. Ceramide-dominant barrier repair lipids alleviate childhood atopic dermatitis: changes in barrier function provide a sensitive indicator of disease activity. J Am Acad Dermatol. 2002;47(2):198-208.

[777] Vlachojannis J, Magora F, Chrubasik S. Willow species and aspirin: different mechanism of actions. Phytother Res. 2011;25(7):1102-4.

[778] Hughes-Formella B, Filbry A, Gassmueller J, Rippke F. Anti-inflammatory efficacy of topical preparations with 10% hamamelis distillate in a UV erythema test. Skin Pharmacol Appl Skin Physiol. 2002;15(2):125-32.

[779] Choi H, Choi J, Han Y, Bae S, Chung H. Peroxynitrite scavenging activity of herb extracts. Phytother Res. 2002;16(4):364-7.

[780] Masaki H, Atsumi T, Sakurai H. Protective activity of hamamelitannin on cell damage of murine skin fibroblasts induced by UVB irradiation. J Dermatol Sci. 1995;10(1):25-34.

[781] Thring T, Hili P, Naughton D. Antioxidant and potential anti-inflammatory activity of extracts and formulations of white tea; rose; and witch hazel on primary human dermal

fibroblast cells. J Inflamm (Lond). 2011;8:27.

782 Trüeb R. North American Virginian Witch Hazel (Hamamelis virginiana): Based Scalp Care and Protection for Sensitive Scalp; Red Scalp; and Scalp Burn-Out. Int J Trichology. 2014;6(3):100-103.

783 Bentley J, Hunt T, Weiss J, Taylor C, Hanson A, Davies G, Halliday B. Peptides from live yeast cell derivative stimulate wound healing. Arch Surg. 1990;125(5):641-6.

784 Bennett C, Lewis L, Karthikeyan G, Lobachev K, Jin Y, Sterling J, Snipe J, Resnick M. Genes required for ionizing radiation resistance in yeast. Nat Genet. 2001;29(4):426-34.

785 Srivastava P, Bajaj A. Ylang-ylang oil Not an Uncommon Sensitizer in India. Indian J Dermatol. 2014;59(2):200-201.

786 Kieć-Swierczyńska M, Krecisz B, Swierczyńska-Machura D. Contact allergy to fragrances. Med Pr. 2006;57(5):431-7.

787 Schwartz J, Marsh R, Draelos Z. Zinc and skin health: overview of physiology and pharmacology. Dermatol Surg. 2005;31(7 Pt 2):837-47.

788 Rostan E, DeBuys H, Madey D, Pinnell S. Evidence supporting zinc as an important antioxidant for skin. Int J Dermatol. 2002;41(9):606-11.

789 van Hoogdalem E. Transdermal absorption of topical anti-acne agents in man; review of clinical pharmacokinetic data. J Eur Acad Dermatol Venereol. 1998;11(S1):@13-9.

790 Ting W, Vest C, Sontheimer R. Practical and experimental consideration of sun protection in dermatology. Int J Dermatol. 2003;42(7):505-13.

791 Lansdown A. Metallothioneins: potential therapeutic aids for wound healing in the skin. Wound Repair Regen. 2002;10(3):130-32.

792 Kootiratrakarn T, Kampirapap K, Chunhasewee C. Epidermal permeability barrier in the treatment of keratosis pilaris. Dermatol Res Pract. 2015;2015:205012.

793 Wei A, Shibamoto T. Antioxidant activities and volatile constituents of various essential oils. J Agric Food Chem. 2007;55(5):1737-42.

794 Miyazawa M, Okuno Y, Fukuyama M, Nakamura S, Kosaka H. Antimutagenic activity of polymethoxyflavonoids from Citrus aurantium. J Agric Food Chem. 1999;47(12):4239-44.

795 Fiume M, Heldreth B, Bergfeld W, Belsito D, Hill R, Klaassen C, Liebler D, Marks Jr J, Shank R, Slaga T, et al. Safety assessment of diethanolamides as used in cosmetics. Int J Toxicol. 2013;32(3S):36S-58S.

796 del Nogal S, Pérez-Pavón J, Moreno Cordero B. Determination of suspected allergens in cosmetic products by headspace-programmed temperature vaporization-fast gas chromatography-quadrupole mass spectrometry. Anal Bioanal Chem. 2010;397(6):2579-91.

797 Rastogi S. Analytical control of preservative labelling on skin creams. Contact Dermatitis. 2000;43(6):339-43.

798 Larsen W, Nakayama H, Fischer T, Elsner P, Frosch P, Burrows D, Jordan W, Shaw S, Wilkinson J, Marks Jr J, et al. Fragrance contact dermatitis: a worldwide multicenter investigation (Part II). Contact Dermatitis. 2001;44(6):344-6.

799 Lajis A, Hamid M, Ariff A. Depigmenting effect of Kojic acid esters in hyperpigmented B16F1 melanoma cells. J Biomed Biotechnol. 2012;2012:952452.

800 Nakatsuji T, Kao M, Fang J, Zouboulis C, Zhang L, Gallo R, Huang C. Antimicrobial property of lauric acid against Propionibacterium acnes: its therapeutic potential for inflammatory acne vulgaris. J Invest Dermatol. 2009;129(10):2480-8.

801 Kejlová K, Jírová D, Bendová H, Gajdoš P, Kolářová H. Phototoxicity of essential oils intended for cosmetic use. Toxicol In Vitro. 2010;24(8):2084-9.

802 Davis E, Callender V. Postinflammatory Hyperpigmentation. J Clin Aesthet Dermatol. 2010;3(7):20-31.

[803] Yosipovitch G, Szolar C, Hui X, Maibach H. Effect of topically applied menthol on thermal, pain and itch sensations and biophysical properties of the skin. Arch Dermatol Res. 1996;288(5-6):245-8.

[804] Travassos A, Claes L, Boey L, Drieghe J, Goossens A. Non-fragrance allergens in specific cosmetic products. Contact Dermatitis. 2011;65(5):276-285.

[805] Lee S, Choi S, Kim H, Hwang J, Lee B, Gao J, Kim S. Mulberroside F isolated from the leaves of Morus alba inhibits melanin biosynthesis. Biol Pharm Bull. 2002;25(8):1045-8.

[806] Callendar V, St Surin-Lord S, Davis E, M. M. Postinflammatory Hyperpigmentation. A J Clin Dermatol. 2012;12(2):87-99.

[807] Jerajani H, Mizoguchi H, Li J, Whittenbarger D, Marmor M. The effects of a daily facial lotion containing vitamins B3 and E and provitamin B5 on the facial skin of Indian women: A randomized; double-blind trial. Indian J Dermatol Venereol Leprol. 2010;76(1):20-26.

[808] Sivapirabu G, Yiasemides E, Halliday G, Park J, Damian D. Topical nicatinamide modulates cellular energy metabolism and provides broad-spectrum protection against ultraviolet radiation-induced immunosuppression in humans. Brit J Dermatol. 2009;161(6):1357-64.

[809] Chiu A, Kimball A. Topical vitamins; minerals and botanical ingredients as modulators of environmental and chronological skin damage. Brit J Dermatol. 2003;149(4):681.

[810] Bissett D, Oblong J, Berge C. Niacinamide: A B Vitamin that Improves Aging Facial Skin Appearance. Dermatol Surg. 2005;31(S1):860-66.

[811] Hayden C, Cross S, Anderson C, Roberts M. Sunscreen Penetration of Human Skin and Related Keratinocyte Toxicity of Topical Application. Skin Pharmacol Appl Skin Physiol. 2005;18(4):170-174.

[812] European Commission Health and Consumers. Substance : 2-Ethylhexyl 4-methoxycinnamate / Octinoxate. [Internet]. 2015 [cited 2015 July]. Available from: http://ec.europa.eu/consumers/cosmetics/cosing/index.cfm?fuseaction=search.details_v2&id=28816.

[813] Travassos A, Claes L, Boey L, Drieghe J, Goossens A. Non-fragrance allergens in specific cosmetic products. Contact Dermatitis. 2011;65(5):276-285.

[814] Verallo-Rowell V, Dillague K, Syah-Tjundawan B. Novel Antibacterial and Emollient Effects of Coconut and Virgin Olive Oils in Adult Atopic Dermatitis. Dermatitis. 2008;19(6):308-15.

[815] Stremnitzer C, Manzano-Szalai K, Willensdorfer A, Starkl P, Pieper M, König P, Mildner M, Tschachler E, Reichart U, Jensen-Jarolim E. Papain Degrades Tight Junction Proteins of Human Keratinocytes In Vitro and Sensitizes C57BL/6 Mice via the Skin Independent of its Enzymatic Activity or TLR4 Activation. J Invest Dermatol. 2015;135(7):1790-1800.

[816] Johnson B, Bolton J, van Breemen R. Screening botanical extracts for quinoid metabolites. Chem Res Toxicol. 2001;14(11):1546-51.

[817] Carlotti M, Ugazio E, Gastaldi L, Sapino S, Vione D, Fenoglio I, Fubini B. Specific effects of single antioxidants in the lipid peroxidation caused by nano-titania used in sunscreen lotions. J Photochem Photobiol B. 2009;96(2):130-5.

[818] Klock J, Ikeno H, Ohmori K, Nishikawa T, Vollhardt J, Schehlmann V. Sodium ascorbyl phosphate shows in vitro and in vivo efficacy in the prevention and treatment of acne vulgaris. Int J Cosmet Sci. 2005;27(3):171-6.

[819] Fitzpatrick R, Rostan E. Double-blind; half-face study comparing topical vitamin C and vehicle for rejuvenation of photodamage. Dermatol Surg. 2002;28(3):231-6.

[820] Wei A, Shibamoto T. Antioxidant activities of essential oil mixtures toward skin lipid squalene oxidized by UV irradiation. Cutan Ocul Toxicol. 2007;26(3):227-33.